# CLINICAL CHEMISTRY

## THIRD EDITION

# CLINICAL CHEMISTRY

## THIRD EDITION

## WILLIAM J MARSHALL
### MA PhD MSc MB BS FRCP FRCPATH

SENIOR LECTURER IN CLINICAL BIOCHEMISTRY
KING'S COLLEGE SCHOOL OF MEDICINE AND DENTISTRY
UNIVERSITY OF LONDON
LONDON, UK

HON. CONSULTANT IN CLINICAL BIOCHEMISTRY
KING'S COLLEGE HOSPITAL
LONDON, UK

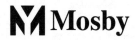 Mosby

| | |
|---|---|
| Project Manager | Louise Crowe |
| Design | Pete Wilder |
| Illustration | Jenni Miller |
| Production | Jane Tozer |
| Publisher | Dianne Zack |

# PREFACE TO THE THIRD EDITION

Although only three years have elapsed since the second edition of this book was published, continuing advances in knowledge and changes in practice have necessitated a complete revision of the text. The aims of the book are unchanged, as is the sequence of chapters. Disorders of water, sodium and potassium homoeostasis are now presented in a single chapter, as are diabetes mellitus and other disorders of carbohydrate metabolism. Despite its increasing importance, I have resisted the temptation to expand the section on molecular genetics; it has never been my intention to discuss analytical techniques, and there are anyway several excellent short textbooks devoted to this topic. These are indicated in the further reading. I have continued to confine this to books which I find useful, major reviews and only occasional papers. Information retrieval is now so simple that readers wishing to delve into the recent literature should have no difficulty doing this on their own.

Bearing in mind the changes being made in undergraduate medical curriculums in the United Kingdom in response to the General Medical Council's document, 'Tomorrow's Doctors', I have tried to ensure that the major part of the text deals with core topics. I have, however, also indicated areas of particular current interest which may be incorporated into special study modules.

In revising the text, I have been fortunate in being able to draw on comments and suggestions made by readers from many countries. I am grateful to all who have written to me, and look forward to continuing correspondence. My own medical students have also made numerous helpful comments.

Many colleagues and friends have generously shared their expertise with me and it is a pleasure to acknowledge their help. They include: Dr Ruth Ayling, Dr Stephen Bangert, Dr David Burnett, Miss Joan Butler, Dr Danielle Freedman, Dr James Hooper, Dr Imogen Morgan and Dr Wassif Wassif.

The publishers of the first two editions, Gower Medical Publishing, have now been swallowed by Mosby, but the good relationships between editors, designers and authors that characterised Gower have not been lost. It has been a pleasure to work with Rachael Miller, Deborah Shipman, Louise Crowe, Pete Wilder and Fiona Foley.

The Marshalls are both writers: Wendy is a poet and continues both to be a source of inspiration and to tolerate my piles of papers which litter the house and my unsocial hours on the word processor.

W J M, 1995

# CONTENTS

# 1. Biochemical Tests in Clinical Medicine

## INTRODUCTION

A central function of the chemical pathology or clinical chemistry laboratory is to provide biochemical information for the management of patients. Such information will be of value only if it is accurate and relevant, and if its significance is appreciated by the clinician so that it can be used appropriately to guide clinical decision-making. This chapter examines how biochemical data are acquired and how they should be used.

## USE OF BIOCHEMICAL TESTS

Biochemical tests are used extensively in medicine, both in relation to diseases that have an obvious metabolic basis (e.g., diabetes mellitus, hypothyroidism) and those in which biochemical changes are a consequence of the disease (e.g., renal failure, malabsorption). Biochemical tests are used in diagnosis, prognosis, monitoring and screening (*Fig. 1.1*).

### Diagnosis
Medical diagnosis is based on the patient's history, if available, the clinical signs found on examination, the results of investigations and sometimes, retrospectively, on the response to treatment. Frequently, a confident diagnosis can be made on the basis of the history combined with the findings on examination. Failing this, it is usually possible to formulate a differential diagnosis, in effect, a short-list of possible diagnoses. Biochemical and other investigations may then be used to distinguish between them.

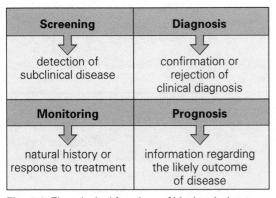

**Fig. 1.1** The principal functions of biochemical tests.

Investigations may be selected to help either confirm or refute a diagnosis and it is important that the clinician appreciates how useful the chosen test is for these purposes. Making a diagnosis, even if incomplete, such as a diagnosis of hypoglycaemia without knowing its cause, may allow treatment to be initiated.

### Prognosis
Tests used primarily for diagnosis may also provide prognostic information and some are used specifically for this purpose; for example, serial measurements of plasma creatinine concentration in progressive renal disease are used to indicate when dialysis may be required. Tests can also indicate the risk of developing a particular condition; for example, the risk of coronary artery disease increases with increasing plasma cholesterol concentration. However, such risks are calculated from epidemiological data and cannot give a precise prediction for a particular individual.

### Monitoring
A major use of biochemical tests is to follow the course of an illness and to monitor the effects of treatment. To do this, there must be a suitable analyte, for instance, glucose in patients with diabetes mellitus. Biochemical tests may also be used to detect complications of treatment, such as hypokalaemia during treatment with diuretics, and are extensively used to screen for possible drug toxicity, particularly in trials, but also in some cases when a drug is in established use.

### Screening
Biochemical tests are widely used to determine whether a condition is present subclinically. The best known example is the mass screening of all newborn babies for phenyl-ketonuria (PKU), which is carried out in many countries, including the United Kingdom and the United States. The use of the 'biochemical profile', a battery of biochemical tests usually performed on a multichannel auto-analyzer, is discussed later in this chapter.

## SAMPLING

### Test request
The sample for analysis must be collected and transported to the laboratory according to a specified procedure if the data are to be of clinical value. This procedure begins with

the test request form which should include:

- Patient's name, sex and date of birth.
- Ward/clinic/address.
- Name of requesting doctor (telephone/page number for urgent requests).
- Clinical diagnosis/problem.
- Test(s) requested.
- Type of specimen.
- Date and time of sampling.
- Relevant treatment (for example, drugs).

In practice, vital information is often omitted and this may either cause delay in analysis and reporting or make it impossible to interpret the results.

Relevant clinical information and details of treatment, especially with drugs, are necessary to allow laboratory staff to assess the results in their clinical context. Drugs may interfere with analytical methods *in vitro* or may cause changes *in vivo* that suggest a pathological process; for instance, oestrogens increase thyroxine-binding globulin and thus total thyroxine concentration. If there is any doubt as to the appropriate test to request or sample to collect, the laboratory should be contacted for advice.

## Patient

Many analytes are little affected by variables such as age and sex, but it may be important to standardize the conditions under which the sample is obtained. Factors of importance in this respect are listed in *Fig. 1.2* and are discussed further in subsequent chapters.

| Factor | Example of variable affected |
|---|---|
| age | alkaline phosphatase |
| sex | gonadal steroids |
| pregnancy | thyroxine (total) |
| posture | proteins |
| exercise | creatine kinase |
| stress | prolactin |
| nutritional status | glucose |
| time | cortisol |

**Fig. 1.2** Important factors which influence biochemical variables.

Even when standardised conditions are used for sampling, the results of repeated quantitative tests (for example, daily measurements of fasting blood glucose concentration) will themselves show a Gaussian distribution, clustering about the 'usual' value for the individual. Typically, the scatter, which can be assessed by determining the standard deviation (SD), is less for analytes subject to strict regulation (e.g., fasting blood glucose and plasma calcium concentrations) than for others (e.g., plasma enzyme activities). Biological variation can be expressed as the coefficient of variation (CV) for repeated tests where $CV = SD \times 100/mean$ value.

## Sample

The sample provided must be appropriate for the test requested. Many biochemical analyses can be made on either plasma or serum but, in some instances, it is of critical importance which of these is used; for example, serum is necessary for protein electrophoresis and plasma for measurement of renin activity. Haemolysis must be avoided when blood is drawn and, if the patient is receiving intravenous therapy, blood must be drawn from a remote site (e.g., the opposite arm) to avoid contamination.

The sample can usually be collected into either a glass or plastic container, but in some circumstances one of these may be preferred or even essential. A preservative may be necessary, such as fluoride to prevent loss of glucose by glycolysis.

All samples must be correctly labelled and transported to the laboratory without delay. The serum or plasma is then separated from blood cells and analyzed. When analysis is delayed, or when samples are sent to distant laboratories for analysis, degradation of labile analytes must be prevented by refrigerating or freezing the serum or plasma.

Equal care is needed with the collection and transportation of other samples, such as urine and spinal fluid. All samples should be regarded as potentially infectious; great care is required with 'high-risk' samples, for example, from patients infected with hepatitis B or human immunodeficiency virus (HIV).

## SAMPLE ANALYSIS AND REPORTING OF RESULTS

### Analysis

The ideal analytical method is accurate, precise, sensitive and specific. It gives a correct result (accurate; *Fig. 1.3*) that is the same if repeated (precise; *Fig.1.3*). It measures low concentrations of the analyte (sensitive) and is not subject to interference by other substances (specific). In addition, it should preferably be cheap, simple and quick to perform.

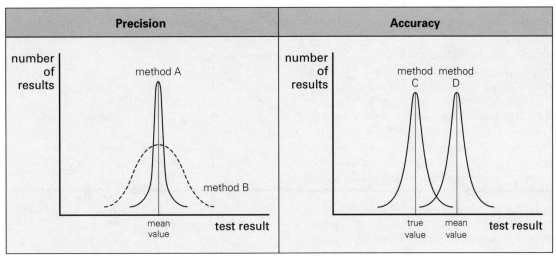

**Fig. 1.3** Precision and accuracy of biochemical tests. Both graphs show the distribution of results for repeated analysis of the same sample by different methods.
**Precision:** the mean value is the same in each case, but the scatter about the mean is less in method A than in method B. Method A is, therefore, more precise.

**Accuracy:** both are equally precise, but in method D, the mean value differs from the true value. The mean for method C is equal to the true value. Both methods are equally precise, but method C is more accurate.

In practice, no test is ideal, but the pathologist must ensure that the results are sufficiently reliable to be clinically useful. Laboratory staff make considerable efforts to achieve this and analytical methods are subject to rigorous quality control.

Nevertheless, there will always be a potential for some degree of imprecision or analytical variation in a result. The extent of this can be assessed by making repeated analyses (using exactly the same method) on the same sample (*cf.* biological variation, above). The results will cluster about a mean for which the SD can be calculated. The imprecision of the analysis can be expressed as the CV where CV = SD × 100/mean result. An understanding of the concepts of both analytical and biological variation is essential to the informed interpretation of laboratory data.

It is important to appreciate that results obtained using different methods may not be strictly comparable. When a comparison between two results is being made, the same analytical method should be used on both occasions.

It is often appropriate to perform a group of related tests on a sample. For example, plasma calcium, phosphate and alkaline phosphatase levels all provide information which may be useful in the diagnosis of bone disease; several liver 'function' tests may usefully be grouped together. Such groupings are sometimes referred to as 'biochemical profiles'.

Labour-saving multichannel auto-analyzers and similar instruments can perform more than 20 assays simultaneously on a single serum sample. However, although it may be tempting to perform all the assays on every sample, this approach generates an enormous amount of information, much of which may be unwanted, ignored or misinterpreted; worst of all, it may actually prevent the clinician from discerning the important results. Discrete analysis, that is, performing only the necessary tests, is to be preferred.

## Reporting results

Once analysis has been completed and the necessary quality control checks made and found to be satisfactory, a report can be issued. Computers are being used increasingly for data processing in laboratory medicine and reports may be generated by computers working on- or off-line to the analyzers. The ability of the computer to store and process data facilitates the production of cumulative reports, allowing trends in the data to be picked out at a glance.

## Near-patient testing

Not all analyses need to be performed in a central laboratory. Reagent sticks for testing urine at the bedside or in the clinic have long been available. Various substances, including glucose, protein, bilirubin, ketones and nitrites (indicative of urinary tract infection) can be tested for using such sticks.

Near-patient or extra-laboratory testing of blood is also feasible, for example, for glucose, cholesterol, hydrogen ion and 'blood gases', certain drugs, etc. This may be more convenient for the patient or the doctor (patients with diabetes can monitor their own blood glucose concentrations at home, for example). Also, the immediate availability of results may allow rapid initiation or change of treatment. However, although the information obtained by near-patient testing may be of considerable benefit to the patient, it is essential that the results are as reliable as, and comparable with, those provided by the main laboratory. This requires adequate training of individuals performing the tests and adherence to protocols designed to ensure quality; both these should ideally be supervised by staff from the main laboratory.

## INTERPRETATION OF RESULTS

When the result of a biochemical test is obtained, the following points must be taken into consideration:
- Is it normal?
- Is it significantly different from previous results?
- Is it consistent with the clinical findings?

### Is it normal?
The use of the word 'normal' is fraught with difficulty. Statistically, it refers to a distribution of values from repeated measurement of the same quantity and is described by the bell-shaped Gaussian curve (*Fig. 1.4*). Many biological variables show a Gaussian distribution; the majority of individuals within a population will have a value approximating to the mean for the whole and the frequency with which any value occurs decreases with increasing distance from the mean.

Skewed distributions are also often found, for example, that of plasma bilirubin concentration, but can often be mathematically transformed to a normal distribution; data distributed with a skew to the right of the mean can often be transformed to a normal distribution if replotted on a semi-logarithmic scale.

If the variable being measured has a normal (Gaussian) distribution in a population, statistical theory predicts that approximately 95% of the values in the population will lie within the range given by the mean ± two standard deviations (*Fig. 1.4*); of the remaining 5%, half the values will be higher and half will be lower than the limits of this range.

When establishing the range of values for a particular variable in healthy people, it is conventional to first exam-

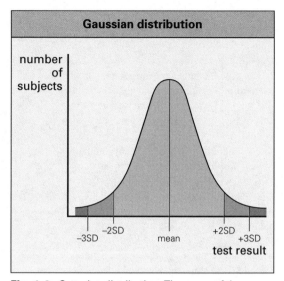

**Fig. 1.4** Gaussian distribution. The range of the mean ± 2 standard deviations (SD) encompasses 95.5% of the total number of test results. The range of the mean ± 3 standard deviations encompasses 99.7% of the total number.

ine a representative sample of sufficient size to determine whether or not the values fall into a Gaussian distribution. The range (mean ± two standard deviations) can then be calculated; this is, in statistical terms, the 'normal range' (NR). Several important points arise from this:
- Although it is assumed that the population is healthy, values from 5% of individuals by definition lie outside the normal range. This suggests that, if the measurement were to be made in a group of comparable individuals, 1 in 20 would have a value outside this range.
- The specialized statistical use of the word 'normal' does not equate with what is generally meant by the word, that is, 'habitual' or 'usually encountered'.
- The statistical 'normal' may not be related to another common use of the word, which is to imply freedom from risk. For example, epidemiological evidence indicates that there is an association between increased risk of coronary heart disease and plasma cholesterol concentrations, even within the normal range as derived from measurements on apparently healthy men.

Thus, the normal range for an analyte, defined and calculated as described, has severe limitations. It only identifies the range of values that can be expected to occur most often in individuals who are comparable to those in the population for whom the range was derived. It is not necessarily normal in terms of being 'ideal', nor is it associated with no risk of having or developing disease. Further, by definition, it will exclude values from some healthy individuals. In all cases, like must be compared with like. When physiological factors affect the concentration of an analyte (*see Fig. 1.2*), an individual's result must be assessed by comparing it with the value expected for comparable healthy people. It may, therefore, be necessary to establish normal ranges for subsets of the population, such as various age groups, or males or females only.

To alleviate the problems associated with the use of the word 'normal', the term 'reference range' (RR) has been widely adopted by laboratory staff using numerical values (reference limits) generally based on the mean ± two SDs. Results can be compared with the RR without assumptions being made about the meaning of normal. In practice, the term 'normal range' is still in general use outside laboratories. It is used synonymously with 'reference range' in this book. Reference ranges for some of the common analytes, as used in the author's laboratory, are given in *Appendix 1*.

In using RRs to assess the significance of a particular result, the individual is being compared with a population. Some analytes show considerable biological variation, but the combined analytical and biological variations will usually be less for an individual than for a population. For example, although the reference range for plasma creatinine concentration is 60–120 µmol/L, the day-to-day variation in an individual is less than this. Thus it is possible for a test result to be abnormal for an individual, yet still be within the accepted 'normal range'.

An abnormal result does not always indicate the presence of a pathological process, nor a normal result its absence. However, the more abnormal a result, that is, the greater its difference from the limits of the reference range, the greater is the probability that it is related to a pathological process.

In practice, there is rarely an absolute demarcation between normal values and those seen in disease; equivocal results must be substantiated by further investigation. If an important decision in the management of a patient is to be based upon a single result, it is vital that the cut-off point, or 'decision level', is chosen to ensure that the test functions efficiently. In screening for PKU, for example, the blood concentration of phenylalanine selected to indicate a positive result must include all infants with the condition; in other words, there must be no false negatives. This means that some normal children will be test-positive (false positives) and will be subjected to further investigation. Generally, it is unusual to have to determine a patient's management on the basis of one result alone.

It has been explained that 5% of healthy people will, by definition, have a value for a given variable that is outside the reference range. If a second and independent variable is measured, the probability that this result will be 'abnormal' is also 0.05 (5%). However, the abnormal results may not arise in the same individuals and the overall probability of an abnormal result from at least one test will be higher than 5%. It follows that the more tests that are performed on an individual, the greater the probability that the result of one of them will be abnormal; for ten independent variables the probability is 0.4, or in other words at least one abnormal result would be expected in 40% of healthy people. For twenty variables, the probability is 0.64.

Although biochemical parameters are frequently, to some extent, interdependent (e.g., albumin and total protein), the use of multichannel auto-analyzers to produce biochemical profiles inevitably generates a number of spuriously 'abnormal' results. Before any decision can be made on the basis of such results, some information is required about their predictive value (PV), that is, the probability that they are related to a pathological process. This topic is discussed *on p. 8*.

## Is it different?

If the result of a previous test is available, the clinician will be able to compare the results and decide whether any difference between them is significant. This will depend upon the precision of the assay itself (a measure of its reproducibility) and the natural biological variation. Some examples of variation in common analytes are given in *Fig. 1.5*.

The probability that the difference between two results is *analytically* significant at a level of $p < 0.05$ is 2.8 times the *analytical* SD. Thus for plasma calcium concentration, with an analytical SD of 0.04 mmol/L, an apparent increase in calcium concentration from 2.54 mmol/L to 2.62 mmol/L ($2 \times SD$) is within the limits of expected analytical variation, whereas an increase from 2.54 to 2.70 ($4 \times SD$) is not. However, to decide whether an analytical change is *clinically* significant it is necessary to consider the extent of natural biological variation. The effects of analytical and biological variation can be assessed by calculating the overall standard deviation of the test given by:

$$SD = \sqrt{SD_A{}^2 + SD_B{}^2}$$

where $SD_A$ and $SD_B$ are the SDs for the analytical and biological variation, respectively. If the difference between two test results exceeds 2.8 times the SD of the test, the difference can be regarded as of potential clinical significance (*see Case History 1.1*).

| Analyte | Analytical variation | Biological variation |
|---|---|---|
| sodium | 1.1 mmol/L | 2.0 mmol/L |
| potassium | 0.1 mmol/L | 0.19 mmol/L |
| bicarbonate | 0.5 mmol/L | 1.3 mmol/L |
| urea | 0.4 mmol/L | 0.85 mmol/L |
| creatinine | 5.0 μmol/L | 4.1 μmol/L |
| calcium | 0.04 mmol/L | 0.04 mmol/L |
| phosphate | 0.04 mmol/L | 0.11 mmol/L |
| total protein | 1.0 g/L | 1.66 g/L |
| albumin | 1.0 g/L | 1.44 g/L |
| aspartate transaminase | 6.0 IU/L | 8.0 IU/L |
| alkaline phosphatase | 4.0 IU/L | 15.0 IU/L |

**Fig 1.5** Analytical and biological variation.

Analytical variation: typical standard deviations for repeated measurements made using a multichannel auto-analyzer on a single quality control serum with concentrations in the normal range.

Biological variation: means of standard deviations for repeated measurements made at weekly intervals in a group of healthy subjects over a period of 10 weeks.

**CASE HISTORY 1.1**

A GP measured the serum creatinine concentration of a 41-year-old man newly diagnosed as having diabetes mellitus and hypertension. The result was 105 μmol/L. Six months later, both conditions were well controlled and the test was repeated.

**Investigation**

serum creatinine 118 μmol/L
The patient was alarmed at the apparent increase, but the GP was uncertain as to whether this was a significant change.

**Comment**

The analytical variation for creatinine is 5.0 μmol/L, the biological variation, 4.1 μmol/L (*Fig. 1.5*). The critical difference is thus:

$$2.8 \times \sqrt{(4.1^2 + 5.0^2)}$$

that is, 18 μmol/L. Thus the apparent increase in creatinine is not significant at a level of p = 0.05.

### Is it consistent with clinical findings?

If the result is consistent with clinical findings, it is evidence in favour of the clinical diagnosis. If it is not consistent, the explanation must be sought. There may have been a mistake in the collection, labelling or analysis of the sample, or in the reporting of the result. In practice, it may be simplest to request a further sample and to repeat the test. If the result is confirmed, the sensitivity and specificity of the test in the clinical context should be considered and the clinical diagnosis itself may have to be reviewed.

## SPECIFICITY, SENSITIVITY AND PREDICTIVE VALUE OF TESTS

In using the result of a test, it is important to know how reliable the test is and how suitable it is for its intended purpose. Thus, the laboratory personnel must ensure, as far as is practicable, that the data are accurate and precise and the clinician should appreciate how specific and sensitive the test is in the context in which it is used.

## Specificity and sensitivity

Specificity is a measure of the incidence of negative results in persons known to be free of a disease, that is 'true negative' (TN). Sensitivity is a measure of the incidence of positive results in patients known to have a condition, that is, 'true positive' (TP). A specificity of 90% implies that 10% of disease-free people would be classified as having the disease on the basis of the test result; 10% would have a 'false positive' (FP) result. A sensitivity of 90% implies that only 90% of people known to have the disease would be diagnosed as having it on the basis of that test alone; 10% would be false negatives (FN).

An ideal diagnostic test would be 100% sensitive, giving positive results in all diseased subjects, and also 100% specific, giving negative results in all subjects free of disease. In reality no tests achieve such high standards; all generate false positives and false negatives. Specificity and sensitivity are calculated as follows :

$$\text{Specificity} = \frac{TN}{\text{all without disease} (FP + TN)} \times 100$$

$$\text{Sensitivity} = \frac{TP}{\text{all with disease} (TP + FN)} \times 100$$

Factors which increase the specificity of a test tend to decrease the sensitivity and vice versa, as there is almost always an overlap between test results seen in health and in disease. To take an extreme example, if it were decided to diagnose thyrotoxicosis only if the plasma free thyroxine concentration were at least 32 pmol/L (the upper limit of the reference range is 26 pmol/L in the author's laboratory), the test would have 100% specificity; positive results (greater than 32 pmol/L) would only be seen in thyrotoxicosis. On the other hand, the test would have a low sensitivity in that many patients with mild thyrotoxicosis would be misdiagnosed. If a concentration of 20 pmol/L were used, the test would be very sensitive (all those with thyrotoxicosis would be correctly assigned) but very non-specific, because many normal people would also be diagnosed as having thyrotoxicosis. These concepts are illustrated in *Fig. 1.6*.

Whether it is desirable to maximize specificity or sensitivity depends on the nature of the condition that the test is used to diagnose and the consequences of making an incorrect diagnosis. For example, sensitivity is paramount in a screening test for a harmful condition, but the inevitable false positive results will have to be investigated further. However, in selecting patients for a trial of a new treatment, a highly specific test is more appropriate to ensure that the treatment is being given only to patients who have a particular condition.

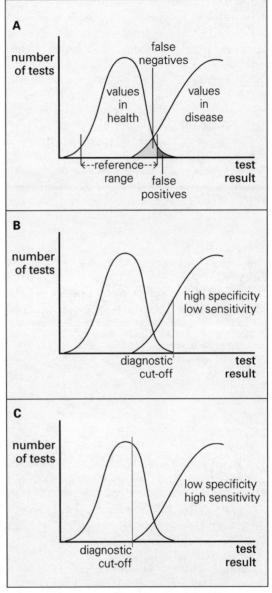

**Fig. 1.6** Because the ranges of values for a test result in health and disease overlap (A), some patients with disease will have results within the reference range (false negatives) while some individuals free of disease will have results outside this range (false positives). If the diagnostic cut-off value for a test is set too high (B), there will be no false positives, but many false negatives; specificity is increased but sensitivity decreases. If the diagnostic cut-off value is set too low (C), the number of false positives, and sensitivity, increases, at the expense of a decrease in specificity.

One way of comparing the sensitivity and specificity of different tests is to construct 'receiver operating characteristic curves' (ROC curves). Each test is performed in each of a series of appropriate individuals. The specificity and sensitivity is calculated using different cut-off values to determine whether a given result is positive or negative (*see* *Fig. 1.7*). The curves can then be assessed to determine which test performs best in the specific circumstances for which it is required.

Readers should be aware that the terms 'sensitivity' and 'specificity' have alternative meanings in biochemistry, in relation to the analytical aspects of diagnostic tests. Thus 'sensitivity' is also used in relation to the ability of a test to measure low concentrations of an analyte; 'specificity' is used to describe the ability of a test to measure only the analyte of interest, and not similar or related substances.

## Efficiency

The efficiency of a test is the number of correct results divided by the total number of tests. Thus efficiency is given by:

$$\frac{TP + TN}{\text{total number of tests}} \times 100$$

When sensitivity and specificity are equally important, the test with the greatest efficiency should be used.

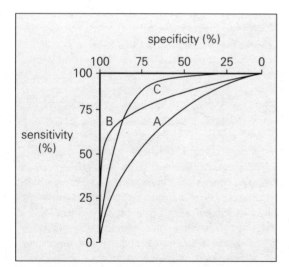

specificity (%)

sensitivity (%)

**Fig. 1.7** ROC curves for three hypothetical tests, A, B, and C. Examination of the curves shows that test A performs less well in terms of both sensitivity and specificity than tests B and C. Test B has better specificity than C, but C has better sensitivity.

## Predictive values (PVs)

A highly specific and sensitive test does not necessarily perform well in a clinical context. This is because the PV of a positive test result is dependent upon the prevalence of the disease. PV(+), the PV for a positive result, is the percentage of all positive results that are TPs, that is:

$$PV(+) = \frac{TP}{TP + FP} \times 100$$

If a condition has a low prevalence and the test is less than 100% specific, many FPs will result.

A high predictive value for a positive test is important if the appropriate management of a true positive (TP) result would be potentially dangerous if applied to a false positive (FP) result. However, when a test is used for screening, the appropriate management is to perform further confirmatory tests, and although these may cause inconvenience for subjects with FP results, they are unlikely to be dangerous.

In order not to miss cases, a screening test should have a very high PV(–), the PV for a negative result, this being the percentage of all negative results which are TNs, that is :

$$PV(-) = \frac{TN}{TN + FN} \times 100$$

This conclusion follows directly from the fact that the test must be highly sensitive.

For clarity, this discussion has centred on the use of single tests for diagnostic purposes but, in practice, the clinician will combine clinical information and, often, the results of several investigations to make the diagnosis. If the tests are used rationally, the PV of positive results will be higher since the tests will be used only in patients who have other features suggesting a particular diagnosis (the prevalence of the disease in question will be much higher than in the general population). For example, although Cushing's disease is rare, making the PV of a positive test for the condition in the general population low, in practice one would only investigate patients suspected on clinical grounds of having the condition and in whom the prevalence will therefore be higher. This may be self-evident, but doctors frequently order tests on flimsy clinical grounds and fail to appreciate how unhelpful, or even misleading, the results may be.

Although most clinicians and pathologists interpret data intuitively, the most efficient approach can be defined mathematically, especially when there are numerous data to consider. With the increasing availability of computers, such mathematical data analysis should become more widely adopted.

Another approach, useful when several tests are performed, is to combine the results mathematically, usually after each result has been weighted by a multiplier, to produce one or more figures called 'discriminant functions' (DFs) or 'indices'. These can then be compared with the range of values calculated for a group of patients shown, by an independent, definitive technique, to have a particular condition. If the DF for an individual falls within this range, there is a high probability that he has the condition in question. This approach has been applied, for example, to the differential diagnosis of hypercalcaemia and obstructive jaundice, but has yet to gain wide acceptance in clinical biochemistry.

## SCREENING

Screening tests are used to detect disease in groups of apparently healthy individuals. Such tests may be applied to whole populations (e.g., the detection of PKU in the newborn); to groups known to be at risk (the detection of hypercholesterolaemia in the relatives of people with premature coronary heart disease), or to groups of people selected for other reasons (biochemical profiling of hospital inpatients and health screening for business executives).

As previously discussed, high sensitivity is essential for screening tests and, to avoid unnecessary further tests of normal people, high specificity is desirable. Screening tests for PKU are designed to maximize sensitivity but are also highly specific. However, PKU has a low incidence so that even with a sensitivity of 100% and specificity of 99.9%, the predictive value of a positive test is only 10%, that is, nine out of ten positive tests will be shown on further investigation to be false positives. These calculations are made as follows:

1. Incidence of PKU = 1 in 10,000 live births

2. Sensitivity = 100% or $\dfrac{1\,TP}{1\,case\ of\ PKU}$

3. Specificity = 99.9% or $\dfrac{9990\,TN}{9999\ without\ PKU}$

4. Number of positive tests per 10,000 infants tested =
$\dfrac{(100 - 99.9)}{100} \times 10\,000 = 10$

5. Numbers of TP and FP results:
TP = 1, FP = 9

6. Predictive value of a positive test =
$\dfrac{1}{10} \times 100 = 10\%$

On the other hand, the predictive value of a negative test will be 100%, confirming that no cases will be missed using the screening test.

Biochemical profiling is based on the use of much less specific or sensitive tests and therefore has a low efficiency for detecting disease. It is also not particularly efficient at detecting minor abnormalities as the more tests that are performed, the greater the probability that one result will be abnormal.

When multichannel auto-analyzers are used to generate biochemical data and an unexpected abnormality is found, a decision must be made as to what action to take. The abnormality may be considered insignificant in some clinical circumstances but, if it is not, further investigations must be made. Although these may be of ultimate benefit to the patient, their cost and economic consequences may be considerable. At the very least, the tests should be repeated to ensure that the abnormality was not due to analytical error.

The ready availability of an investigation often leads to it being used unnecessarily or inappropriately. Doctors should be encouraged to be selective in making test requests. They should also join with laboratory staff in critically examining all current tests and investigative techniques to ensure that they are using these tests to their best advantage in medical practice.

## SUMMARY

Biochemical tests are used in diagnosis, monitoring patients' progress, screening for disease and for prognosis. The results of some biochemical tests provide specific diagnostic information but, in many instances, biochemical changes reflect pathological processes which are common to a number of diseases.

In selecting a test or tests, it is essential to consider what type of information is required and whether the test is capable of providing it. Samples for analysis must be collected under appropriate conditions and the analytical methods must be reliable. In assessing the significance of a test result, the clinical circumstances and the possible contribution of any analytical or biological variation must be considered. When a test result is assessed by comparison with a reference range of values expected for healthy people, this reference range should be based on analyses of subjects who are comparable in, for example, age and sex.

Since there is rarely a clear distinction between test results which can occur in health and in disease, it is essential to appreciate the statistical basis on which such comparisons can be made. This is also necessary when a result is compared with one obtained previously.

## PLASMA AND SERUM

Plasma is the aqueous phase of blood. For technical reasons, many biochemical measurements are more conveniently made on serum, but the concentrations of most analytes are effectively the same in both fluids. In this book, the term 'serum' is used only where actual measurements made in serum are referred to (e.g., in the Case Histories) and in the few instances where serum must be used for analysis.

## FURTHER READING

Fraser C G (1986) *Interpretation of Clinical Chemistry Laboratory Data*. Oxford: Blackwell Scientific Publications.

Fraser C G & Fogarty Y (1989) Interpreting Laboratory Results. *British Medical Journal*, **298**, 1659–1660.

Galen R S & Gambino S R (1975) *Beyond Normality: The Predictive Value and Efficiency of Medical Diagnosis*. New York: John Wiley.

Henderson A R (1993) Assessing test accuracy and its clinical consequences: a primer for receiver operating characteristic curve analysis. *Annals of Clinical Biochemistry*, **30**, 521–539.

# 2. Water, Sodium and Potassium

## INTRODUCTION

### Water distribution

Water accounts for approximately 60% of body weight in men and 55% in women, reflecting a greater body fat content in women. Approximately 66% of this water is in the intracellular fluid (ICF) and 33% in the extracellular fluid (ECF); only 8% of body water is in the plasma (*Fig. 2.1*). Water is not actively transported in the body. It is, in general, freely permeable through the ICF and ECF and its distribution is determined by the osmotic contents of these compartments. Except in the kidney, the osmotic concentrations, or osmolalities, of these compartments are always equal; they are isotonic. Any change in the solute content of a compartment engenders a shift of water which restores isotonicity.

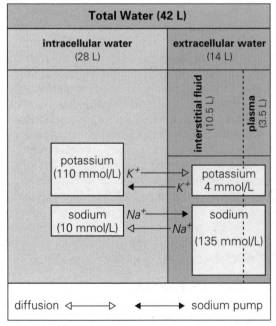

**Fig. 2.1** Distribution of water, sodium and potassium in the body of a 70 kg man. The distribution is similar in women although the amount of water as a percentage of body weight is less. In children and infants, total body water is 75–80% of body weight, with a higher ECF:ICF volume ratio than in adults, but the proportion of the total body water contained in the plasma is the same.

The major contributors to the osmolality of the ECF are sodium and its associated anions, mainly chloride and bicarbonate; in the ICF, the predominant cation is potassium. Other determinants of ECF osmolality include glucose and urea. Protein makes a numerically small contribution of approximately 0.5%. However, since the capillary endothelium is relatively impermeable to protein and since the protein concentration of interstitial fluid is much less than that of plasma, the osmotic effect of the protein is an important factor in determining water distribution between these two compartments. The contribution of protein to the osmotic pressure of plasma is known as the colloid osmotic pressure or oncotic pressure (*see Chapter 13*).

Under normal circumstances, the amounts of water taken into the body and lost from it are equal over a period of time. Water is obtained from the diet and oxidative metabolism and is lost through the kidneys, skin, lungs and gut (*Fig. 2.2*). The minimum volume of urine necessary for normal excretion of waste products is about 500 mL/24 h but, as a result of obligatory losses by other routes, the minimum daily water intake necessary for the maintenance of water balance is approximately 1100 mL. This increases if the losses are abnormally large, for example, with excessive sweating or diarrhoea. Water intake is usually considerably greater than this minimum requirement but the excess is easily removed by the kidneys.

### Sodium distribution

The body of an adult man contains approximately 3000 mmol of sodium, 70% of which is freely exchangeable, with the remainder complexed in bone. The majority of the exchangeable sodium is extracellular; the normal ECF sodium concentration is 135–145 mmol/L while that of the ICF is only 4–10 mmol/L. Most cell membranes are relatively impermeable to sodium but some leakage into cells occurs and the gradient is maintained by active pumping of sodium from the ICF to the ECF, by $Na^+$, $K^+$-ATPase.

As with water, sodium input and output normally are balanced. The normal intake of sodium in the Western world is 100–200 mmol/24 h but the obligatory sodium loss, via the kidneys, skin and gut, is less than 10 mmol/24 h. Thus, the sodium intake necessary to maintain sodium balance is much less than the normal intake and excess sodium is excreted in the urine. Despite this, excessive sodium intake may be harmful, being a contributory factor in some cases of hypertension.

| Obligatory losses | Sources | |
|---|---|---|
| skin   500 mL | | |
| lungs   400 mL | | |
| gut   100 mL | water from oxidative metabolism | 400 mL |
| kidneys   500 mL | minimum in diet | 1100 mL |
| total      1500 mL | total | 1500 mL |

Fig. 2.2 Daily water balance in an adult. The minimum intake necessary to maintain balance is approximately 1100 mL. Actual water intake in food and drink is usually greater than this, and the excess over requirements is excreted in the urine.

It is important to appreciate that there is a massive internal turnover of sodium. Sodium is secreted into the gut at a rate of approximately 1000 mmol/24 h and filtered by the kidneys at a rate of 25,000 mmol/24 h, the vast majority being regained by reabsorption in the gut and renal tubules. If there is even a partial failure of this reabsorption, sodium homoeostasis will be compromised.

## Potassium distribution

Potassium is the predominant intracellular cation. Ninety percent of the total body potassium is free and therefore exchangeable, whilst the remainder is bound in red blood cells, bone and brain tissue. However, only approximately 2% (50–60 mmol) of the total is located in the extracellular compartment (see Fig. 2.1) where it is readily accessible for measurement. As a consequence, the concentration of potassium in the plasma is not an accurate index of total body potassium status. The potassium concentration of serum is 0.2–0.3 mmol/L higher than that of plasma, due to the release of potassium from platelets during clot formation, but this difference is not of practical significance.

There is a constant tendency for potassium to diffuse down its concentration gradient from the intra- to the extracellular fluid, opposed by the action of $Na^+$, $K^+$ ATPase (the sodium pump), which transports potassium into cells.

Potassium homoeostasis and its disorders are described later in this chapter.

## WATER AND SODIUM HOMOEOSTASIS

### Water and ECF osmolality

Changes in body water content independent of the amount of solute will alter the osmolality (Fig. 2.3). The osmolality of the ECF is normally maintained in the range 282–295 mmol/kg of water. Any loss of water from the ECF, such as occurs with water deprivation, will increase its osmolality and result in movement of water from the ICF to the ECF. However, a slight increase in ECF osmolality will

still occur, stimulating the hypothalamic thirst centre, which promotes a desire to drink, and the hypothalamic osmoreceptors, which causes the release of vasopressin (antidiuretic hormone or ADH).

Vasopressin renders the renal collecting ducts permeable to water, permitting water reabsorption and concentration of the urine; the maximum urine concentration that can be achieved in humans is about 1200 mmol/kg. The osmoreceptors are highly sensitive to osmolality, responding to a change of as little as 1%. Vasopressin is undetectable in the plasma at a plasma osmolality of 282 mmol/kg, but its concentration rises sharply if the plasma osmolality increases above this level (Fig. 2.4).

If the ECF osmolality falls, there is no sensation of thirst and vasopressin secretion is inhibited. A dilute urine is produced, allowing water loss and restoration of the ECF osmolality to normal. If an increase in ECF osmolality occurs as a result of the presence of a solute, such as urea, which diffuses readily across cell membranes, the ICF osmolality is also increased and osmoreceptors are not stimulated.

Other stimuli affecting vasopressin secretion (Fig. 2.5) include angiotensin II, arterial and venous baroreceptors and volume receptors. If there is a decrease in plasma volume of more than 10%, hypovolaemia becomes a powerful stimulus to vasopressin release (see Fig. 2.4) and osmolar controls are overridden. In other words, ECF volume is defended at the expense of a decrease in osmolality.

### Sodium and ECF volume

The volume of the ECF is directly dependent upon the total body sodium content since water intake and loss are regulated to hold the concentration of sodium in the ECF constant and because sodium is virtually confined to the ECF.

Sodium balance is maintained by regulation of its renal excretion. Sodium excretion is dependent upon glomerular filtration, but the glomerular filtration rate (GFR) appears to become an important limiting factor in sodium excretion only at extremely low rates of filtration (sodium retention

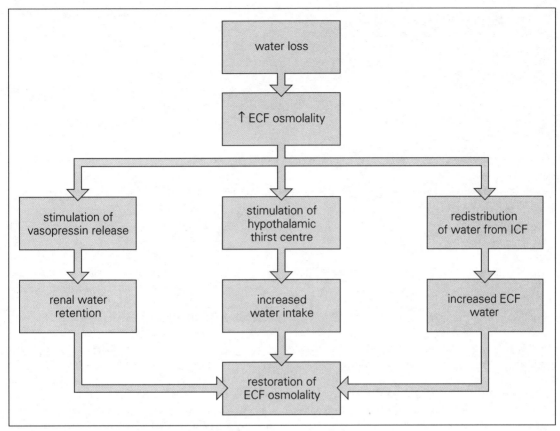

**Fig. 2.3** Physiological responses to water loss.

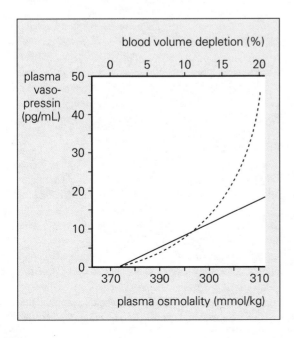

**Fig. 2.4** Vasopressin concentration in relation to blood volume and osmolality. Vasopressin secretion increases linearly (solid line) with increasing plasma osmolality if blood volume remains constant. A small decrease in blood volume under iso-osmotic conditions has little effect on the secretion of vasopressin (broken line) whereas a fall of more than 10% results in a massive increase in vasopressin secretion.

| Control of vasopressin secretion | |
|---|---|
| **Stimulating factors** | **Inhibiting factors** |
| increased ECF osmolality | decreased ECF osmolality |
| severe hypovolaemia (via angiotensin II and arterial and venous volume receptors) | hypervolaemia |
| | alcohol |
| stress, including pain | |
| exercise | |
| drugs: narcotic analgesics, nicotine, some sulphonylureas, carbamazepine, clofibrate and vincristine | |

**Fig. 2.5** Factors affecting vasopressin secretion. ECF osmolality is normally the most important of these.

is a late feature of chronic renal failure). Normally, approximately 70% of filtered sodium is actively reabsorbed in the proximal convoluted tubules, with further reabsorption in the loops of Henle. Less than 5% of filtered sodium reaches the distal convoluted tubules. Aldosterone, released from the adrenal cortex in response to activation of the renin–angiotensin system, stimulates sodium reabsorption in the distal convoluted tubules and collecting ducts and is the major factor controlling renal sodium excretion.

Other factors must however be involved in the control of sodium reabsorption since patients with adrenal insufficiency, on a fixed replacement dose of mineralocorticoids, maintain sodium balance even though their plasma mineralocorticoid levels are not controlled by sodium status. In such subjects, chronic loading with mineralocorticoids causes sodium retention only for a short period; thereafter, sodium balance is regained, albeit with an increased ECF volume.

This response may be mediated by atrial natriuretic hormone. This is a 28 amino acid peptide, secreted by the cardiac atria in response to atrial stretch following a rise in atrial pressure (for example, due to ECF volume expansion). It appears to have a role, as yet imperfectly understood, in regulating blood volume and blood pressure. It is natriuretic, acting by reducing basal renin activity and

angiotensin converting enzyme activity and by antagonizing the actions of aldosterone, and also antagonizes the pressor actions of noradrenaline and angiotensin II. Atrial natriuretic hormone can be measured in plasma by immunoassay, but its measurement has not yet found an established role in routine clinical practice. Two other structurally similar peptides have been described. One, found in the brain and the cardiac ventricles, has similar properties to the atrial hormone; the other, found in vascular endothelium, causes vasodilatation but apparently not natriuresis.

There is also evidence for a natriuretic factor with a low molecular weight (less than 500 daltons), possibly having a structure resembling a cardiac glycoside and acting through the inhibition of $Na^+$, $K^+$-ATPase. However, this substance has yet to be purified and characterized.

In general, the control mechanisms for ECF volume respond less rapidly and are less precise than the control mechanisms for ECF osmolality. Except at extremes of hypovolaemia, maintenance of osmolality takes precedence.

## WATER AND SODIUM DEPLETION

Water depletion or combined water and sodium depletion will occur if losses are greater than intake. Pure water depletion is seen much less frequently than depletion of both water and sodium. As sodium cannot be excreted from the body without water, sodium loss never occurs alone but is always accompanied by some loss of water. The fluid may be isotonic or hypotonic with respect to the plasma.

The clinical and biochemical features of pure water depletion and of isotonic sodium and water loss are quite different, as are the physiological responses. In clinical practice, however, states of fluid depletion encompass the whole spectrum between these two extremes and the clinical and biochemical features will reflect this. Further, it should be appreciated that they may have been modified by previous treatment.

### Water depletion

Water depletion will occur if water intake is inadequate or if losses are excessive (*Fig. 2.6*). Excessive loss of water without any sodium loss is unusual, except in diabetes insipidus, but provided that the sodium loss is small the clinical consequences will be related primarily to the water depletion (*Fig. 2.6*).

Loss of water from the ECF causes an increase in osmolality which in turn causes movement of water from the ICF to the ECF, thus lessening the increase. Nevertheless, ECF osmolality will be higher than normal; this stimulates the thirst centre and vasopressin secretion. Patients are

| Water depletion | |
|---|---|
| **Causes** | **Clinical features** |
| **Increased loss**<br>*from kidneys:*<br>    renal tubular disorders<br>    diabetes insipidus<br>    increased osmotic load due to diabetes mellitus,<br>    osmotic diuretics or high protein intake<br>*from skin:*<br>    sweating<br>*from lungs:*<br>    hyperventilation<br>*from gut:*<br>    diarrhoea (in infants) | **Symptoms**<br>thirst<br>dryness of mouth<br>difficulty in swallowing<br>weakness<br>confusion<br><br>**Signs**<br>weight loss<br>dryness of mucus membranes<br>decreased saliva secretion<br>loss of skin turgor<br>decreased urine volume (early) |
| **Decreased intake**<br>  infancy          dysphagia<br>  old age         restriction of<br>  unconsciousness    oral intake | |

**Fig. 2.6** Causes and clinical features of predominant water depletion. In infantile gastroenteritis and in acclimatization to high temperatures, some sodium is lost from the gut and skin, but the effects of water loss may predominate.

hypernatraemic; plasma protein concentration and the haematocrit are usually only slightly elevated. Unless water depletion is due to uncontrolled loss through the kidneys, the urine becomes highly concentrated and there is a rapid decrease in its volume (*see Fig. 2.9*). Because water loss is borne by the total body water, and not just the ECF (*Fig. 2.7*), signs of a reduced ECF volume are not usually present. Furthermore, the increased colloid osmotic pressure of the plasma tends to hold extracellular water in the vascular compartment. Circulatory failure may be a very late feature of water depletion; it is much more likely to occur if sodium depletion is also present.

Severe water depletion induces cerebral dehydration which may cause cerebral haemorrhage through tearing of blood vessels. Such damage can also occur if rehydration is too rapid. If dehydration persists, the brain cells synthesize osmotically active compounds and cerebral oedema may then follow rapid fluid replacement.

The management of water depletion involves treatment of the underlying cause and replacement of the fluid deficit. Water should preferably be given either orally or via a nasogastric tube. If this is not possible, either 5% dextrose or, if there is also some sodium depletion, hypotonic saline, should be given intravenously. The aim should be to correct approximately two-thirds of the deficit in the first 24 hours and the remainder in the next 24 hours.

## Sodium depletion

Sodium depletion is seldom due to inadequate oral intake alone, but sometimes inadequate parenteral input is responsible. More often, sodium depletion is a consequence of excessive sodium loss (*Fig. 2.8*). Sodium can be lost from the body in either isotonic or hypotonic fluid. In each case, there will be a decrease in ECF volume (*see Fig. 2.7*), but this will be less with hypotonic loss since some of the water loss will then be shared with the ICF. The clinical features of sodium depletion (*Fig. 2.8*) are primarily a result of the decrease in ECF volume.

The normal responses to hypovolaemia are an increase in aldosterone secretion, stimulating renal sodium reabsorption in the distal convoluted tubules, and a fall in urine volume as a consequence of a decreased GFR. Increased vasopressin secretion, which stimulates the production of a highly concentrated urine, only occurs with severe ECF volume depletion (*see Fig. 2.4*).

The decrease in GFR may lead to prerenal uraemia (*see Case History 4.1*). In contrast to the effects of pure water depletion, plasma protein concentration and the haematocrit are usually clearly increased in sodium depletion, unless this is due to the loss of plasma or blood. Furthermore, because the fluid loss is borne mainly by the ECF, signs of a reduced ECF volume are usually present and peripheral circulatory failure is more likely to occur than in

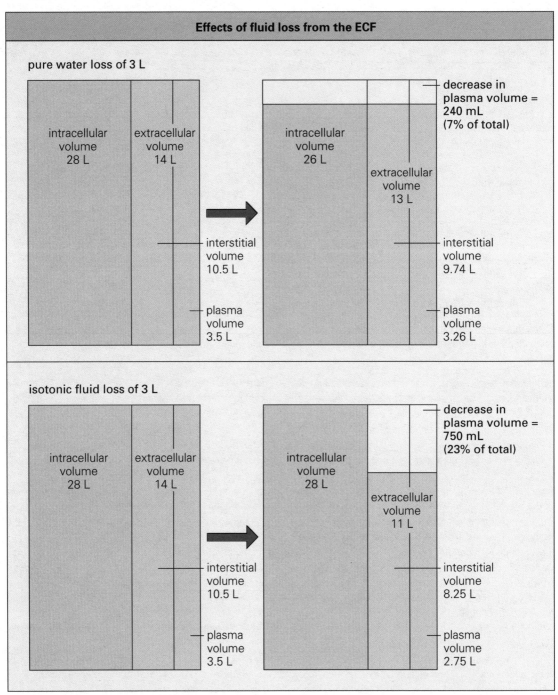

**Fig. 2.7** Comparison of the effects of water loss and isotonic fluid loss from the extracellular compartment. When only water is lost from the ECF, the increase in osmolality causes water to move from the ICF to minimize the decrease in plasma volume. When isotonic fluid is lost from the ECF, no osmotic imbalance is produced, there is no movement of water from the ICF and the effect on plasma volume is, therefore, much greater.

| Sodium depletion | |
|---|---|
| **Causes** | **Clinical features** |
| **Excessive loss**<br>*from kidneys:*<br>    diuretic phase of 'acute tubular necrosis'<br>    diuretic therapy<br>    mineralocorticoid deficiency<br>    other salt-losing states<br>*from skin:*<br>    massively increased sweating<br>    cystic fibrosis<br>    widespread dermatitis<br>    burns<br>*from gut*<br>    vomiting, diarrhoea<br>    fistulae<br>    ileus<br>    intestinal obstruction | **Symptoms**<br>weakness<br>apathy<br>postural dizziness<br>syncope<br><br>**Signs**<br>weight loss<br>related to decreased plasma volume:<br>    tachycardia<br>    hypotension<br>    peripheral circulatory failure<br>    oliguria<br>related to decreased interstitial fluid:<br>    decreased intraocular pressure<br>    decreased skin turgor |
| **Inadequate intake**<br>sodium depletion will occur whenever<br>    intake is inadequate to balance excessive<br>    losses; inadequate intake alone is rarely<br>    a cause of depletion | |

**Fig. 2.8** Causes and clinical features of predominant sodium depletion. Thirst is usually absent. The clinical signs are due to hypovolaemia. Oliguria develops gradually; it is primarily due to the decrease in GFR, rather than to vasopressin.

| Clinical and laboratory findings in sodium and water depletion | | |
|---|---|---|
| | **Sodium depletion** | **Water depletion** |
| plasma [Na$^+$] | normal or ↓ | ↑ |
| haematocrit | ↑↑↑* | normal or slightly ↑ |
| ECF volume | ↓↓↓ | usually normal |
| plasma [urea] | ↑ | high normal |
| urine volume | ↓ | ↓↓↓ |
| urine concentration | ↑ | ↑↑↑ |
| thirst | late | early |
| tachycardia hypotension | early | late |

**Fig. 2.9** Clinical and laboratory findings in sodium and water depletion.   * unless due to loss of blood

water depletion. The features of sodium and water depletion are compared in *Fig. 2.9*.

The plasma sodium concentration can give an indication of the relative amounts of water and sodium that have been lost; the plasma sodium will be normal if fluid is lost isotonically and increased if it is lost hypotonically. With severe sodium depletion, increased vasopressin secretion secondary to the resulting hypovolaemia may cause water retention; plasma volume is then maintained at the expense of osmolality and hyponatraemia develops. Thus the plasma sodium concentration in a sodium depleted patient may be low, normal or high (*Fig. 2.10*).

Management of sodium depletion involves treatment of the underlying cause and, if necessary, restoration of the intravascular volume by giving isotonic fluid ('normal saline', plasma or blood) by intravenous infusion. This can usually be done rapidly, but any associated free water deficit requires more cautious correction.

## WATER AND SODIUM EXCESS

Excess of water and sodium may result from a failure of normal excretion or from excessive intake. The latter is

| Mechanism of sodium depletion | Plasma sodium concentration |
|---|---|
| sodium and water loss, water loss predominating; e.g., excessive sweating | increased |
| isotonic sodium and water loss; e.g., burns, haemorrhage | normal |
| sodium loss with water retention; e.g., treatment of isotonic sodium depletion with low sodium fluids | decreased |

**Fig. 2.10** Plasma sodium concentration with various causes of sodium depletion. The plasma sodium concentration alone is a poor guide to ECF sodium status.

often iatrogenic. As with the syndromes of depletion, pure water excess and sodium excess with isotonic retention of water can be considered as separate conditions although, in practice, there is often a degree of overlap.

## Water excess

This is usually related to an impairment of water excretion (*Fig. 2.11*). However, the limit to the ability of the healthy kidney to excrete water is about 20 mL/min and, occasionally, excessive intake is alone sufficient to cause water intoxication. Hyponatraemia is invariably present. The increased water load is shared by the ICF and ECF.

The clinical features of water overload (*Fig. 2.11*) are related to cerebral over-hydration, the incidence and severity depending upon the extent of the water excess and its time course. A patient with a plasma sodium concentration of 120 mmol/L, in whom water retention has occurred gradually over several days, may be asymptomatic while another, in whom this is an acute phenomenon, may show signs of severe water intoxication.

| Excess body water | |
|---|---|
| **Causes** | **Clinical features** |
| **Increased intake**<br>compulsive water drinking<br>excessive parenteral fluid administration<br>water absorption during bladder irrigation<br><br>**Decreased excretion**<br>renal failure (severe)<br>cortisol deficiency<br>inappropriate or ectopic secretion of vasopressin<br>drugs:<br>    stimulating vasopressin release<br>    potentiating the action of vasopressin,<br>      e.g., chlorpropamide<br>    agonists of vasopressin,<br>      e.g., oxytocin<br>    interfering with renal diluting capacity,<br>      e.g., diuretics | behavioural disturbances<br>confusion<br>headache<br>convulsions<br>coma<br>muscle twitching<br>extensor plantar responses |

**Fig. 2.11** Causes and clinical features of excess body water.

The management of water overload is discussed with that of hyponatraemia, *on p. 22*.

## Sodium excess

Sodium excess can be due to increased intake or decreased excretion. The clinical features are related primarily to expansion of ECF volume. When related to excessive intake (for example the inappropriate use of hypertonic saline), a rapid shift of water from the intracellular compartment may cause cerebral dehydration in addition. When sodium overload is due to excessive intake, hypernatraemia is usual (see *Case History 2.6*).

Sodium overload is more usually due to impaired excretion than to excessive intake. Intrinsic renal disease is a relatively uncommon cause (*Fig. 2.12*). Increased mineralocorticoid secretion, due to primary adrenal disease, is also uncommon. Sodium overload is most frequently due to secondary aldosteronism. This is seen in patients who, despite clinical evidence of increased ECF volume (e.g., peripheral oedema), appear to have a decreased effective plasma volume, due for example to venous pooling or a disturbance in the normal distribution of extracellular fluid between the vascular and extravascular compartments.

Many such patients with sodium excess are, paradoxically, hyponatraemic, implying the coexistence of a defect in free water excretion. This is probably in part due to an increase in vasopressin secretion as a result of the decreased plasma volume. Also, the decrease in GFR and consequent increase in proximal tubular sodium reabsorption decreases the delivery of sodium and chloride to the loops of Henle and distal convoluted tubules. This reduces the kidneys' diluting capacity, thereby compromising water excretion. The 'sick cell syndrome' (see below) may also contribute to the hyponatraemia in such patients.

The management of sodium excess should be directed towards the cause, where possible. In addition, diuretics may be used to promote sodium excretion and sodium intake must be controlled. Dialysis may be necessary if renal function is poor and is occasionally necessary in acute sodium overload associated with the use of hypertonic fluids.

## LABORATORY ASSESSMENT OF WATER AND SODIUM STATUS

The plasma sodium concentration is dependent upon the relative amounts of sodium and water in the plasma. In

| Sodium excess | |
|---|---|
| **Causes** | **Clinical features** |
| Increased intake<br>excessive parenteral administration<br>absorption from saline emetics | peripheral oedema<br>dyspnoea<br>pulmonary oedema<br>venous congestion |
| Decreased excretion<br>decreased glomerular filtration:<br>  acute and chronic renal failure | hypertension<br>effusions<br>weight gain |
| increased tubular reabsorption:<br>  primary mineralocorticoid excess:<br>    Cushing's syndrome<br>    Conn's syndrome<br>  secondary mineralocorticoid excess:<br>    congestive cardiac failure<br>    nephrotic syndrome<br>    hepatic cirrhosis with ascites<br>    renal artery stenosis | |

**Fig. 2.12** Causes and clinical features of predominant sodium excess.

isolation, therefore, plasma sodium concentration provides no information about the sodium content of the ECF. It may be raised, normal or low, in states of sodium excess or depletion, according to the amount of water in the ECF. The plasma sodium concentration is one of the most frequent measurements made in clinical chemistry laboratories but valid indications for its measurement are few and results are often misinterpreted. Plasma sodium concentration should be measured in the following:

- Patients with dehydration or excessive fluid loss, as a guide to appropriate replacement.
- Patients on parenteral fluid replacement who are unable to indicate or respond to thirst (e.g., the comatose, infants and the elderly).
- Patients with unexplained confusion, abnormal behaviour or signs of CNS irritability.

In the assessment of a patient's water and sodium status, clinical observations, such as the measurements of central venous pressure, fluid balance and body weight, may all provide vital information. An increase in the concentration of plasma proteins or in the haematocrit suggests haemoconcentration. Other abnormal results may suggest specific conditions; for example, hyperkalaemia in a hyponatraemic patient with clinical evidence of sodium depletion suggests adrenal failure.

Analysis of urine can provide valuable information but results may be misleading. It should be established whether the urine volume and composition are physiologically appropriate for the patient's water and sodium status. If they are not, the reason should be sought. Thus, a low urinary sodium excretion is an appropriate response in a patient with hyponatraemia who is sodium depleted. Natriuresis in such a patient would imply either a failure of aldosterone secretion or a failure of the kidney to respond to the hormone (see Case History 2.1).

## Sodium measurement

Sodium concentration has traditionally been measured by flame photometry, which determines the number of sodium atoms in a defined volume of solution. Sodium is now usually measured by ion-selective electrodes, which determine the activity of sodium; that is, the number of atoms which act as true ions in a defined volume of water.

Under most circumstances the two techniques give results that are, for practical clinical purposes, the same. However, as activity is a measure of sodium in the water fraction of plasma (normally 93% by volume), significant discrepancies between activity and concentration may arise if the fractional plasma water content is decreased, such as in severe hyperlipidaemia and hyperproteinaemia. The sodium concentration, measured by flame photometry in millimoles per litre of plasma, will be less than the concentration inferred from the activity. This is because, although the concentration of sodium in plasma water is unchanged, there is less water and thus less sodium in a given volume of plasma. Analyzers employing electrodes for which the plasma is diluted before measurement also give a spuriously low result. This effect, known as pseudohyponatraemia, is only seen with massive hyperlipidaemia when the plasma will usually appear turbid to the naked eye (see Case History 14.2) and with large increases in total protein due to paraproteinaemia. If it is suspected, the plasma osmolality should be measured; it is osmolality that is regulated by the hypothalamus through the release of vasopressin. Plasma osmolality should be normal in a patient with pseudohyponatraemia.

## Osmolality and osmolarity measurement

Given that it is osmolality, rather than sodium concentration, that is controlled by the hypothalamus, it might appear logical to measure plasma osmolality rather than sodium concentration. The measurement of osmolality is, however, less precise than that of sodium and is not easily automated. It is nevertheless useful under certain circumstances.

Measurement of osmolality may help in the interpretation of a low plasma sodium concentration and is necessary in water deprivation tests. It can also be useful in the investigation of patients suspected of having ingested substances such as ethanol or ethylene glycol (see Case History 20.3) since if present, these increase the osmolality. This can be revealed by comparing the measured osmolality with the approximate expected osmolarity calculated from the formula:

$$\text{osmolarity (expected)} = 2 \times [Na^+] + [\text{urea}] + [\text{glucose}]$$

where all concentrations are measured in mmol/L.

Osmolality is a measure of concentration per kilogram of solvent; osmolarity is a measure of concentration per litre of solution. They are normally numerically very similar. Significant discrepancies (an 'osmolar gap') occur when abnormal osmotically active species are present in plasma (as may occur in poisoning) or when the fractional water content of plasma is reduced, as in severe hyperlipidaemia or hyperproteinaemia.

## Anion measurement

A change in plasma sodium concentration must be matched by a change in anion concentration. The major anions of the ECF are chloride and bicarbonate. Bicarbonate (strictly, total carbon dioxide) is frequently measured since it reflects the extracellular buffering capacity, but the measurement of plasma chloride rarely adds to the information that can be derived from knowledge of the sodium concentration alone, and few laboratories in the United Kingdom now measure plasma chloride concentration routinely for this reason. However, it may occasionally be helpful in the diagnosis of patients with non-respiratory acidosis and those with rare chloride-losing states.

# HYPONATRAEMIA

A slightly low plasma sodium concentration is a frequent finding. The mean plasma sodium concentration of hospital in-patients is 5 mmol/L lower than in healthy controls. Mild hyponatraemia is seen with a wide variety of illnesses and is most probably a result of the 'sick cell syndrome' (*see p. 24*). It is essentially a secondary phenomenon which merely reflects the presence of disease; treatment should be directed at the underlying cause and not at the hyponatraemia. Severe hyponatraemia does sometimes warrant primary treatment, but usually only when it is associated with clinical features of water intoxication (*see Fig. 2.11*).

## Causes

It has been emphasized that plasma sodium concentration depends upon the amounts of both sodium and water in the plasma, and so a low sodium concentration does not necessarily imply sodium depletion. Water excess is also an important cause of hyponatraemia. In the majority of cases, one of three mechanisms is usually primarily responsible for the development and maintenance of hyponatraemia, although in individual patients, more than one factor may be involved. These are:

- Depletion of sodium.
- Excess of water.
- Excess of water and sodium.

### Depletion of sodium

Sodium is never lost without water and isotonic or hypotonic loss would not be expected to cause a fall in plasma sodium concentration. However, hyponatraemia can occur in sodium-depleted patients, and is due to either inappropriate replacement of fluid (e.g., containing insufficient sodium) or, in severe sodium depletion, to the hypotonic stimulus to vasopressin secretion which overrides the osmotic control and permits water retention at the expense of a decrease in osmolality. A case of adrenal failure with hyponatraemia as a result of sodium depletion is presented in *Case History 8.1*.

**CASE HISTORY 2.1**

A 50-year-old woman with a long history of rheumatoid disease complained of fainting episodes following an attack of gastroenteritis and, on examination, was found to have postural hypotension.

**Investigations**

| serum: | sodium | 118 mmol/L |
|---|---|---|
| | potassium | 3.9 mmol/L |
| | urea | 9.1 mmol/L |

| short Synacthen test: normal cortisol response to ACTH | |
|---|---|
| plasma aldosterone (recumbent) | 720 pmol/L |
| 24 h urine sodium excretion | 118 mmol |

**Comment**
Postural hypotension may be due to hypovolaemia, autonomic neuropathy or hypotensive drugs. This patient was not taking such medication and there was no other evidence of neuropathy. The hyponatraemia with a slightly raised urea is consistent with sodium depletion producing hypovolaemia. The Synacthen test is normal, excluding adrenal failure, and indeed the aldosterone is appropriately raised. The patient's urinary sodium excretion is excessive; although the input was not assessed, normal kidneys should retain sodium in a sodium depleted patient with hypovolaemia.

It was concluded that the patient had a renal salt-losing state such that the kidneys could not respond to the normal physiological stimuli to retain sodium. She only became symptomatic when diarrhoea and vomiting caused further fluid loss. This was later confirmed by sodium balance studies and the patient was found to have renal papillary necrosis, an occasional complication of the use of certain analgesic drugs, which principally affects renal tubular function.

It should be noted that in patients with hyponatraemia due to sodium depletion, clinical signs of sodium depletion (*see Fig. 2.8*) may be expected. Unless the sodium loss is occurring through the kidneys, increased aldosterone secretion will cause maximal renal sodium retention and the urinary sodium concentration will be low (usually <20 mmol/L). This finding is a valuable aid to the diagnosis of sodium depletion as a cause of hyponatraemia.

The management of hyponatraemia associated with sodium depletion involves correction of the underlying cause, and appropriate fluid replacement, e.g., physiological saline or plasma expanders.

Plasma sodium concentration is usually normal in patients treated with diuretics, but these drugs have complex effects on sodium and water homoeostasis. Although primarily tending to cause sodium depletion, the blocking of sodium reabsorption in the cortical diluting segment of the nephron may impair free water excretion. This, perhaps exacerbated by the effect of vasopressin secretion secondary to hypovolaemia and an increase in water intake due to thirst, can result in hyponatraemia.

### Water excess

This gives rise to a dilutional hyponatraemia with reduced plasma osmolality. It can occur acutely purely due to excessive water intake, but this is rare. Normal kidneys are capable of excreting one litre of water per hour and water intoxication and hyponatraemia will thus be seen only when very large quantities of fluid are ingested rapidly, as in some psychotics and heavy beer drinkers. More frequently, water excess and hyponatraemia develop acutely because of a combination of excessive hypotonic fluid intake and impairment of diuresis.

---

## CASE HISTORY 2.2

Blood was taken for biochemical tests from a man who had undergone major abdominal surgery 36 hours earlier.

### Investigations

serum: sodium      127 mmol/L
       urea        4.0 mmol/L

Serum potassium and bicarbonate were normal. The patient was alert and appeared neither under- nor over-hydrated.

### Comment

Hyponatraemia is a very common finding in postoperative patients on intravenous drips. It is usually a reflection of excessive administration of hypotonic fluids (5% dextrose or 'dextrose–saline') at a time when the ability of the body to excrete water is

---

depressed as part of the normal metabolic response to trauma. It may also be due, in part, to the sick cell syndrome. If, as is usually the case, there are no clinical features of water intoxication, the only action necessary is adjustment of the fluid input. This patient had been given a total of 3.5 L of dextrose–saline since his operation and a check on the fluid balance chart showed that he had a positive balance of 2 L.

---

Reduction of water intake is usually sufficient treatment in acute cases of hyponatraemia with water overload, although occasionally treatment of features of water intoxication (e.g., fits) may be required.

Since osmolality is normally precisely controlled, the persistence of dilutional hyponatraemia implies either a failure of diuresis, which must be due to either continued (and inappropriate) production of vasopressin, or an impairment of the renal diluting mechanism.

---

## CASE HISTORY 2.3

An elderly man was admitted to hospital in an acute confusional state. No history was available but the nicotine stains on his fingers indicated that he was a heavy smoker. Physical examination revealed he had digital clubbing and signs of a right-sided pleural effusion but no other obvious abnormality was detected. He was neither dehydrated nor oedematous.

### Investigations

| | | |
|---|---|---|
| serum: | sodium | 114 mmol/L |
| | potassium | 3.6 mmol/L |
| | bicarbonate | 22 mmol/L |
| | urea | 2.5 mmol/L |
| | glucose | 4.0 mmol/L |
| | total protein | 48 g/L |
| | osmolality | 236 mmol/kg |
| | | |
| urine: | osmolality | 350 mmol/kg |
| | sodium | 50 mmol/L |

A chest radiograph confirmed the presence of the effusion and showed a mass in the right lower zone with an appearance typical of a carcinoma.

## Comment

There is severe hyponatraemia. The patient is not clinically dehydrated and the low serum protein and urea concentrations suggest that the hyponatraemia is dilutional. The serum osmolality is equal to the calculated osmolarity, militating against the presence of additional solute in the plasma. The normal response should be for vasopressin secretion to be inhibited, resulting in the production of a dilute urine. However, in this case, the urine is inappropriately concentrated in relation to the serum, indicating continuing vasopressin secretion. The chest radiograph indicates the likely source: ectopic secretion of vasopressin by a bronchial carcinoma, an example of the syndrome of inappropriate antidiuretic hormone secretion (SIADH). The diagnostic features of SIADH are:

- Hyponatraemia.
- Decreased plasma osmolality.
- Inappropriately concentrated urine.
- Continued natriuresis (>20 mmol/L).
- No oedema.
- Normal renal function.
- Normal adrenal function.
- Clinical and biochemical response to fluid restriction.

In SIADH, there is a continued natriuresis despite the low plasma sodium concentration because plasma volume is maintained by water retention and there is therefore no hypovolaemic stimulus to aldosterone secretion. Hyponatraemia with natriuresis can also occur in adrenal failure and in renal disorders and these must be excluded before a diagnosis of SIADH can be made.

Water intoxication should always be considered as a possible cause of a confusional state, especially in the elderly, and this is one of the few situations in which emergency measurement of plasma sodium concentration is genuinely indicated.

The diagnosis of SIADH is frequently made on insufficient evidence without regard to other possible causes of hyponatraemia. It is difficult to measure vasopressin in the plasma and the diagnosis is usually made on clinical and other laboratory data. It is essential to measure urine and plasma osmolalities; the urine may not be more concentrated than the plasma but must be less than maximally dilute (osmolality >50 mmol/kg). Oedema is not a feature of SIADH; the excess of water is shared by the ICF and the ECF and the effect on ECF volume is insufficient to cause oedema.

There is undoubtedly more than one type of SIADH. Tumours may produce the hormone (ectopic production) but patients with many other conditions (*Fig. 2.13*) can also fulfil the criteria for SIADH. In some of these there may be an inappropriate stimulus to vasopressin release, such as stimulation of volume receptors during artificial ventilation, and in others the 'osmostat' appears to be reset, so that osmolality is still controlled but at a lower level. Intracellular solute (especially potassium) depletion may be one mechanism whereby the osmostat can be reset.

Patients have been described in whom suppression of vasopressin release when osmolality falls is incomplete (a 'vasopressin leak') while in others, the production of vasopressin is entirely normal and antidiuresis must be

---

### Conditions associated with SIADH

**Ectopic secretion**
bronchial carcinomas

other tumours, e.g., thymus and
    prostrate

**Inappropriate secretion**
pulmonary diseases:
    pneumonia
    tuberculosis
    positive pressure mechanical
        ventilation

cerebral diseases:
    head injury
    encephalitis
    tumours
    aneurysms

miscellaneous:
    pain, e.g., postoperative
    intermittent acute porphyria
    Guillain-Barré syndrome
    hypothyroidism
    drugs, e.g., narcotics,
        chlorpropamide, carbamazepine,
        oxytocin and vinca alkaloids

**Fig. 2.13** Conditions associated with the syndrome of inappropriate antidiuretic hormone secretion (SIADH).

presumed to reflect an abnormal response to the hormone. Finally, certain drugs either stimulate vasopressin release (*see Fig. 2.5*) or have a vasopressin-like action on the kidneys. Clearly, inappropriate secretion of the hormone is not always present in patients satisfying the criteria for the diagnosis of SIADH, and because of this the term 'syndrome of inappropriate antidiuresis' may be preferable.

The logical treatment of this condition is to reduce the patient's water intake to less than that required to maintain normal water balance, to 400 mL/24 h, for example. This form of treatment is unpleasant and is impractical in chronic cases. An alternative is to administer the drug, demeclocycline, which antagonizes the action of vasopressin on the renal collecting ducts, although it is potentially nephrotoxic and should be used with care, particularly in the elderly. Occasionally, in severe water intoxication, it may be necessary to infuse hypertonic saline with a diuretic. This is potentially dangerous, since the ECF can become overloaded, and must be done cautiously with careful monitoring.

### Combined water and sodium excess

This is a frequent cause of hyponatraemia. It underlies the hyponatraemia of congestive cardiac failure, hypoproteinaemic states and some cases of renal failure. The mechanism is discussed on p. 19.

The fact that there is sodium excess is indicated by signs of increased extracellular fluid volume, for example peripheral oedema. The logical treatment in these patients involves measures to treat the underlying cause and remove the excess sodium and water (e.g., with diuretics). Despite the hyponatraemia, saline should not be given as they are already sodium overloaded.

Other, less common, causes of hyponatraemia include:

- Decreased fractional water content of plasma (pseudo-hyponatraemia).
- Addition of a solute to the plasma which is confined to the ECF.
- Decreased total negative charge on plasma proteins.

*Decreased fractional water content of plasma* can occur with severe hyperproteinaemia and hyperlipidaemia, *see p. 20*.
*Addition of a solute to the plasma which is confined to the ECF* will tend to increase ECF osmolality. Acutely, this will cause a shift of water from the ICF to the ECF, lowering the ECF sodium concentration, and stimulation of vasopressin secretion, leading to water retention. The resulting increase in ECF volume inhibits aldosterone secretion, leading to natriuresis.

---

**CASE HISTORY 2.4**

An insulin-dependent diabetic patient woke up feeling hypoglycaemic and drank two glasses of a sugar-rich drink which abolished the symptoms. She had a hospital appointment that morning and, worried that she might become hypoglycaemic while driving, decided to omit her usual injection of insulin. She felt quite well on arrival at the hospital. Blood was taken for biochemical tests.

**Investigations**

| | | |
|---|---|---|
| blood: | glucose | 28 mmol/L |
| serum: | sodium | 126 mmol/L |
| | osmolality | 290 mmol/kg |

serum urea, potassium and bicarbonate concentrations were normal.

**Comment**
The hyponatraemia is dilutional. It is the result of a movement of water from the ICF to the ECF to maintain isotonicity as the plasma glucose concentration rose. In that short time, there was no significant osmotic diuresis and thus no dehydration.

Hyponatraemia may occur for the same reason when glucose is administered intravenously at a rate greater than it can be metabolized, for example, during parenteral nutrition. It can also occur following mannitol infusion. Mannitol may be given to patients with cerebral oedema, to reduce intracellular water content, and is also used as an osmotic diuretic.

---

Movement of water from the ICF to the ECF does not occur in uraemia. In renal failure, the rate of increase in plasma urea concentration is slow, allowing time for urea to equilibrate between the ECF and the ICF, and thus preventing an osmotic imbalance.
*A decrease in the total negative charge on plasma proteins*, which contributes to the anion gap, can displace sodium from the plasma. This is unusual, but it may contribute to hyponatraemia in severe hypoalbuminaemia and in paraproteinaemias if the paraprotein is positively charged.

## The sick cell syndrome

Hyponatraemia is frequently observed in patients with either acute or chronic illness without any obvious cause. The term 'sick cell syndrome' has been used to describe this phenomenon, which used to be attributed to an increase in the permeability of cell membranes to sodium with or without a decrease in the activity of the sodium pump. However, any trans-membrane shift of sodium would be expected to be accompanied by an iso-osmotic movement of water, which should not affect plasma sodium concentration, although it is possible that sodium could become bound to intracellular macromolecules, thus nullifying its effect on osmolality.

Many sick patients may have a degree of stress-related increased vasopressin secretion or another cause of SIADH. Resetting of the osmostat, for example due to depletion of intracellular solutes, may also be contributory.

In practice, however, the mechanism of the hyponatraemia of the 'sick cell syndrome' is relatively unimportant. The hyponatraemia reflects the presence of the underlying disease, and it is this that should be treated, not the hyponatraemia.

## Investigation of hyponatraemia

It should be apparent from the previous section that, in many instances, the cause of hyponatraemia can often be recognized clinically and that additional investigation adds nothing to the management of the patient. Even in apparently obscure cases, careful clinical evaluation and study of fluid balance charts (if reliable) will often indicate the underlying mechanism or mechanisms, and thus point the way to a diagnosis.

As has been indicated, hyponatraemia due to sodium depletion may be accompanied by physical signs of a decrease in extracellular fluid volume whereas this is normal in patients with water excess, and in combined water and sodium excess, the signs will be of extracellular fluid expansion.

An algorithm for the diagnosis of hyponatraemia is given in *Fig. 2.14*. Some of the commoner causes of hyponatraemia are indicated in *Fig. 2.15* and some investigations which may help in elucidating its cause are shown in *Fig. 2.16*. It must be emphasized that an appreciation of the underlying principles is vital for correct interpretation of their results.

## Management of hyponatraemia

Hyponatraemia is essentially a sign of a disturbance or a disorder involving water or sodium or both. Measures to treat the causative condition may have to be supplemented by direct measures to correct the imbalance of sodium and water. It is essential to understand the pathogenesis of the hyponatraemia if the measures are to be appropriate. Hyponatraemia itself usually only requires treatment if features of water intoxication are present.

## HYPERNATRAEMIA

Hypernatraemia is much less common than hyponatraemia, but is much more frequently of clinical significance. The causes include pure water depletion, combined sodium and water depletion, with water loss predominating, or sodium excess; of these, excess sodium is the least common.

---

### CASE HISTORY 2.5

Following surgery for major abdominal injuries sustained in a knife-fight, a young man was fed parenterally and artificially ventilated. On the fifth day after his operation, serum biochemical results, which had been normal the day before, were as follows:

**Investigations**

serum:
| | |
|---|---|
| sodium | 150 mmol/L |
| potassium | 4.2 mmol/L |
| urea | 10.2 mmol/L |
| glucose | 25 mmol/L |

During the previous 24 hours he had become pyrexial and positive blood cultures were subsequently obtained. His fluid intake had been 3000 mL, urine output had been steady at 90–100 mL/h and 300 mL of fluid had been aspirated via a nasogastric tube. The sodium intake had been 70 mmol.

---

**Comment**

Sodium input is not excessive; water depletion is the more likely cause of the hypernatraemia. His measured net fluid intake is only 400 mL. This is insufficient to balance insensible losses, which will have been increased by the pyrexia and possibly by ventilation. The urine output has not decreased and there has therefore also been an excessive renal water loss. This is due to an osmotic diuresis as a result of glycosuria and a high urea output.

Glucose intolerance may be a problem in patients receiving parenteral nutrition and can be exacerbated by sepsis, which causes insulin resistance. Parenteral administration of excessive nitrogen will result in increased formation of urea which will also contribute to an osmotic diuresis; this patient was receiving amino acids equivalent to over 100 g of protein per day, more than his probable requirements. Inadequate humidification of inspired air may also be a causative factor in water depletion in such circumstances.

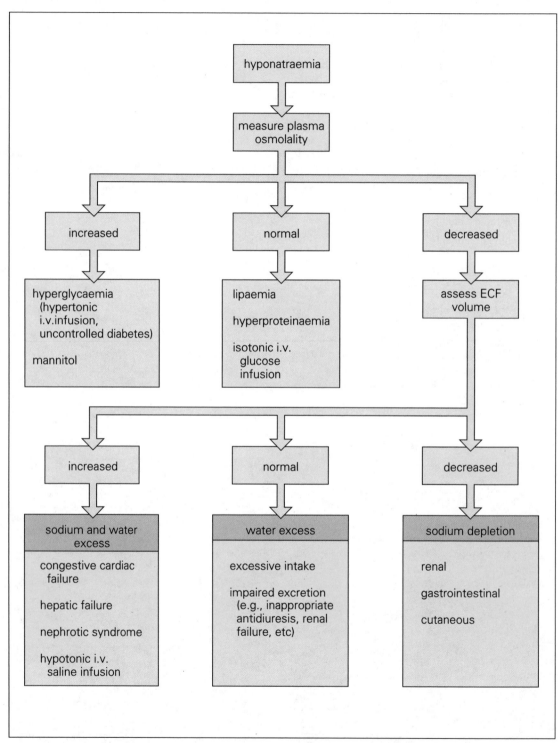

**Fig. 2.14** A simple algorithm for the diagnosis of hyponatraemia. In practice, hyponatraemia is often multifactorial but one cause may predominate and determine the clinical features.

| Some common causes of hyponatraemia | | |
|---|---|---|
| **Cause** | **Mechanism** | **ECF volume** |
| inappropriate i.v. fluids | water excess | normal or increased |
| diuretic therapy | sodium depletion water retention (*see text*) | decreased |
| non-specific ('sick cell syndrome') | *see text* | normal |
| congestive cardiac failure & hypo-proteinaemic states | sodium retention water retention | increased |
| carcinoma of bronchus | water excess | normal |
| hyperglycaemia, parenteral feeding | isotonic redistribution | normal |

**Fig. 2.15** Some common causes of hyponatraemia.

---

**CASE HISTORY 2.6**

A male infant aged 15 weeks was admitted to hospital for the investigation of recurrent diarrhoea. He had been well until 8 weeks of age, when the first episode had occurred. Since then, there had been several further attacks, he had lost weight and on admission was dehydrated.

**Investigations**

| serum: | sodium | 167 mmol/L |
|---|---|---|
| | potassium | 4.9 mmol/L |
| | urea | 2.6 mmol/L |
| urine: | sodium | 310 mmol/L |

**Comment**

Hypernatraemia is a feature of hypotonic fluid loss such as can occur with diarrhoea, but with chronic diarrhoea hyponatraemia is more usual, due to the loss of salt. In dehydration, however, the kidneys should conserve sodium. The combination of high urine sodium excretion together with hypernatraemia in this case suggests salt overload. Stool chromatography revealed the presence of an abnormal sugar which was identified as lactulose. Lactulose is a non-absorbed osmotic laxative. Careful observation confirmed the suspicion that the child's mother was adding salt and lactulose to his feeds. She was not allowed to stay with him unattended and the diarrhoea and electrolyte abnormalities resolved rapidly.

---

In most cases of hypernatraemia, the cause is obvious from the history and clinical observations. Diabetes insipidus is an important cause and the investigation of patients suspected of having this condition is considered *in Chapter 7.*

| Investigations for hyponatraemia |
|---|
| inspection of serum for lipaemia |
| serum: osmolality potassium urea creatinine total protein TSH & free T4 |
| haematocrit |
| Synacthen test |
| urine: sodium osmolality |

**Fig. 2.16** Some laboratory investigations of value in the investigation of hyponatraemia.

Regardless of its cause, hypernatraemia should be treated by administration of hypotonic fluids such as water (orally) or 5% dextrose (parenterally). In patients with sodium overload, measures to remove excess sodium may have to be considered. As already emphasized, it is important not to correct too rapidly hypernatraemia due to water depletion.

## POTASSIUM HOMOEOSTASIS

Extracellular potassium balance is controlled primarily by the kidneys and, to a lesser extent, by the gastrointestinal tract. In the kidneys, filtered potassium is almost completely reabsorbed in the proximal tubules. Some active potassium secretion takes place in the most distal part of the distal convoluted tubules but potassium excretion is primarily a passive process. The active reabsorption of sodium generates a membrane potential which is neutralized by the movement of potassium and hydrogen ions from tubular cells into the lumen. Thus, urinary potassium excretion depends upon several factors:

- The amount of sodium available for reabsorption in the distal convoluted tubules and the collecting ducts.
- The relative availability of hydrogen and potassium ions in the cells of the distal convoluted tubules and the collecting ducts.
- The ability of these cells to secrete hydrogen ions.
- The circulating concentration of aldosterone.
- The rate of flow of tubular fluid. A high flow rate (e.g., osmotic diuresis, treatment with diuretics) favours the transfer of potassium into the tubular lumen.

Aldosterone stimulates potassium excretion both indirectly, by increasing the active reabsorption of sodium in the distal convoluted tubules and the collecting ducts, and directly, by increasing active potassium secretion in the distal part of the distal convoluted tubules. Aldosterone secretion from the adrenal cortex is stimulated indirectly, by activation of the renin–angiotensin system in response to hypovolaemia (*see pp 121 & 122*), and directly, by hyperkalaemia.

Since both hydrogen and potassium ions can neutralize the membrane potential generated by active sodium reabsorption, there is a close relationship between potassium and hydrogen ion homoeostasis. In a state of acidosis, hydrogen ions will tend to be secreted in preference to potassium; in alkalosis, fewer hydrogen ions will be available for excretion and there will be an increase in potassium excretion. Thus, there is a tendency to hyperkalaemia in acidosis and to hypokalaemia in alkalosis. An exception to this tendency is renal tubular acidosis caused by defec-

tive renal hydrogen ion excretion (*see p. 68*). In this condition, because of the decrease in hydrogen ion excretion, potassium secretion must increase to balance sodium reabsorption. The result is the unusual combination of hypokalaemia with acidosis.

The relationship between the excretion of hydrogen and potassium ions also explains why potassium depletion tends to produce alkalosis. If there is insufficient potassium available for excretion as sodium is reabsorbed, then the excretion of hydrogen ions will be increased.

The healthy kidneys are less efficient at conserving potassium than sodium; even on a potassium-free intake, urinary excretion remains at 10–20 mmol/24 h. Since there is also an obligatory loss from the skin and gut of approximately 15–20 mmol/24 h the kidneys cannot compensate if intake falls much below 40 mmol/24 h. The average diet contains more potassium than this. However, potassium depletion can occur, even on a normal diet, if there are increased losses from the body.

Potassium is secreted in gastric juice and much of this, along with dietary potassium, is reabsorbed in the small intestine. In the colon and rectum, potassium is secreted in exchange for sodium, partly under the control of aldosterone. Stools normally contain some potassium, but considerable amounts may be lost in patients with fistulae or chronic diarrhoea, or in patients who are losing gastric secretions through persistent vomiting or nasogastric aspiration.

Movement of potassium between the intracellular and extracellular compartments can have a profound effect on the plasma potassium concentration. The cellular uptake of potassium is stimulated by insulin. Potassium ions move passively into cells from the ECF in exchange for sodium which is actively excluded by a membrane-bound, energy-dependent sodium pump. Hyperkalaemia may result either if the activity of this sodium pump is impaired or if there is damage to cell membranes.

Transcellular shifts of hydrogen ion can cause reciprocal shifts in potassium. In a systemic acidosis, intracellular buffering of hydrogen ions results in the displacement of potassium into the ECF. In alkalosis, there is a shift of hydrogen ions from the ICF to the ECF and a net movement of potassium ions in the opposite direction which tends to produce hypokalaemia.

## POTASSIUM DEPLETION AND HYPOKALAEMIA

Potassium depletion occurs when output exceeds intake. Potassium is available in many foods (normal dietary intake is 60–200 mmol/24h) and except in patients who are fasting, inadequate intake is rarely the sole cause of potassium depletion. However, increased loss of potassium is a frequent occurrence. Such loss can be from the gut or through the kidneys. Drug therapy is often implicated in the pathogenesis of potassium depletion.

Hypokalaemia (*Fig. 2.17*) may be due to potassium depletion but can also be a result of redistribution of potassium from the extra- to the intracellular compartment.

probably unnecessary unless the plasma concentration is below 3.0 mmol/L and they are potentially dangerous in patients with renal impairment since hyperkalaemia may result.

---

**CASE HISTORY 2.7**

A 67-year-old woman presented with severe muscular weakness. She had been in the habit of taking large amounts of purgatives and recently had been prescribed a thiazide diuretic for mild heart failure.

**Investigations**

serum:  potassium      2.4 mmol/L
        bicarbonate    36 mmol/L

**Comment**
The patient is severely hypokalaemic and the high serum bicarbonate concentration reflects the associated extracellular alkalosis.

Purgative abuse can cause considerable potassium loss from the gut. Thiazides act by decreasing chloride reabsorption, and thus sodium reabsorption, in the distal part of the ascending limbs of the loops of Henle and in the first part of the distal convoluted tubules. As a result, there is an increase in the amount of sodium delivered to and available for reabsorption from the distal tubules; this will tend to increase potassium excretion from the kidneys. Loop diuretics similarly increase renal potassium excretion, though to a lesser extent. With either type of diuretic, however, plasma potassium concentrations tend to stabilize unless, as in this case, other causes of hypokalaemia are present.

Potassium supplements are often prescribed at the same time as diuretics; combined preparations are widely used but they are generally expensive and typically provide less than 10 mmol of potassium per tablet. Hypokalaemia potentiates digoxin toxicity and this is an important practical consideration since diuretics and digoxin are very often prescribed together. However, in general, the routine use of potassium supplements is to be deprecated. They are

---

**CASE HISTORY 2.8**

A 60-year-old man underwent total gastrectomy for a carcinoma. He was malnourished prior to surgery and it was decided to provide parenteral nutrition postoperatively. On the fifth day, his serum potassium concentration was 3.0 mmol/L despite the provision of 60 mmol potassium per 24 h in the intravenous feed.

**Comment**
The patient is hypokalaemic in spite of the provision of sufficient potassium to cover normal obligatory losses.

Potassium excretion increases during the metabolic response to trauma but once a patient becomes anabolic, the body's requirements increase as potassium is taken up into cells. Furthermore, during total parenteral nutrition, glucose is often the predominant energy source and thus provides a considerable stimulus to insulin release. Potassium requirements may, therefore, be much greater than normal because insulin stimulates its uptake into cells.

This patient had recently undergone abdominal surgery and an ileus is usual in these circumstances. This will result in decreased reabsorption of any potassium secreted into the gut and may also contribute to the loss of potassium from the ECF.

---

## Clinical features

Even severe hypokalaemia may be asymptomatic. When symptoms are present, they are related primarily to disturbances of neuromuscular function (*Fig. 2.18*); muscular weakness, constipation and paralytic ileus are common problems.

## Management

Although the plasma potassium concentration is a poor guide to total body potassium, a plasma concentration of

| Causes of hypokalaemia |
| --- |
| **Decreased K⁺ intake**<br>oral (rare)<br>parenteral |
| **Transcellular K⁺ movement**<br>alkalosis<br>insulin administration<br>β-adrenergic agonists<br>rapid cellular proliferation |
| **Increased K⁺ loss**<br>renal:<br>   diuretics<br>   diuretic phase of acute renal failure<br>   mineralocorticoid excess:<br>      primary aldosteronism<br>      secondary aldosteronism<br>      Cushing's syndrome<br>      carbenoxolone, liquorice<br>      renal tubular acidosis (types 1 & 2)<br>extrarenal:<br>   diarrhoea<br>   purgative abuse<br>   villous adenoma of the rectum<br>   vomiting, gastric aspiration<br>   enterocutaneous fistulae<br>   excessive sweating |

**Fig. 2.17** Causes of hypokalaemia. Carbenoxolone and liquorice are aldosterone agonists.

| Clinical features of hypokalaemia | |
| --- | --- |
| **Disorder** | **Feature** |
| neuromuscular | weakness<br>constipation, ileus<br>hypotonia<br>depression<br>confusion |
| cardiac | arrhythmias<br>potentiation of digoxin toxicity<br>ECG changes (ST depression,<br>   T depression/inversion,<br>   prolonged P-R interval,<br>   prominent U wave) |
| renal | impaired concentrating ability<br>   leading to polyuria and<br>   polydipsia |
| metabolic | alkalosis |

**Fig. 2.18** Clinical features of hypokalaemia. The resting potential of excitable membranes is reduced in hypokalaemia, thereby decreasing excitability. The effect on the kidneys is due to increased synthesis of prostaglandins which antagonize the action of ADH.

3.0 mmol/L generally implies a deficit of the order of 300 mmol. However, since this deficit is almost entirely from the ICF and since administered potassium first enters the ECF, replacement must be undertaken with care, particularly when the intravenous route is used.

As a guide, the following potassium dosages should not be exceeded without good reason: a rate of 20 mmol/h, a concentration of 40 mmol/L in the intravenous fluid or a total of 140 mmol/24 h. Thorough mixing with the bulk of the fluid to be infused is vital. Plasma concentrations should be monitored during treatment. If unusually large amounts of potassium are necessary and particularly if there is impaired renal function, electrocardiograph (ECG) monitoring is useful since characteristic changes in the waveform occur with changing plasma potassium concentrations (*Fig. 2.19*).

## POTASSIUM EXCESS AND HYPERKALAEMIA

Potassium excess can be due to excessive intake or decreased excretion. A normal intake may be excessive if excretion is decreased (e.g., in renal failure). Excessive intake is otherwise virtually always iatrogenic and parenteral.

Hyperkalaemia (*Fig. 2.20*) may be due to potassium excess but can also be a result of redistribution of potassium from the intra- to the extracellular compartment. This mechanism can sometimes give rise to hyperkalaemia even in a patient who is potassium depleted (e.g., in diabetic ketoacidosis). As with hypokalaemia, more than one cause of hyperkalaemia is often present. Spurious hyperkalaemia, due to the leakage of potassium from blood cells, often occurs. If hyperkalaemia is found unexpectedly, the possibility that it is spurious should be explored by repeating the measurement on a fresh sample. Spurious hyperkalaemia may be present in the absence of frank haemolysis.

### hyperkalaemia

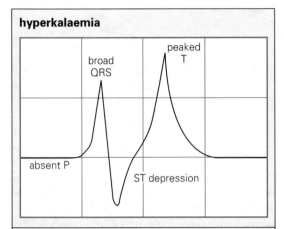

### normal

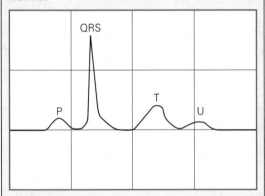

### hypokalaemia

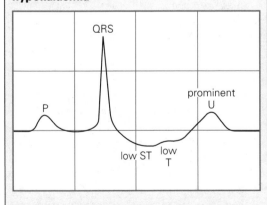

**Fig. 2.19** Characteristic ECG changes in hyper- and hypokalaemia. Each sinus discharge produces atrial depolarization (P wave) followed by ventricular depolarization (QRS complex) and ventricular repolarization (T wave). The U wave, of unknown cause, is present in most normal ECGs.

## CASE HISTORY 2.9

A young man was admitted to hospital after sustaining a fractured femur and ruptured spleen in a motorcycle accident. He underwent splenectomy and was put in traction. Twenty-four hours after admission, he had passed only 300 mL of urine.

### Investigations

serum: urea           21.5 mmol/L
       potassium     6.5 mmol/L

### Comment

Since the patient is oliguric with a high serum urea he is by definition in renal failure; this might be reversible, that is, pre-renal (*see p. 58*). The hyperkalaemia is due to a combination of decreased renal perfusion (hypovolaemic shock), and the release of potassium either from cells damaged directly by trauma or from cells whose membrane integrity is impaired by hypoxaemia.

Similar results may be seen in patients who have sustained a gastrointestinal haemorrhage. This may itself cause hypovolaemic shock, affecting renal function. In addition, there will be absorption of potassium from red blood cells undergoing lysis in the gut and increased synthesis of urea from the amino acids released.

## CASE HISTORY 2.10

Blood from an outpatient being treated with diuretics was received in the laboratory for biochemical analysis. The serum potassium concentration was 6.7 mmol/L. There was no visible haemolysis and the blood was freshly drawn.

### Comment

The patient was recalled and asked to bring all her tablets with her. It transpired that she had initially been prescribed a loop diuretic and potassium supplements for congestive cardiac failure. However, at an outpatient attendance she had been prescribed spironolactone, a potassium-sparing diuretic which is an antagonist of aldosterone, instead of the potassium supplements. She had misunderstood the instructions given to her and continued to take both the supplements and the diuretic.

She surrendered the potassium supplements and her serum potassium concentration was normal when checked one week later.

### Causes of hyperkalaemia

**Spurious**
haemolysis
delayed separation of serum
contamination

**Excessive K+ intake**
oral (rare except with K+-sparing
    diuretics taken simultanously)
parenteral infusion
transfusion of stored blood

**Transcellular K+ movement**
tissue damage
catabolic states
systemic acidosis
insulin lack

**Decreased K+ loss**
acute renal failure
chronic renal failure
K+-sparing diuretics
angiotensin converting enzyme
    (ACE) inhibitors

mineralocorticoid deficiency:
    Addison's disease
    adrenalectomy

**Fig. 2.20** Causes of hyperkalaemia.

### Clinical features

Hyperkalaemia can kill without warning. It lowers the resting membrane potential, shortens the cardiac action potential and increases the speed of repolarization. Cardiac arrest with ventricular fibrillation may be the first sign of hyperkalaemia. It is therefore necessary to be alert for this disorder in appropriate circumstances, for instance, in acute renal failure, to ensure that effective early management is instituted. Characteristic ECG changes precede the onset of ventricular fibrillation (*Fig. 2.19*). Peaking of T waves occurs first, followed by loss of P waves and, finally, the development of abnormal QRS complexes.

### Management

Intravenous calcium gluconate (10 mL of a 10% solution given over one minute and repeated as necessary) affords some degree of immediate protection to the myocardium by antagonizing the effect of hyperkalaemia on myocardial excitability. Intravenous glucose and insulin, for example, 500 mL of 20% dextrose with 20 units of soluble insulin given over 30 minutes, promotes intracellular potassium uptake. Salbutamol, which activates $Na^+$, $K^+$-ATPase, has a similar effect. In the acidotic patient, hyperkalaemia can be controlled temporarily by bicarbonate infusion.

In acute renal failure and in other circumstances where the hyperkalaemia is uncontrollable, dialysis or haemofiltration will be required. In chronic renal failure restriction of potassium intake and the administration of oral ion-exchange resins are often successful in preventing dangerous hyperkalaemia until such time as dialysis becomes necessary for other reasons.

ECG monitoring can be valuable in patients with hyperkalaemia. Changes in the plasma potassium concentration are reflected by changes in the ECG waveform more rapidly than could be determined by biochemical measurement.

### SUMMARY

Sodium, potassium and water homoeostasis are closely linked. Sodium is the principal extracellular cation and the amount of sodium in the body is the major determinant of ECF volume. Potassium is the major intracellular cation.

Both ions are transported actively in the body; water moves passively in response to changes in the solute contents of the body's fluid compartments. Sodium excretion is primarily controlled by aldosterone; this hormone is released in response to a decrease in ECF volume and causes sodium retention and loss of potassium. Water excretion is controlled by vasopressin (antidiuretic hormone); this is secreted in response to an increase in ECF osmolality and a decrease in ECF volume and promotes water retention. Potassium excretion is regulated in part by aldosterone, but also depends on extracellular hydrogen ion concentration and sodium and water excretion.

Primary disturbances of either water or sodium homoeostasis produce characteristic clinical and biochemical features but combined disturbances are common and the features may then be less clear-cut. Changes in plasma sodium concentration require careful interpretation since they can be due to changes in the amounts of extracellular sodium or water or both. Hyponatraemia may occur as a non-specific consequence of disease or be an appropriate physiological response to disease. Hyponatraemia may not require treatment (particularly in asymptomatic patients) but when necessary, treatment must be based on knowledge of the cause. Hypernatraemia is less common than hyponatraemia and usually is related to predominant loss of water. This should be treated cautiously and appropriate measures taken to treat the underlying cause.

Plasma potassium concentration is a poor guide to the body's overall potassium status. Depletion is not always associated with hypokalaemia, or hypokalaemia due to potassium depletion, and the same applies to potassium excess and hyperkalaemia.

Hypokalaemia is most frequently due to excessive gastrointestinal or renal loss of potassium and may be exacerbated by a poor intake. It can also be due to increased cellular uptake of potassium from the plasma. Hypokalaemia results in skeletal and smooth muscle weakness and impairment of myocardial contractility and renal concentrating ability. It also potentiates digoxin toxicity.

Hyperkalaemia is most frequently due to decreased renal excretion or to loss of potassium from cells; excessive intake should be avoidable, since it is usually iatrogenic. Spurious hyperkalaemia, due to release of potassium from cells *in vitro*, is common. The danger of true hyperkalaemia is that it can cause cardiac arrest; this can occur in the absence of any warning clinical symptoms or signs.

## FURTHER READING

Anon (1989) Hyperkalaemia – silent and deadly *Lancet*, **1**, 1240.

Arieff A I (1993) Management of hyponatraemia. *British Medical Journal* **307**, 305–308.

Beck L H (1981) Body fluid and electrolyte disorders. *The Medical Clinics of North America*, **65**, 247–451.

Gill G V & Flear C T G (1985) Hyponatraemia. *Recent Advances in Clinical Biochemistry*, **3**, 149–159.

Morgan D B (ed.) (1984) Electrolyte disorders. *Clinics in Endocrinology and Metabolism*, **13**, 231–434.

# 3. Hydrogen Ion Homoeostasis and Blood Gases

## INTRODUCTION

The normal processes of metabolism result in the net formation of 40–80 mmol of hydrogen ion per 24 h, principally from the oxidation of sulphur-containing amino acids. This burden of hydrogen ion is excreted by the kidneys in the urine. In addition there is a considerable endogenous turnover of hydrogen ion as a result of normal metabolic processes. Incomplete oxidation of energy substrates generates acid (e.g., lactic acid by glycolysis, ketoacids from triglycerides) while further metabolism of these intermediates consumes it (e.g., gluconeogenesis from lactate, oxidation of ketones). Temporary imbalances between the rates of production and consumption may arise in health (e.g., the accumulation of lactic acid during anaerobic exercise), but in general they are in balance and so make no contribution to net hydrogen ion excretion. In disease states, however, imbalances can occur. As will be seen, increased hydrogen ion production is an important cause of acidosis.

Potentially far more acid is generated as carbon dioxide during energy-yielding oxidative metabolism. In excess of 15,000 mmol per 24 h of carbon dioxide is produced in this way, and is normally excreted by the lungs. Although carbon dioxide itself is not an acid, in the presence of water it can undergo hydration to form a weak acid, carbonic acid (*Equation 3.1*).

$$(3.1) \quad CO_2 + H_2O \rightleftharpoons H_2CO_3$$

Carbon dioxide is removed from the body in expired air. Since hydrogen ions can be generated stoichiometrically from carbon dioxide, the normal daily production of carbon dioxide is potentially equivalent to at least 15 mol of hydrogen ion. Not surprisingly, impaired excretion of carbon dioxide is an important cause of acidosis. In health, however, the mechanisms controlling pulmonary ventilation respond in such a way that the rate of carbon dioxide excretion is adjusted to meet the rate of production.

The homoeostatic mechanisms for hydrogen ion and carbon dioxide are very efficient. Temporary imbalances can be absorbed by buffering and, as a result, the hydrogen ion concentration of the body is maintained within narrow limits (36–43 nmol/L, (pH 7.35–7.46) in extracellular fluid (ECF)). The intracellular hydrogen ion concentration is slightly higher but is also rigorously controlled. In disease, an imbalance between the rates of production and excretion may occur; the hydrogen ion concentration then becomes abnormal and a state of acidosis or alkalosis results.

## Buffering of hydrogen ions

As hydrogen ions are generated they are buffered, thus limiting the rise in hydrogen ion concentration which would otherwise occur. A buffer system consists of a weak acid, that is, one which is incompletely dissociated, and its conjugate base. If hydrogen ions are added to a buffer, some will combine with the conjugate base and convert it to the undissociated acid. Thus, the addition of hydrogen ions to the bicarbonate–carbonic acid system (*Equation 3.2*) drives the reaction to the right, increasing the amount of carbonic acid and consuming bicarbonate ions.

$$(3.2) \quad H^+ + HCO_3^- \rightleftharpoons H_2CO_3$$

Conversely, if the hydrogen ion concentration falls, carbonic acid dissociates, thereby generating hydrogen ions.

The efficacy of any buffer is limited by its concentration and by the position of the equilibrium. A buffer operates most efficiently at hydrogen ion concentrations which result in approximately equal concentrations of undissociated acid and conjugate base. The bicarbonate buffer system is the most important in the ECF, yet at normal ECF hydrogen ion concentrations the concentration of carbonic acid is about 1.2 mmol/L while that of bicarbonate is 20 times greater. However, the capacity of the bicarbonate system in the body is greatly enhanced by the fact that carbonic acid can readily be formed from carbon dioxide or disposed of by conversion into carbon dioxide and water (*Equation 3.1*).

For every hydrogen ion buffered by bicarbonate, a bicarbonate ion is consumed (*Equation 3.2*). To maintain the capacity of the buffer system, the bicarbonate must be regenerated. Yet, when bicarbonate is formed from carbonic acid (indirectly from carbon dioxide and water), equimolar amounts of hydrogen ion are formed simultaneously (*Equation 3.2*). Bicarbonate formation can only continue if these hydrogen ions are removed. This process occurs in the cells of the renal tubules, where hydrogen ions are secreted into the urine while bicarbonate is generated and retained in the body.

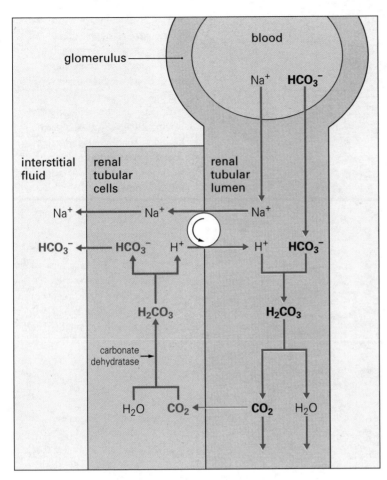

**Fig. 3.1** Reabsorption of filtered bicarbonate by renal tubular cells. Bicarbonate cannot be reabsorbed directly. Hydrogen and bicarbonate ions are generated in renal tubular cells and the hydrogen ions are secreted in exchange for sodium into the tubular lumen where they combine with filtered bicarbonate to form carbon dioxide and water. Bicarbonate ions are secreted with sodium from the tubular cells into the extracellular space.

Proteins, including intracellular proteins, are also involved in buffering. The proteinaceous matrix of bone is an important buffer in chronic acidosis. Phosphate is a minor buffer in the ECF but is of fundamental importance in the urine. The special role of haemoglobin is considered *on p. 37.*

## Bicarbonate reabsorption and hydrogen ion excretion

The glomerular filtrate contains the same concentration of bicarbonate ions as the plasma. If this bicarbonate were not reabsorbed, copious amounts would be excreted in the urine, depleting the body's buffering capacity and causing an acidosis to develop. In health, at normal plasma bicarbonate concentrations, virtually all the filtered bicarbonate is reabsorbed.

The luminal surface of renal tubular cells is impermeable to bicarbonate and therefore direct reabsorption cannot occur. Within the renal tubular cells, carbonic acid is formed from carbon dioxide and water (*Fig. 3.1*). This reaction (*Equation 3.1*) is catalyzed in the kidney by the enzyme carbonate dehydratase (carbonic anhydrase). The carbonic acid thus formed dissociates to give hydrogen and bicarbonate ions. The bicarbonate ions pass across the basal border of the cells into the interstitial fluid. The hydrogen ions are secreted across the luminal membrane in exchange for sodium ions, which accompany bicarbonate into the interstitial fluid (*Fig. 3.1*). The formation of bicarbonate and hydrogen ions is promoted by their continuous removal and by the presence of carbonate dehydratase.

In the tubular fluid, hydrogen ions combine with bicarbonate to form carbonic acid, most of which dissociates into carbon dioxide and water. Some of the carbon dioxide diffuses back into the renal tubular cells while the remainder is excreted in the urine. This whole process effectively results in the reabsorption of filtered bicarbonate.

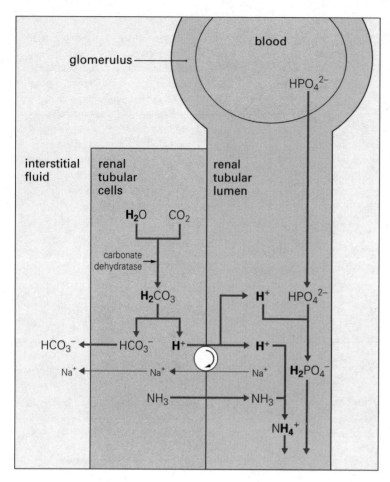

**Fig. 3.2** Renal hydrogen ion excretion. Hydrogen and bicarbonate ions are generated in renal tubular cells from carbon dioxide and water by the reversal of the buffering reaction. The hydrogen ions are excreted in the urine buffered by phosphate and ammonia while the bicarbonate enters the extracellular fluid replacing that which was consumed in buffering.

Although hydrogen ions are secreted into the tubular fluid, there is no net hydrogen ion excretion, as the formation of hydrogen ions provides the means for the reabsorption of bicarbonate. Hydrogen ion excretion depends upon the same reactions occurring in the renal tubular cells but, in addition, requires the presence of a suitable buffer system in the urine. The minimum urinary pH that can be generated, 4.6, is equivalent to a hydrogen ion concentration of approximately 25 μmol/L. Given a normal urine volume of 1.5 L/24 h, free hydrogen ion excretion can account for less than a thousandth of the total amount that has to be excreted. The principal urinary buffer is phosphate. This is present in the glomerular filtrate, approximately 80% being in the form of the divalent anion, $HPO_4^{2-}$. This combines with hydrogen ions and is converted to $H_2PO_4^-$ (*Equation 3.3*).

**(3.3)**   $HPO_4^{2-} + H^+ \rightleftharpoons H_2PO_4^-$

At the minimum urinary pH, virtually all the phosphate is in the $H_2PO_4^-$ form. About 30–40 mmol of hydrogen ions are normally excreted in this way every 24 h.

Ammonia, produced by the deamination of glutamine in renal tubular cells, is also an important urinary buffer. The enzyme which catalyzes this reaction, glutaminase, is induced in states of chronic acidosis, allowing increased ammonia production and, hence, increased hydrogen ion excretion via ammonium ions. Ammonia can readily diffuse across cell membranes but ammonium ions, formed when ammonia buffers hydrogen ions (*Equation 3.4*), cannot. Passive reabsorption of ammonium ions is therefore prevented.

**(3.4)**   $NH_3 + H^+ \rightleftharpoons NH_4^+$

At normal intracellular hydrogen ion concentrations, most ammonia is present as ammonium ions. Diffusion of ammonia out of the cell disturbs the equilibrium, causing more ammonia to be formed. The simultaneous production of hydrogen ions would seem to negate the process. However, these ions can be used up in gluconeogenesis when they combine with glutamate formed by the deamination of glutamine. Urinary hydrogen ion excretion is summarized in *Fig. 3.2.*

It will be apparent that hydrogen and bicarbonate ions are generated in equimolar amounts in renal tubular cells. This is essential for the reabsorption of filtered bicarbonate but also means that when a hydrogen ion is excreted in the urine, a bicarbonate ion is produced and retained. This process effectively regenerates the bicarbonate ions consumed when hydrogen ions are buffered.

## Transport of carbon dioxide

Carbon dioxide, produced by aerobic metabolism, diffuses out of cells and dissolves in the ECF. A small amount combines with water to form carbonic acid, thereby increasing the hydrogen ion concentration of the ECF.

In red blood cells, metabolism is anaerobic and little carbon dioxide is produced. Carbon dioxide thus diffuses into red cells down a concentration gradient and carbonic acid is formed, facilitated by carbonate dehydratase (*Fig. 3.3*). Haemoglobin buffers the hydrogen ions formed when the carbonic acid dissociates. Haemoglobin is a more powerful buffer when in the deoxygenated state and the proportion in this state increases during the passage of blood through capillary beds as oxygen is lost to the tissues.

The overall effect of this process is that carbon dioxide is converted to bicarbonate in red blood cells. This bicarbonate diffuses out of the red cells because a concentration gradient develops and electrochemical neutrality is maintained by inward diffusion of chloride ions (the chloride shift). In the lungs, the reverse process occurs because of the low partial pressure of carbon dioxide in the alveolar capillaries. Carbon dioxide is produced from bicarbonate and diffuses into the alveoli to be excreted in the expired air.

Most of the carbon dioxide in the blood is present in the form of bicarbonate. Dissolved carbon dioxide, carbonic acid and carbamino compounds (compounds of carbon dioxide and protein) account for less than 2.0 mmol/L in a total carbon dioxide concentration of approximately 26 mmol/L. The terms 'bicarbonate' and 'total carbon dioxide' are frequently used synonymously. They are not strictly the same but may be considered to be for most practical clinical purposes. It is technically difficult to measure bicarbonate concentration alone; most analytical techniques for bicarbonate actually measure total carbon dioxide.

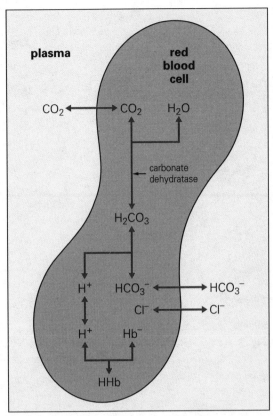

**Fig. 3.3** Transport of carbon dioxide in the blood. In capillary beds, carbon dioxide diffuses into red blood cells and combines with water to form carbonic acid; the reaction is catalyzed by carbonate dehydratase. The carbonic acid dissociates to form hydrogen ions, which are buffered by haemoblogin, and bicarbonate, which diffuses out of the cell; chloride diffuses in to maintain electrochemical neutrality. In the alveoli, the process reverses; carbon dioxide is produced from bicarbonate and is excreted in the expired air.

## CLINICAL AND LABORATORY ASSESSMENT OF HYDROGEN ION STATUS

As will be seen, many conditions are associated with abnormalities of blood hydrogen ion concentration and partial pressure of carbon dioxide ($P_{CO_2}$). The clinical features associated with these abnormalities and those with an altered partial pressure of oxygen ($P_{O_2}$) are shown in *Fig. 3.4.*

It is usual to measure hydrogen ion concentration [$H^+$] in arterial blood, anticoagulated with heparin. The arteriovenous

|  | Increase | Decrease |
|---|---|---|
| $P_{CO_2}$ | peripheral vasodilation<br>headache<br>bounding pulse<br>papilloedema ⎤<br>flapping tremor ⎬ late signs<br>drowsiness, coma ⎦ | paraesthesiae<br>dizziness<br>muscle cramps<br>headache<br>tetany |
| $P_{O_2}$ | pulmonary and retinal<br>  fibrosis (only with<br>  prolonged use of high<br>  inspiratory $P_{O_2}$,<br>  particularly in infants) | breathlessness<br>cyanosis<br>drowsiness, confusion and coma<br>pulmonary hypotension (in<br>  chronic hypoxaemia) |
| $[H^+]$ | hyperventilation<br>increased catecholamine release<br>hyperkalaemia<br>decreased myocardial ⎤<br>  contractility ⎬ severe acidosis only<br>  CNS depression ⎦ | hyperventilation<br>paraesthesiae<br>muscle cramps<br>dizziness<br>headache<br>tetany<br>drowsiness, confusion and coma |

**Fig. 3.4** Effects of increased or decreased values of $P_{CO_2}$, $P_{O_2}$ and $[H^+]$ in the blood. Paraesthesiae, dizziness, muscle cramps and tetany are related to a decrease in ionized calcium.

difference for $[H^+]$ is small (<2 nmol/L), but the difference is significant for $P_{CO_2}$ (approximately 1.1 kPa (8 mmHg) higher in venous blood) and $P_{O_2}$ (approximately 7.5 kPa (56 mmHg) lower in venous blood).

It is vital that air is excluded from the syringe, both before and after drawing blood, and that, if possible, analysis is performed immediately. If the blood sample has to be transported, the syringe, capped with a blind hub and enclosed in a plastic bag, should be chilled in ice-water. Analytical instruments measure $[H^+]$ (strictly, activity), $P_{CO_2}$ and $P_{O_2}$ using specific electrodes; these measurements are together known colloquially as 'blood gases'.

By the law of mass action it follows, from the equations describing the dissociation of carbonic acid (*Equations 3.1 and 3.2*), that $[H^+]$ is directly proportional to $P_{CO_2}$ and inversely proportional to bicarbonate concentration; that is, it is determined by the ratio of $P_{CO_2}$ to bicarbonate (*Equation 3.5*).

$$(3.5) \quad [H^+] = K \frac{PCO_2}{[HCO_3^-]} \times 100$$

The constant, K, embraces the dissociation constants for *Equations 3.1 and 3.2* and the solubility coefficient of carbon dioxide, which governs the concentration of the gas in solution at a given partial pressure. When $[H^+]$ is measured in nmol/L, bicarbonate in mmol/L and $P_{CO_2}$ in kilopascals (kPa), the value of K is approximately 180 at 37°C; if $P_{CO_2}$ is measured in mmHg, the value of K is 24.

It follows that it is possible to calculate the bicarbonate concentration from the $[H^+]$ and $P_{CO_2}$ alone. In blood gas analyzers, the bicarbonate concentration is derived by calculation in this way and is not measured. It is not the same as the bicarbonate (strictly, total carbon dioxide) measured by autoanalyzers. There has been considerable argument over whether it is valid to derive a bicarbonate concentration in this way, given that the values of the constants involved are based upon observations in supposedly ideal solutions, which biological fluids are not. However, for most practical purposes the derivation is an acceptable one.

An appreciation of the relationship between $[H^+]$, bicarbonate concentration and $P_{CO_2}$ is of fundamental importance to an understanding of the pathophysiology of hydrogen ion homoeostasis. It will be apparent from

*Equation 3.5* that the relationships between [H$^+$] and $P\text{co}_2$ and between bicarbonate concentration and $P\text{co}_2$ are linear. These relationships have been quantified by measurements made *in vivo* and it is therefore possible to predict the effect of a change in one variable on another; for example, the effect of an acute rise in $P\text{co}_2$ on [H$^+$]. This information is an important aid in the interpretation of acid–base data.

The relationships between [H$^+$], $P\text{co}_2$ and bicarbonate concentration are plotted in *Fig. 3.5*. This may be useful as an *aide-mémoire* to the interpretation of acid–base data but should not be used as a substitute for a full understanding of the underlying principles.

Many instruments for blood gas analysis generate other data such as standard bicarbonate and base excess. The meanings, uses and misuses of these terms are described later.

## DISORDERS OF HYDROGEN ION HOMOEOSTASIS

There are four components in the pathophysiology of hydrogen ion disorders (acid–base disorders):

- Generation.
- Buffering.
- Compensation.
- Correction.

It is helpful to consider these separately although in reality they occur concurrently, albeit with different time courses.

Acid–base disorders are classified as either respiratory or non-respiratory (metabolic) according to whether or not there is a primary (causative) change in $P\text{co}_2$. The term 'acidosis' signifies a tendency for the [H$^+$] to be above normal and 'alkalosis' for it to be below normal.

Primary mixed acid–base disorders, that is, disorders of combined respiratory and non-respiratory origin, are common. However, the secondary, or compensatory, responses to a primary disorder of hydrogen ion homoeostasis may produce changes indistinguishable from those seen in primary mixed disorders.

### Non-respiratory (metabolic) acidosis

The primary abnormality in non-respiratory acidosis is either increased production or decreased excretion of hydrogen

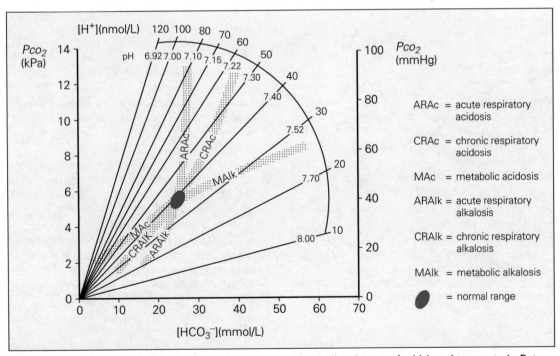

**Fig. 3.5** The relationship between $P\text{co}_2$, hydrogen ion concentration and bicarbonate concentration. The shaded areas represent the ranges of values found in simple disturbances of acid–base homoeostasis. Data falling outside these areas indicate mixed disturbances.

ions. In some cases, both of these may contribute. Loss of bicarbonate from the body can also, indirectly, cause an acidosis. Common causes of non-respiratory acidosis are given in *Fig. 3.6*. Excess hydrogen ions are buffered by bicarbonate (*Equation 3.2*) and other buffers. The carbonic acid thus formed dissociates (*Equation 3.1*) and the carbon dioxide is lost in the expired air. This buffering limits the potential rise in hydrogen ion concentration at the expense of a reduction in bicarbonate concentration.

Compensation is effected by hyperventilation, which increases the removal of carbon dioxide and lowers the $P_{CO_2}$. The $P_{CO_2}/[HCO_3^-]$ ratio is reduced, thus reducing the $[H^+]$ (*Equation 3.5*). Hyperventilation is a direct result of the increased $[H^+]$ stimulating the respiratory centre. Respiratory compensation cannot completely normalize the $[H^+]$ since it is the high concentration itself that stimulates the compensatory hyperventilation. Furthermore, the increased work of the respiratory muscles produces carbon dioxide, thereby limiting the extent to which the $P_{CO_2}$ can be lowered.

If the cause of the acidosis is not corrected, a new steady state may be attained, with a raised $[H^+]$, low bicarbonate and low $P_{CO_2}$. In the steady rate, the decrease in $P_{CO_2}$ attributable to respiratory compensation is approximately 0.17 kPa (1.3 mmHg) for each 1 mmol/L decrement in bicarbonate concentration. The extent to which compensation can take place will be limited if respiratory function is compromised. Even with normal respiratory function, it is exceptional for a $P_{CO_2}$ of less than 1.5 kPa (11.3 mmHg) to be recorded, however severe the non-respiratory acidosis.

In a healthy person, hyperventilation would produce a respiratory alkalosis. In general, the compensatory mechanism for any acid–base disturbance involves the generation of a second, opposing disturbance. In the case of a metabolic acidosis, compensation is through the generation of a respiratory alkalosis; in a respiratory acidosis, it is through the generation of a metabolic alkalosis (*see below*).

If renal function is normal in a patient with non-respiratory acidosis, excess hydrogen ions can be excreted by the kidneys. However, in many cases there is impairment of renal function, although this is not necessarily the primary cause of the acidosis.

The complete correction of a non-respiratory acidosis requires reversal of the underlying cause, for example, rehydration and insulin for diabetic ketoacidosis (*see Case History 11.2*) and removal of salicylate in salicylate overdose. It is important to maintain adequate renal perfusion to maximize renal hydrogen ion excretion. The use of exogenous bicarbonate to buffer hydrogen ions is discussed below and on p. 169.

### Increased production of hydrogen ions

This is the cause of the acidosis in ketoacidosis (diabetic, alcoholic), lactic acidosis and acidosis seen in poisoning, for example, with salicylates and ethylene glycol.

---

**Causes of non-respiratory acidosis**

**Increased H⁺ formation**
ketoacidosis (usually diabetic, also alcoholic)
lactic acidosis
poisoning: e.g., ethanol, methanol,
    ethylene glycol and salicylate
inherited organic acidosis

**Acid ingestion**
acid poisoning
excessive parenteral administration of
    amino acids: e.g., arginine, lysine
    and histidine

**Decreased H⁺ excretion**
renal tubular acidosis
generalized renal failure
carbonate dehydratase inhibitors

**Loss of bicarbonate**
diarrhoea
pancreatic, intestinal and biliary fistulae
    or drainage

**Fig. 3.6** Principal causes of non-respiratory (metabolic) acidosis.

---

**CASE HISTORY 3.1**

A 60-year-old man was admitted to hospital with severe abdominal pain which had begun two and a half hours earlier. He was not taking any drugs. On examination, he was shocked and had a distended, rigid abdomen; neither femoral pulse was palpable.

**Investigations**

| | | |
|---|---|---|
| arterial blood: hydrogen ion | 90 nmol/L (pH 7.05) | |
| $P_{CO_2}$ | 3.5 kPa (26.3 mmHg) | |
| $P_{O_2}$ | 12 kPa (90 mmHg) | |
| bicarbonate (derived) | | 7 mmol/L |

## Comment

The patient is acidotic (raised [H$^+$]) and this must be non-respiratory in origin since the $P\text{co}_2$ is not raised. Indeed, $P\text{co}_2$ is decreased, reflecting compensatory hyperventilation. The hyperventilation may be clinically obvious (Kussmaul's respiration, *see Case History 11.2*). An even lower $P\text{co}_2$ might have been expected as a result of respiratory compensation, but, in this case, splinting of the abdominal muscles (the abdomen is rigid) has restricted respiratory movements. The low bicarbonate concentration reflects the primary abnormality; bicarbonate is consumed as hydrogen ions are buffered. If there is no respiratory component to the acidosis, the plasma bicarbonate concentration is a good guide to the severity of a metabolic acidosis.

The clinical diagnosis (confirmed at laparotomy) is a ruptured abdominal aortic aneurysm. The patient is severely shocked following extravasation of blood from the aneurysm. Impaired tissue perfusion has led to inadequate oxygenation, despite the normal arterial $P\text{o}_2$, with consequently increased anaerobic metabolism of glucose to lactic acid, rather than oxidative metabolism.

Lactic acid is a normal metabolite of muscle and is converted back to glucose in the liver (the Cori cycle). However, with greatly increased production and possible impairment of hepatic metabolism due to poor perfusion, lactic acid accumulates. If renal function is compromised, for instance, by hypoperfusion, the ability of the kidneys to excrete excess hydrogen ions is also impaired.

Other causes of lactic acidosis are given in *Fig. 3.7*.

---

### Causes of lactic acidosis

tissue hypoxia:
    decreased perfusion
    reduced arterial $P\text{o}_2$

drugs, etc:
    ethanol, methanol
    phenformin
    fructose, sorbitol

congenital:
    glucose 6-phosphatase deficiency
    other inherited diseases with defective
        gluconeogenesis or pyruvate oxidation

**Fig. 3.7** Causes of lactic acidosis. Lactic acidosis is sometimes classified as type A (tissue hypoxia) and type B (all other causes).

---

### Decreased excretion of hydrogen ions

Acidosis occurs in renal glomerular failure, when the decreased glomerular filtration causes a reduction in the amount of sodium that is filtered and therefore available for exchange with hydrogen ions. The amount of phosphate filtered and available for buffering also decreases (*see Case History 4.2*). Renal tubular acidosis is discussed in *Chapter 4*.

### Loss of bicarbonate

Loss of bicarbonate and retention of hydrogen ions may result in acidosis in patients losing alkaline secretions from the small intestine, for example through fistulae. In the stomach, bicarbonate generated from carbon dioxide and water is retained and hydrogen ions are secreted into the lumen (*Fig 3.8*). In the pancreas and small intestine, the movements of bicarbonate and hydrogen ions occur in the opposite directions (*Fig 3.8*). Therefore, hydrogen ions which are secreted into the stomach lumen are neutralized by bicarbonate in the small intestine.

Under normal circumstances, since most of the fluid and ions secreted into the gut are reabsorbed, the gut is effectively a closed system with regard to acid–base balance. If, however, alkaline secretions are lost, the patient is at risk of becoming acidotic. Increased renal hydrogen ion excretion (with generation and retention of bicarbonate) may prevent this, but excessive fluid loss from the gut may deplete the ECF to such an extent that the glomerular filtration rate falls and the kidneys are no longer able to compensate.

### The anion gap

When the bicarbonate concentration falls in a non-respiratory acidosis, electrochemical neutrality must be maintained by other anions. In many cases, anions are produced simultaneously and equally with hydrogen ions, for example, acetoacetate and β-hydroxybutyrate in diabetic ketoacidosis, and lactate in lactic acidosis. When this does not occur, the deficit is met by chloride ions.

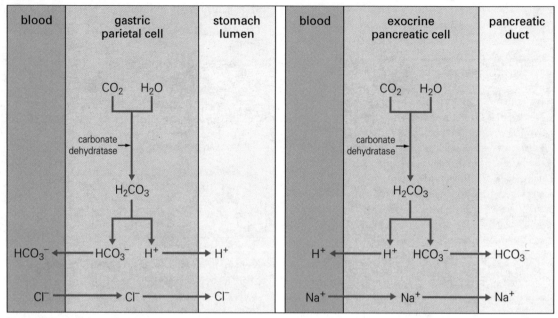

**Fig. 3.8** Generation of acidic gastric and alkaline pancreatic secretions. Hydrogen and bicarbonate ions are generated from carbon dioxide and water, catalyzed by carbonate dehydratase. In the stomach, the hydrogen ions are secreted while bicarbonate is retained. The reverse process occurs in the pancreas.

The difference between the sums of the concentrations of the principal cations (sodium and potassium) and of the principal anions (chloride and bicarbonate) is known as the 'anion gap', *Equation 3.6.*

**(3.6)**   Anion gap = $([Na^+] + [K^+]) - ([Cl^-] + [HCO_3^-])$

In health, the anion gap has a value of 14–18 mmol/L and mainly represents the unmeasured net negative charge on plasma proteins.

In an acidosis in which anions other than chloride are increased, the anion gap is increased. In contrast, in an acidosis due to loss of bicarbonate, for example, renal tubular acidosis, the plasma chloride concentration is increased and the anion gap is normal. It has therefore been suggested that calculation of the anion gap is of value in the diagnosis of acidosis. In the majority of cases of acidosis, however, the cause is obvious clinically and can be confirmed by the results of simple tests. The anion gap may be useful in the analysis of complex acid–base disorders, as shown by *Case History 3.7*, but some laboratories do not routinely measure chloride and the anion gap cannot then be calculated.

The characteristic biochemical changes seen in the blood in non-respiratory acidosis can be summarized as follows:

Non-respiratory acidosis

| | |
|---|---|
| $[H^+]$ | ↑ |
| pH | ↓ |
| $P_{CO_2}$ | ↓ |
| $[HCO_3^-]$ | ↓ |

The decrease in $P_{CO_2}$ is a compensatory change; the decrement in $P_{CO_2}$ is approximately 0.17 kPa (1.3 mmHg) per millimole decrease in the concentration of bicarbonate.

Changes due to the underlying condition will also be present. Hyperkalaemia is common in acidotic patients, except in bicarbonate-wasting conditions, for reasons discussed in *Chapter 2*.

### Management

The management of non-respiratory acidosis must be directed at reversal of the underlying cause. Where this is not immediately possible, bicarbonate may be given to buffer hydrogen ions although there is no general agreement as to when bicarbonate should be used. Many would consider it prudent to give bicarbonate when the arterial $[H^+]$ is greater than 100 nmol/L (pH < 7) and there is no immediate prospect of lowering it by other means, particularly in a patient whose clinical condition is generally poor. However, when bicarbonate is used it should be given in small quantities and the effect on the arterial [H⁺] measured. Large amounts of bicarbonate, given rapidly in an attempt to correct an acidosis, may be dangerous.

## Respiratory acidosis

Some of the many conditions associated with the development of respiratory acidosis are shown in *Fig. 3.9*. They are all characterized by an increase in $P_{CO_2}$. For every hydrogen ion that is produced a bicarbonate ion is generated. The majority of the hydrogen ions are buffered by intracellular buffers, particularly haemoglobin. With an acute rise in $P_{CO_2}$, every 1 kPa (7.5 mmHg) increase is associated with a concomitant increase in bicarbonate concentration of just under 1 mmol/L and [H⁺] of approximately 5.5 nmol/L. In chronic carbon dioxide retention, when renal compensation is maximal, the [H⁺] is increased by only 2.5 nmol/L for each 1 kPa (7.5 mmHg) rise in $P_{CO_2}$.

A respiratory acidosis can only be corrected by means which restore the $P_{CO_2}$ to normal but, if a high $P_{CO_2}$ persists, compensation occurs through increased renal hydrogen ion excretion.

In acute respiratory acidosis, unless very severe, the bicarbonate concentration, although increased, is usually within the reference range. If the bicarbonate concentration is clearly elevated in a respiratory acidosis, either a more chronic course with renal compensation (*see Case History 3.3*) or a coexisting non-respiratory alkalosis is suggested. A low bicarbonate would suggest a coexisting non-respiratory acidosis.

---

### Causes of respiratory acidosis

**Airway obstruction**
chronic obstructive airway disease
  (e.g., bronchitis, emphysema)
bronchospasm, e.g., in asthma
aspiration

**Depression of respiratory centre**
anaesthetics
sedatives
cerebral trauma
tumours

**Neuromuscular disease**
poliomyelitis
Guillain-Barré syndrome
motor neuron disease
tetanus, botulism
neurotoxins, curare

**Pulmonary disease**
pulmonary fibrosis
severe pneumonia
respiratory distress syndrome

**Extrapulmonary thoracic disease**
flail chest
severe kyphoscoliosis

**Fig. 3.9** Major causes of respiratory acidosis.

---

**CASE HISTORY 3.2**

A young man sustained injury to the chest in a road traffic accident. Effective ventilation was compromised by a large flail segment.

**Investigations**
arterial blood:  $P_{O_2}$        8 kPa (60 mmHg)
                $P_{CO_2}$       8 kPa (60 mmHg)
                hydrogen ion 58 nmol/L (pH 7.24)
                bicarbonate (derived)    25 mmol/L

**Comment**
There is a severe acidosis and the raised $P_{CO_2}$ indicates that it is respiratory in origin. The magnitude of the increase in [H⁺] suggests that no renal compensation has occurred. Such compensation can take several days to become fully effective, in contrast to the rapid respiratory compensation in non-respiratory disorders.

---

**CASE HISTORY 3.3**

A 70-year-old man, known to suffer from chronic obstructive airways disease, was admitted to hospital with an acute exacerbation of his illness. Arterial blood analysis was carried out on admission (results A). In spite of vigorous physiotherapy and medical treatment his condition deteriorated (results B) and it was decided to start artificial ventilation. Analysis was repeated after six hours (results C). After 12 hours he had a generalized fit (results D).

## Investigations

| arterial blood: | A | B | C | D |
|---|---|---|---|---|
| $P\text{co}_2$ (kPa) | 9.5 | 11.0 | 7.7 | 5.7 |
| (mmHg) | 71.3 | 82.5 | 58.5 | 42.8 |
| hydrogen ion (nmol/L) | 50 | 58 | 40 | 29 |
| pH | 7.30 | 7.24 | 7.40 | 7.54 |
| bicarbonate (mmol/L) | | | | |
| (derived) | 35 | 35 | 34 | 35 |

## Comment

The results on admission (A) indicate an acidosis. This is of respiratory origin since the $P\text{co}_2$ is raised. However, the [H+] is only slightly elevated, indicating that renal compensation is occurring as would be expected in a case of chronic carbon dioxide retention. The raised bicarbonate, which suggests a non-respiratory alkalosis, is the result of the compensatory increase in renal hydrogen ion excretion. Indeed, the commonest causes of raised plasma bicarbonate concentration in the elderly are chronic carbon dioxide retention and diuretic-induced potassium depletion (see p. 29).

A more severe acidosis (B) subsequently develops, commensurate with the rise in $P\text{co}_2$. This is a result of further carbon dioxide retention with no corresponding increase in renal hydrogen ion excretion.

Artificial ventilation lowers the $P\text{co}_2$ rapidly (C); the [H+] is now normal although the $P\text{co}_2$ is still elevated. This represents this patient's normal steady state, in which there is an almost complete renal compensation of the acidosis.

Continued ventilation reduces the $P\text{co}_2$ (D) to within the normal range for a healthy subject but to below this patient's normal. He has become alkalotic and suffers a fit as a consequence. The alkalosis is due to the continued high rate of renal hydrogen ion excretion in response to the chronically raised $P\text{co}_2$. Adaptation of renal hydrogen ion excretion in response to a change in $P\text{co}_2$ takes several days. Thus, rapid reduction of the $P\text{co}_2$ exposes the compensatory, secondary response, which then appears to be the sole acid–base abnormality. The compensatory mechanism in respiratory acidosis involves the generation of a metabolic alkalosis.

## Management

The aim when treating respiratory acidosis is to improve alveolar ventilation and lower the $P\text{co}_2$. In acute alveolar hypoventilation, however, it is usually hypoxaemia rather than hypercapnia that poses the main threat to life, unless the $P\text{o}_2$ is being maintained by the supply of additional oxygen. If ventilation ceases abruptly, death from hypoxaemia will occur in approximately four minutes; the $P\text{co}_2$ by comparison rises at such a rate that it would take more than ten minutes for it to reach a lethal level.

In chronic respiratory acidosis, it is seldom possible to correct the underlying cause and treatment is directed at maximizing alveolar ventilation by, for example, utilizing physiotherapy, bronchodilators and antibiotics. If artificial ventilation becomes necessary, it is vital to monitor the patient's arterial blood gases and hydrogen ion in order to avoid over-correction of the respiratory acidosis.

Oxygen may safely be used at high concentrations in patients with acute respiratory failure. In many patients with chronic carbon dioxide retention, however, the respiratory centre becomes insensitive to carbon dioxide and hypoxaemia provides the main stimulus to respiration. Oxygen administration in such patients must be carefully controlled to prevent abolition of this stimulus.

It is important to appreciate that, on the basis of the data alone, it would not be possible to tell whether results 'C' in Case History 3.3 represent a state of either compensated chronic carbon dioxide retention or acute carbon dioxide retention developing in a patient with a pre-existing metabolic alkalosis. The management of these two states would not be the same.

The characteristic biochemical changes in arterial blood in acute and chronic acidosis can be summarized as follows:

Respiratory acidosis

| | acute | chronic |
|---|---|---|
| [H+] | ↑ | slight ↑ or normal |
| pH | ↓ | slight ↓ or normal |
| $P\text{co}_2$ | ↑ | ↑ |
| [HCO$_3$−] | slight ↑ | ↑ |

## Non-respiratory (metabolic) alkalosis

Non-respiratory alkalosis is characterized by a primary increase in the ECF bicarbonate concentration, with a consequent reduction in the [H+] (see Equation 3.5 ). In a normal subject, an increase in plasma bicarbonate concentration leads to incomplete renal tubular bicarbonate reabsorption and excretion of bicarbonate in the urine.

Massive quantities of bicarbonate must be ingested to produce a sustained alkalosis.

Since the body is a net producer of acid, it might be supposed that non-respiratory alkalosis should be corrected by normal acid production. In practice, and in contrast to non-respiratory acidosis and to respiratory disorders of acid–base balance, a non-respiratory alkalosis may persist even after the primary cause has been corrected. It is thus necessary to consider both the mechanisms which cause non-respiratory alkalosis and those which can perpetuate it.

Causes of non-respiratory alkalosis are shown in *Fig. 3.10*. Alkali loading causes only a transient alkalosis unless there are additional factors operating to sustain it. Disproportionate loss of chloride, for example, during diuretic-induced mobilization of oedema fluid when little bicarbonate is excreted in the urine, can cause a non-respiratory alkalosis but, if this is the sole mechanism, the disturbance is always mild.

The maintenance of a non-respiratory alkalosis requires inappropriately high (as far as hydrogen ion homoeostasis is concerned) renal bicarbonate reabsorption. Factors which may be responsible for this include a decrease in ECF volume, mineralocorticoid excess and potassium depletion.

In hypovolaemia, there is an increased stimulus to renal sodium reabsorption (*see p. 15*). Sodium reabsorption is dependent upon the availability of adequate anions. If there is a relative deficit of chloride as, for example, with loss of gastric juice and treatment with some diuretics, electrochemical neutrality during sodium reabsorption is maintained by increased bicarbonate reabsorption and by hydrogen and potassium ion excretion. In states of mineralocortoid excess, alkalosis is perpetuated by the increased hydrogen ion excretion in the nephron which occurs secondarily to the increased sodium reabsorption.

The correction of a non-respiratory alkalosis requires reversal both of the primary cause and of the mechanism responsible for its perpetuation. The expected compensatory change would be an increase in $P_{CO_2}$ which would increase the ratio $P_{CO_2}/[HCO_3^-]$ and thus $[H^+]$ (*see Equation 3.5*). A low arterial $[H^+]$ inhibits the respiratory centre, causing hypoventilation, and thus an increase in $P_{CO_2}$. However, since an increase in $P_{CO_2}$ is itself a powerful stimulus to respiration, this compensation, particularly in acute non-respiratory alkalosis, may be self-limiting. In more chronic disorders, significant compensation may occur, presumably because the respiratory centre becomes less sensitive to carbon dioxide. Should hypoventilation lead to significant hypoxaemia, however, this will provide a powerful stimulus to respiration and prevent further compensation.

## Causes of non-respiratory alkalosis

### Loss of unbuffered hydrogen ion

gastrointestinal:
 gastric aspiration
 vomiting with pyloric stenosis
 congenital chloride-losing diarrhoea

renal:
 mineralocorticoid excess:
  Cushing's syndrome
  Conn's syndrome
 drugs with mineralocorticoid activity,
  e.g., carbenoxolone
 diuretic therapy (not K+-sparing)
 rapid correction of chronically raised $P_{CO_2}$
 potassium depletion

### Administration of alkali

inappropriate treatment of acidotic states
chronic alkali ingestion

**Fig. 3.10** Causes of non-respiratory alkalosis.

**CASE HISTORY 3.4**
A 45-year-old man was admitted to hospital with a history of persistent vomiting. He had a long history of dyspepsia but had never sought advice for this, preferring to treat himself with proprietary remedies. On examination he was obviously dehydrated and his respiration was shallow.

**Investigations**
arterial blood:

| | | |
|---|---|---|
| hydrogen ion | 28 nmol/L (pH 7.56) | |
| $P_{CO_2}$ | 7.2 kPa (54 mmHg) | |
| bicarbonate (derived) | | 45 mmol/L |
| serum: sodium | | 146 mmol/L |
| potassium | | 2.8 mmol/L |
| urea | | 34.2 mmol/L |

A barium meal, performed after this metabolic imbalance had been corrected, showed pyloric stenosis, thought to be due to scarring caused by peptic ulceration.

**Comment**

The patient is alkalotic and since the $P_{CO_2}$ is high, this must be non-respiratory in origin. The increase in $P_{CO_2}$ is a result of compensatory hypoventilation leading to carbon dioxide retention. In chronic non-respiratory alkalosis, as in this case, each increment of 1mmol/L in bicarbonate concentration typically gives rise to an increase in $P_{CO_2}$ of approximately 0.1 kPa (0.8 mmHg).

The alkalosis is a result of loss of unbuffered hydrogen ions in gastric juice with a concomitant retention of bicarbonate. The raised urea is consistent with the clinical signs of dehydration resulting from fluid loss. Fluid loss stimulates renal sodium reabsorption, but sodium can only be reabsorbed either with chloride or in exchange for hydrogen and potassium ions. Gastric juice has a high concentration of chloride and patients losing gastric secretions become hypochloraemic. This means that less sodium than usual can be reabsorbed with chloride. However, it appears that the defence of ECF volume takes precedence over acid–base homoeostasis and further sodium reabsorption occurs in exchange for hydrogen ions (perpetuating the alkalosis) and potassium ions (leading to potassium depletion). This explains the apparently paradoxical findings of an acidic urine in patients with severe non-respiratory alkalosis. Potassium is also lost in the gastric juice, and thus patients frequently become potassium-depleted and yet are losing potassium in the urine.

A non-respiratory alkalosis due to loss of gastric acid may also occur in patients undergoing nasogastric aspiration. It is not usually a feature of vomiting if the pylorus is patent, since the additional loss of alkaline secretions from the upper small intestine counteracts the effect of the retention of bicarbonate ions generated by gastric parietal cells. Vomiting with pyloric stenosis is an unusual cause of non-respiratory alkalosis; other causes rarely result in such a severe disturbance.

*Management*

The management of a non-respiratory alkalosis depends upon the severity of the condition and upon the cause. When hypovolaemia and hypochloraemia are present, they can be simultaneously corrected by an infusion of isotonic sodium chloride solution ('normal saline') which will also improve renal perfusion and allow excretion of the bicarbonate load. In such cases, it is common practice to provide potassium supplements although often this is not necessary. It is very rarely

necessary to attempt rapid correction of non-respiratory alkalosis, for example, by administration of ammonium chloride.

The mild alkalosis commonly associated with potassium depletion which may, for example, be diuretic induced, rarely requires treatment *per se* although the hypokalaemia may require correction. The management of a state of mineralocorticoid excess is considered in *Chapter 8*.

The biochemical features of non-respiratory alkalosis can be summarized as follows:

Non-respiratory alkalosis

| | |
|---|---|
| $[H^+]$ | ↓ |
| pH | ↑ |
| $P_{CO_2}$ | ↑ |
| $[HCO_3^-]$ | ↑ |

## Respiratory alkalosis

The main causes of respiratory alkalosis are shown in *Fig. 3.11*. The common feature and cause of the alkalosis is a fall in $P_{CO_2}$, which reduces the ratio of $P_{CO_2}$ to bicarbonate concentration (*see Equation 3.5*, page 38). In acute respiratory alkalosis, the $[H^+]$ falls by approximately 5.5 nmol/L for each 1.0 kPa (7.5 mmHg) fall in $P_{CO_2}$.

The fall in $P_{CO_2}$ causes a small decrease in bicarbonate concentration. Compensation occurs through a reduction in renal hydrogen ion excretion, which further decreases the plasma bicarbonate concentration. Renal compensation in a respiratory alkalosis develops slowly, as it does in a respiratory acidosis. If a steady $P_{CO_2}$ is maintained, maximal compensation with a new steady state develops within 36–72 hours.

**CASE HISTORY 3.5**

As part of a class experiment in physiology, a medical student volunteered to have a sample of arterial blood taken. The demonstrator took some time to explain the procedure to the class, during which time the student became increasingly anxious. As the blood was being drawn she complained of tingling in her fingers and toes.

**Investigations**

arterial blood:

| | |
|---|---|
| hydrogen ion | 30 nmol/L(pH 7.52) |
| $P_{CO_2}$ | 3.5 kPa(26.3 mmHg) |
| bicarbonate (derived) | 22 mmol/L |

**Comment**

The student is alkalotic with a low $P\text{co}_2$, thus the disturbance is respiratory in origin. The extent of the decrease in [H⁺] indicates that there is neither compensation nor additional acid–base disturbance. The low $P\text{co}_2$ is a result of anxiety-induced hyperventilation and no compensation would be expected to have occurred in this short time. The symptoms are a result of a decrease in the concentration of ionized calcium, an effect of alkalosis.

**CASE HISTORY 3.6**

A young woman was admitted to hospital unconscious, following a head injury. A skull fracture was demonstrated on radiography and a computerized tomography (CT) scan revealed extensive cerebral contusions. The respiratory rate was 38/min. Three days after admission, the patient's condition was unchanged and arterial blood was analyzed.

**Investigations**
arterial blood:

| | |
|---|---|
| hydrogen ion | 36 nmol/L(pH 7.44) |
| $P\text{co}_2$ | 3.6 kPa(29.3 mmHg) |
| bicarbonate (derived) | 19 mmol/L |

**Comment**

This is a compensated respiratory alkalosis. The $P\text{co}_2$ is reduced as a result of hyperventilation. The hydrogen ion concentration is at the lower limit of normal. Abnormalities of respiration (hypo- and hyperventilation) are common in patients with head injuries. Hyperventilation can occur with injuries involving the brain stem and as a result of raised intracranial pressure. Even though a low $P\text{co}_2$ is also characteristic of the respiratory compensation in non-respiratory acidosis, the history and normal [H⁺] preclude this diagnosis. Also, a much lower bicarbonate concentration would be expected in a non-respiratory acidosis.

*Management*

As with other disturbances of acid–base homoeostasis, the management of patients with respiratory alkalosis should be directed towards the underlying cause although this is frequently not possible. Fortunately, a chronic compensated respiratory alkalosis is not, in itself, dangerous. Increasing the inspired $P\text{co}_2$ by making the patient re-breathe into a paper bag may abort the clinical features of acute hypocapnia in acute hyperventilation, but is only a temporary measure.

The biochemical features of respiratory alkalosis can be summarized as follows:

Respiratory alkalosis

| | acute | chronic |
|---|---|---|
| [H⁺] | ↓ | slight ↓ or normal |
| pH | ↑ | slight ↑ or normal |
| $P\text{co}_2$ | ↓ | ↓ |
| [HCO₃⁻] | slight ↓ | ↓ |

## INTERPRETATION OF ACID–BASE DATA

A thorough understanding of the pathophysiology of acid–base homoeostasis is essential for the correct interpretation of laboratory data, but these data should always be considered in the clinical context.

**Causes of respiratory alkalosis**

**Hypoxia**
high altitude
severe anaemia
pulmonary disease

**Increased respiratory drive**
respiratory stimulants, e.g., salicylates
cerebral disturbances, e.g., trauma,
    infection and tumours
hepatic failure
Gram-negative septicaemia
primary hyperventilation syndrome
voluntary hyperventilation

**Pulmonary disease**
pulmonary oedema
pulmonary embolism

**Mechanical overventilation**

**Fig. 3.11** Major causes of respiratory alkalosis.

The starting point in any evaluation should be the hydrogen ion concentration or pH. This will indicate whether the predominant disturbance is an acidosis or an alkalosis. However, a normal value does not exclude an acid–base disorder. There may be either a fully compensated disturbance or two primary disturbances, where effects on hydrogen ion concentration cancel each other out.

If the $Pco_2$ is abnormal, there must be a respiratory component to the disturbance; if the $Pco_2$ is raised in an acidosis, the acidosis is respiratory and comparison of the hydrogen ion concentration with that predicted for an acute change in $Pco_2$ will indicate whether there is an additional metabolic component; this may be compensatory. If the $Pco_2$ is low in an acidosis, the acidosis is non-respiratory and there is an additional, often compensatory, respiratory component. A similar rationale applies to alkalotic states. An algorithm for the analysis of acid–base data is given in *Fig. 3.12.*

Since the derived bicarbonate is calculated from the $Pco_2$ and [H⁺], it does not provide any more information than these two measurements alone. However, knowledge of the bicarbonate level may simplify the interpretation of acid–base data. Its concentration is always decreased in non-respiratory acidosis and increased in non-respiratory alkalosis, regardless of whether or not there is compensation.

---

**CASE HISTORY 3.7**

A young woman was admitted to hospital, eight hours after she had taken an overdose of aspirin.

**Investigations**
arterial blood:

| | |
|---|---|
| hydrogen ion | 30 nmol/L (pH 7.53) |
| $Pco_2$ | 2.0 kPa (15 mmHg) |

**Comment**
The patient is alkalotic and the low $Pco_2$ indicates a respiratory origin. However, the [H⁺] is not as low as would have been expected as a result of an acute fall in $Pco_2$. The data would be appropriate for a chronic, compensated respiratory alkalosis, but such a low $Pco_2$ would be exceptional and this interpretation is not compatible with the history. The alternative is that there is an acute respiratory alkalosis with a coexistent non-respiratory acidosis. This combination is characteristic of salicylate poisoning where initial respiratory stimulation causes a respiratory alkalosis

but later the metabolic effects of salicylate tend to predominate, producing an acidosis.

This case history illustrates the importance of considering the clinical setting when analyzing acid–base data. Calculation of the anion gap might have been helpful here. It would have been increased by the presence of organic anions, indicating a coexisting non-respiratory acidosis, but is normal in compensated respiratory alkalosis.

---

**CASE HISTORY 3.8**

An elderly man was admitted to hospital in a confused state. He was dyspnoeic and had a cough productive of sputum. He was unable to give a coherent history but one of the casualty officers knew him to be an insulin-dependent diabetic patient with a long history of chronic bronchitis.

**Investigations**
arterial blood:

| | |
|---|---|
| hydrogen ion | 66 nmol/L (pH 7.18) |
| $Pco_2$ | 7.4 kPa (55.5 mmHg) |

**Comment**
The patient is acidotic and the raised $Pco_2$ indicates a respiratory component. However, the [H⁺] is higher than would be expected in an acute respiratory acidosis with a $Pco_2$ at this level. Therefore, there must be a non-respiratory component to the acidosis.

On the basis of these data alone, it is not possible to determine whether the respiratory disturbance is acute or chronic. These results could, for example, represent the results of the concurrent development of an acute respiratory and a non-respiratory acidosis. On the other hand, they are also compatible with the presence of severe non-respiratory acidosis in a patient with chronic carbon dioxide retention. Given that the patient is known to suffer from chronic bronchitis, the second interpretation is more likely.

---

Mixed acid–base disturbances occur frequently and appear complex. Correct diagnosis requires a logical approach and a clear understanding both of the relevant

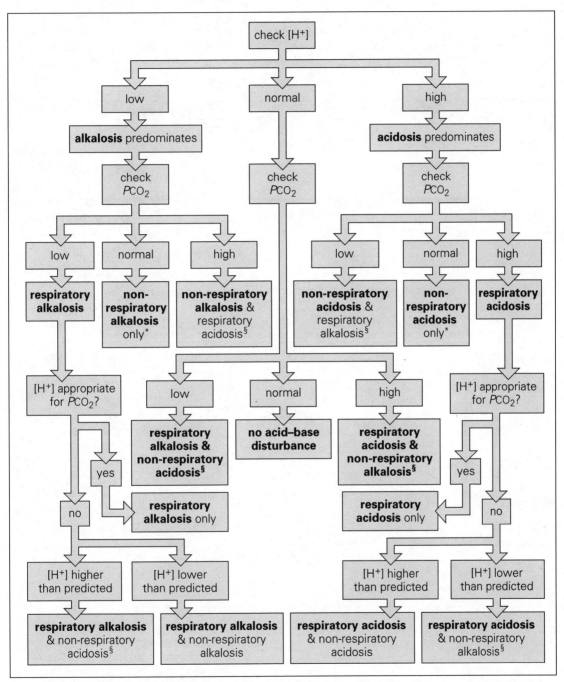

**Fig. 3.12** An algorithm for the analysis of acid–base data. Where two disturbances are shown, the predominant one is in bold type.
§ Indicates a disturbance that would be expected to develop as a result of physiological compensation, but could be a coexisting pathological process.

* Because compensation for non-respiratory disorders develops so rapidly, 'pure', i.e., uncompensated non-respiratory disorders do not occur unless the normal respiratory response is prevented, e.g., in a ventilated patient. Acutely, compensation for non-respiratory alkalosis is less efficient than for acidosis.

pathophysiology and of the quantitative relationships between [H⁺] and $P_{CO_2}$. The biochemical changes which are characteristic of the various acid–base disturbances are shown in *Fig. 3.13*. With this physiological approach, cal-

culated parameters such as 'standard bicarbonate' and 'base excess' are obsolete.

The standard bicarbonate is a calculated estimate of the bicarbonate concentration that would be present if the

| | Acidosis | | | Alkalosis | | |
|---|---|---|---|---|---|---|
| | Non-respiratory | Respiratory | | Non-respiratory | Respiratory | |
| | | acute | chronic | | acute | chronic |
| [H⁺] | ↑ | ↑ | slight ↑ or normal | ↓ | ↓ | slight ↓ or normal |
| pH | ↓ | ↓ | slight ↓ or normal | ↑ | ↑ | slight ↑ or normal |
| $P_{CO_2}$ | ↓ | ↑ | ↑ | ↑ | ↓ | ↓ |
| [HCO₃⁻] | ↓ | slight ↑ | ↑ | ↑ | slight↓ | ↓ |

**Fig. 3.13** Biochemical changes characteristic of disturbances of acid–base homoeostasis.

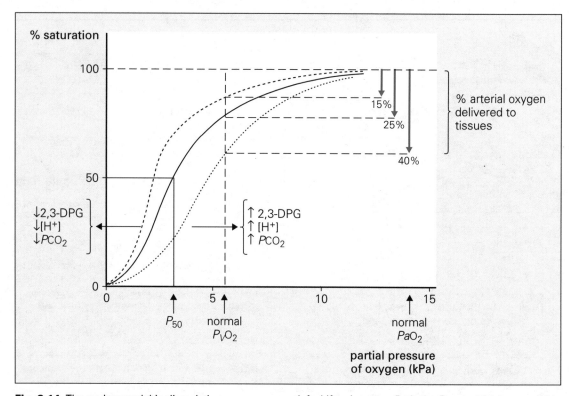

**Fig. 3.14** The oxyhaemoglobin dissociation curve. Normal arterial and venous $P_{CO_2}$ are shown. The effect of a right or left shift in the amount of oxygen delivered to tissues is indicated. A right shift causes an increase, a left shift a decrease. $P_{50}$ is the $P_{O_2}$ at which haemoglobin is 50% saturated with oxygen. 2,3-DPG is 2,3-diphosphoglycerate.

$P_{CO_2}$were normal and thus reflects only the non-respiratory influences on bicarbonate. The base excess is a calculated estimate of the non-respiratory influences on total buffering capacity. These parameters were introduced with a view to distinguishing between the respiratory and non-respiratory components in acid–base disorders, but they take no account of normal physiological responses. An abnormal standard bicarbonate or base excess indicates the presence of a non-respiratory acidosis or alkalosis. It does not, however, indicate whether this is either part of a mixed disturbance of acid–base homoeostasis or related to normal physiological compensation.

## OXYGEN TRANSPORT AND ITS DISORDERS

In patients with respiratory disorders, a disturbance of the partial pressure of oxygen ($P_{O_2}$) may be of greater clinical significance than either an abnormal $P_{CO_2}$ or abnormal [$H^+$]. Although both oxygen and carbon dioxide are transported between the alveoli and the bloodstream, albeit in opposite directions, their respective partial pressures do not necessarily change in a reciprocal fashion. There are two reasons for this: first, carbon dioxide is generally more diffusible than oxygen, with the result that, in pulmonary oedema and interstitial lung disease, hypoxaemia develops but the $P_{O_2}$ may not increase; and secondly, very little oxygen is carried in physical solution in the blood, while haemoglobin is normally nearly fully saturated with oxygen. Hyperventilation cannot, therefore, increase the arterial $P_{O_2}$ significantly, but can reduce the $P_{CO_2}$. A raised $P_{O_2}$ is only seen in patients given supplementary oxygen, which results in an increased inspired $P_{O_2}$ .

The oxyhaemoglobin dissociation curve, which relates $P_{O_2}$ to the percentage of the maximum saturation of haemoglobin with oxygen, is sigmoid (*Fig. 3.14*). As a consequence, a considerable drop in $P_{O_2}$ can occur without a significant effect on the amount of oxygen carried in the blood. Saturation only falls below 90% when $P_{O_2}$ falls below about 8 kPa, but if $P_{O_2}$ decreases further, saturation declines rapidly.

There are many causes of hypoxaemia (*Fig. 3.15*). The reasons for the hypoxaemia associated with hypoventilation, venous-to-arterial shunting and impaired diffusion are self-evident. However, in many respiratory diseases, such as lung collapse and pneumonia, there is an imbalance between ventilation and perfusion of the alveoli. Blood leaving poorly ventilated, well perfused alveoli will have a low $P_{O_2}$ and a raised $P_{CO_2}$. The effect on $P_{CO_2}$ can be compensated in normally perfused and ventilated alveoli by hyperventilation. This removes additional carbon dioxide,

| Hypoxaemia | |
|---|---|
| **Cause** | **Mechanism** |
| **Low inspired oxygen** low baromeric pressure low % oxygen in inspired air | low alveolar $P_{O_2}$ |
| **Alveolar hypoventilation** respiratory depression neuromuscular disease | low alveolar $P_{O_2}$ |
| **Venous-to-arterial shunt** cyanotic congenital heart disease | admixture of arterial blood (high $P_{O_2}$) with venous blood (low $P_{O_2}$) |
| **Impaired diffusion** pulmonary fibrosis | inadequate arterial oxygenation despite normal alveolar $P_{O_2}$ |
| **Ventilation/perfusion imbalance** chronic obstructive airways disease | blood perfuses non-aerated parts of lung and is not oxygenated |

**Fig. 3.15** Causes and mechanisms of hypoxaemia.

but cannot compensate for the low $P_{O_2}$ since the haemoglobin will be fully saturated and thus the amount of oxygen carried cannot be increased. The poorly perfused alveoli are effectively dead space. With moderate degrees of ventilation/perfusion imbalance, the $P_{O_2}$ is reduced and the $P_{CO_2}$ is either normal or even reduced. With severe imbalance, hyperventilation cannot compensate through increased removal of carbon dioxide from normally ventilated and perfused alveoli and the $P_{CO_2}$ becomes elevated.

Although an adequate arterial $P_{O_2}$ is essential for normal tissue oxygenation, it is not the only factor involved. The amount of oxygen delivered to tissues depends upon arterial oxygen *content* and their blood supply.

Oxygen content depends on haemoglobin concentration and on its saturation, which is a function of the affinity of haemoglobin for oxygen and the $P_{O_2}$. Haemoglobin saturation can be measured using an oximeter. Various factors can affect the affinity of haemoglobin for oxygen, and thus the percentage saturation at a given $P_{O_2}$. 2,3-Diphosphoglycerate (2,3-DPG) is an important physiological regulator. An increase in red cell 2,3-DPG causes a shift in the oxyhaemoglobin dissociation curve to the right and this facilitates oxygen uptake by tissues (*Fig. 3.14*). 2,3-DPG levels are increased in chronic hypoxia. Acidosis and an increase in $P\text{CO}_2$ also shift the curve to the right.

Tissue blood supply depends on the cardiac output and local vascular resistance. Thus tissue hypoxia can be caused not only by hypoxaemia, but also by anaemia, impaired haemoglobin function, decreased cardiac output or vasoconstriction. Even if oxygen delivery to tissues is adequate, utilization may be impaired by poisons such as cyanide.

## SUMMARY

The body is a net producer of hydrogen ions and also of carbon dioxide which can be hydrated to form carbonic acid. Hydrogen ion homoeostasis depends upon buffering in the tissues and bloodstream, excretion of hydrogen ions in urine and removal of carbon dioxide through the lungs in the expired air. The [H$^+$] of the blood is directly proportional to the partial pressure of carbon dioxide, $P\text{CO}_2$, and inversely proportional to the concentration of bicarbonate, the principal extracellular buffer.

In an acidosis, the [H$^+$] is greater than normal; in an alkalosis it is below normal. Both acidosis and alkalosis can be either primarily respiratory or non-respiratory in origin. Thus respiratory acidosis is the result of carbon dioxide retention and respiratory alkalosis of excessive carbon dioxide loss. A non-respiratory, or metabolic, acidosis is the result of either increased hydrogen ion production or decreased excretion or both, while a non-respiratory or metabolic alkalosis is usually a result of excessive hydrogen ion excretion from the body.

Compensatory mechanisms may counteract a tendency to acidosis or alkalosis. Compensation in effect results from the physiological generation of an opposing disturbance. Therefore, in a respiratory acidosis, compensation is through increased renal hydrogen ion excretion which, in a normal subject, would produce a non-respiratory alkalosis. Ultimate correction of a disturbance of hydrogen ion homoeostasis usually requires correction of the underlying cause.

Mixed disturbances, with respiratory and non-respiratory components, occur frequently. Even in these cases, a diagnosis can be made based on clinical assessment and logical consideration of the arterial hydrogen ion concentration and partial pressure of carbon dioxide.

## FURTHER READING

Cohen J J & Hassiven J P (1982) *Acid-Base*. Boston: Little Brown & Company.

Kurtzman N A & Batalle D C (eds) (1983) Acid-base disorders. *The Medical Clinics of North America*, **67**, 751–932.

Riley L J Jr, Ilson B E & Natrins R G (1987) Acute metabolic acid-base disorders. *Critical Care Clinics*, **5**, 699–724.

# 4. The Kidneys

## INTRODUCTION

The kidneys have three major functions: (i) excretion of waste, (ii) maintenance of extracellular fluid (ECF) volume and composition and (iii) hormone synthesis. Each kidney consists of approximately one million functional units, the nephrons.

The kidneys have a rich blood supply and normally receive about 25% of the cardiac output. Most of this is distributed initially to the capillary tufts of the glomeruli which act as high pressure filters. Blood is separated from the lumen of the nephron by three layers: the capillary endothelial cells, the basement membrane and the epithelial cells of the nephron (*Fig. 4.1*). The endothelial and epithelial cells are in intimate contact with the basement membrane; the endothelial cells are fenestrated and contact between the epithelial cells and the membrane is discontinuous so that the membrane is exposed to blood on one side and to the lumen of the nephron on the other.

The glomerular filtrate is an ultrafiltrate of plasma, that is, it has a similar composition to plasma except that it is almost free of proteins. This is because the endothelium provides a barrier to red and white blood cells and the basement membrane, though permeable to water and low molecular weight substances, is largely impermeable to macromolecules. This impermeability is related to both molecular size and electrical charge. Proteins with molecular weights lower than that of albumin (68,000 daltons) are filterable; negatively charged molecules are less easily filtered than those bearing a positive charge. Almost all the protein in the glomerular filtrate is reabsorbed and catabolized by proximal convoluted tubular cells with the result that normal urinary protein excretion is less than 150 mg/24h.

Filtration is a passive process. The total filtration rate of the kidneys is mainly determined by the difference between the blood pressure in the glomerular capillaries and the hydrostatic pressure in the lumen of the nephron, by the nature of the glomerular basement membrane and by the number of glomeruli. The normal glomerular filtration rate (GFR) is approximately 120 mL/min, equivalent to a volume of about 170 L/24h. However, urine production is only 1–2 L/24h, depending on fluid intake; the bulk of the filtrate is reabsorbed further along the nephron.

The glomerular filtrate passes into the proximal convoluted tubule where much of it is reabsorbed. Under normal circumstances, all the glucose, amino acids, potassium and

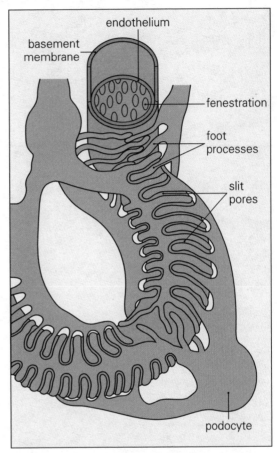

**Fig. 4.1** Diagram of a glomerular capillary, showing fenestrations in endothelial cells, basement membrane and epithelial cells (podocytes) with slit pores between interdigitating foot processes.

bicarbonate, and about 75% of the sodium, is reabsorbed isotonically here by energy-dependent mechanisms.

Medullary hyperosmolality, which is vital for the further reabsorption of water, is generated by the counter-current system, summarized in *Fig. 4.2*. Chloride ions, accompanied by sodium, are pumped out of the ascending limb of the loop of Henle into the surrounding interstitial fluid, and thence diffuse into the descending limb. Since the ascending limb of the loop of Henle is impermeable to water, the net effect is an exchange of sodium and chloride ions

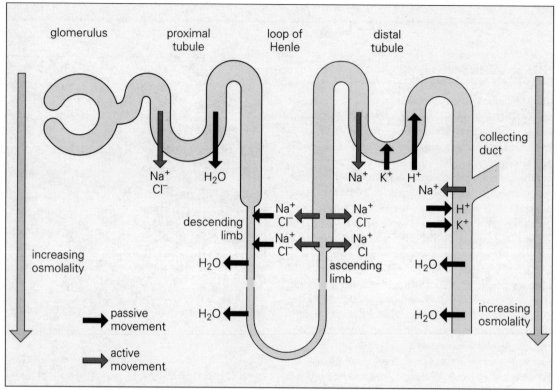

**Fig. 4.2** Movements of major ions, passive movement of water and changes in osmolality in the nephron. In the ascending loop of Henle, chloride ions are actively transported and sodium ions accompany them to maintain electrochemical neutrality.

between the ascending and descending limbs. This alters the osmolality of both the fluid within the nephron and the surrounding interstitial fluid. A gradient of osmolality is set up between the isotonic cortico-medullary junction and the extremely hypertonic (approximately 1200 mmol/L) deep medulla. Diffusion of urea from the collecting duct into the interstitium and thence into the loop of Henle also makes an important contribution to medullary hypertonicity. It is noteworthy that urinary concentrating ability is impaired in malnourished children but can be restored by increasing their dietary protein intake or even adding urea to their diets.

The tubular fluid becomes increasingly dilute as it passes up the ascending limb of the loop of Henle, as a result of the continued removal of chloride and sodium ions. Fluid entering the distal convoluted tubule is hypotonic (approximately 150 mmol/L) with respect to the glomerular filtrate.

Approximately 90% of the filtered sodium and 80% of the filtered water has been reabsorbed from the glomeru-

lar filtrate by the time it reaches the beginning of the distal convoluted tubule. In the distal tubule, further sodium reabsorption takes place, controlled by aldosterone; this generates an electrochemical gradient which engenders the secretion of potassium and hydrogen ions. Ammonia is also secreted in the distal tubule and buffers hydrogen ions, being excreted as ammonium ions (*see page 36*).

Whereas the proximal tubule is responsible for bulk reabsorption of the glomerular filtrate, the distal tubule exerts fine control over the composition of the tubular fluid, depending upon the requirements of the body.

Tubular fluid then passes into the collecting ducts which extend through the hypertonic renal medulla and discharge urine into the renal pelvis. The cells lining the collecting ducts are normally impermeable to water. Vasopressin (antidiuretic hormone, ADH) renders them permeable and allows water to be reabsorbed passively in response to the osmotic gradient between the duct lumen and the interstitial fluid. Thus, in the absence of vasopressin, a dilute urine is produced; in its presence, the urine is concentrated. Some reabsorption of sodium also occurs in the collecting ducts under the stimulus of aldosterone.

Since the normal GFR is approximately 120 mL/min, a volume of fluid equivalent to the entire ECF is filtered every two hours. Disease processes affecting the kidney therefore have an enormous potential for affecting water, salt and hydrogen ion homoeostasis and the excretion of waste products.

The kidneys are also important endocrine organs, producing renin, erythropoietin and calcitriol. The secretion of these hormones may be altered in renal disease. In addition, several other hormones are either inactivated or excreted by the kidneys and hence their concentrations in the blood can also be affected by renal disease.

# BIOCHEMICAL TESTS OF RENAL FUNCTION

Diseases affecting the kidneys can selectively damage glomerular or tubular function, but isolated disorders of tubular function are relatively uncommon. In acute and chronic renal failure, there is effectively a loss of function of whole nephrons and since the process of filtration is essential to the formation of urine, tests of glomerular function are almost invariably required in the investigation and management of any patient with renal disease. The principal function of the glomeruli is to filter water and low molecular weight components of the blood while retaining cells and high molecular weight components. Tests of glomerular function are divided into those that assess the rate of filtration (the GFR) and those that assess permeability.

It should be noted that the GFR declines with age (to a greater extent in males than in females) and this must be taken into account when interpreting results.

## Measurement of glomerular filtration rate (GFR)

### Clearance

An estimate of the GFR can be made by measuring the urinary excretion of a substance which is completely filtered from the blood by the glomeruli and which is not secreted, reabsorbed or metabolized by the renal tubules. Experimentally, inulin has been found to meet these requirements. The volume of blood from which inulin is cleared or completely removed in one minute is known as the inulin clearance and is equal to the GFR.

Measurement of inulin clearance requires the infusion of inulin into the blood and is therefore not suitable for routine clinical use. The clearance of creatinine, an endogenous substance normally present in the blood and excreted

after glomerular filtration, can be measured instead (Equation 4.1).

**(4.1)** Clearance = $\dfrac{U \times \dot{V}}{P}$ mL/min

U = urinary creatinine concentration (µmol/L)
$\dot{V}$ = urine flow rate [mL/min or (L/24 h)/1.44]
P = plasma creatinine concentration (µmol/L)

Creatinine is derived largely from the turnover of creatine phosphate in muscle and the daily production is relatively constant, being a function of total muscle mass. A small amount is derived from meat in the diet. Creatinine clearance in adults is normally of the order of 120 mL/min, corrected to a standard body surface area of 1.73m².

The accurate measurement of creatinine clearance is difficult, especially in outpatients, since it is necessary to obtain a complete and accurately timed sample of urine. The usual collection time is 24 hours, but patients may forget the time or forget to include some urine in the sample. Incontinent patients may find it impossible to make a urine collection. Patients have been known to add water or some other person's urine to their own collection, hoping to gain the doctor's approval for having been so prolific.

It may be more convenient and reliable to base the collection period on a patient's normal habits. Thus the time at which the bladder is emptied before retiring to bed is noted; any urine passed during the night is collected as is the urine voided when the patient rises. The time is noted and a blood sample is taken that morning for the measurement of plasma creatinine. As long as the time over which the urine collection is made is known, and the collection is complete, any suitable time period can be used.

Creatinine is actively secreted by the renal tubules and, as a result, the creatinine clearance is higher than the true GFR. The difference is of little significance when the GFR is normal but when the GFR is low (< 10 mL/min), tubular secretion makes a major contribution to creatinine excretion and the creatinine clearance significantly overestimates the GFR. The effect of creatinine breakdown in the gut also becomes significant when the GFR is very low. Lastly, in the calculation of creatinine clearance, two measurements of creatinine concentration and one of urine volume are required. Each of these has an inherent imprecision which can affect the accuracy of the overall result. Even in well-motivated subjects, studied under ideal conditions, the coefficient of variation of measurements of creatinine clearance can be as high as 10%, and it can be two or three times greater than this in ordinary patients.

Thus, although measurements of creatinine clearance are made frequently in clinical chemistry laboratories, they are potentially unreliable and should not be carried out unless there is a definite indication. In fact, accurate measurement of the GFR is required infrequently. Indications for its measurement include: assessment of potential kidney donors; investigation of patients with minor abnormalities of renal function, and calculation of the initial dose of a potentially toxic drug that is eliminated from the body by renal excretion. The majority of patients with established renal disease do not require repeated measurements of creatinine clearance. In most cases, their renal function can be more reliably monitored by serial measurements of the plasma creatinine concentration (*see below*).

In hospitals with facilities for handling radioactive isotopes and measuring radioactivity, the technique of choice for measuring GFR is based on the injection of $^{51}$Cr-labelled EDTA (ethylenediaminetetra-acetic acid) or $^{99m}$Tc-labelled DTPA (diethylenetriaminepenta-acetic acid). These substances are completely filtered by the glomeruli and are neither secreted nor reabsorbed by the tubules. Serial blood samples are taken after injection of the isotope and the GFR can be calculated from the rate of fall of plasma radioactivity as the isotope is cleared.

### Plasma Creatinine

The plasma creatinine concentration is the most reliable simple biochemical test of glomerular function. Ingestion of stewed meat can increase the plasma creatinine concentration by as much as 30% seven hours after a meal and ideally blood samples should be collected after an overnight fast. Strenuous exercise also causes a transient, slight increase in plasma creatinine concentration. Plasma creatinine concentration is related to muscle bulk and therefore a concentration of 120 μmol/L could be normal for an athletic young man but would suggest renal functional impairment, though not necessarily of clinical significance, in a thin, 70-year-old woman. Although muscle bulk tends to decline with age, so too does the GFR and hence plasma creatinine concentrations remain fairly constant.

The reference range for plasma creatinine in the adult population is 60–120 μmol/L, but the day-to-day variation in an individual is much less than this range. In the clearance formula (see *Equation 4.1*), the GFR is inversely related to the plasma creatinine concentration. Consequently, a normal plasma creatinine does not necessarily imply normal renal function, although a raised creatinine does usually indicate impaired renal function (*Fig. 4.3*). Furthermore, a change in creatinine concentration, provided that it is outside the limits of normal biological and analytical variation,

does suggest a change in GFR, even if both values are within the population reference range (see *Case History 1.1*).

Changes in plasma creatinine concentration can occur, independently of renal function, due to changes in muscle mass. Thus a decrease can occur as a result of starvation and in wasting diseases, immediately after surgery and in patients treated with corticosteroids; an increase can occur during re-feeding. However, changes in creatinine concentration for these reasons rarely lead to diagnostic confusion.

In pregnancy the GFR increases. This usually more than balances the effect of increased creatinine synthesis during pregnancy and results in a decrease in plasma creatinine concentration.

### Plasma urea

Urea is synthesized in the liver, primarily as a by-product of the deamination of amino acids. Its elimination in the urine represents the major route for nitrogen excretion. It is filtered from the blood at the glomerulus but passive tubular reabsorption occurs to a significant extent, especially at low rates of urine flow.

Although plasma urea concentration is often used as an index of renal glomerular function, measurement of plasma creatinine provides a more accurate assessment. Urea production is increased by a high protein intake, in catabolic states, and by the absorption of amino acids and peptides after gastrointestinal haemorrhage. Conversely, production is decreased in patients with a low protein

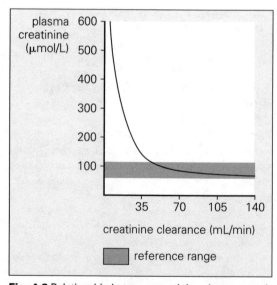

**Fig. 4.3** Relationship between creatinine clearance and plasma creatinine concentration.

| Causes of abnormal plasma urea to creatinine ratio | |
|---|---|
| **Increased** | **Decreased** |
| high protein intake<br>gastrointestinal bleeding<br>hypercatabolic state<br>dehydration<br>urinary stasis<br>muscle wasting*<br>amputation* | low protein intake<br>dialysis<br>severe liver diseae |

**Fig. 4.4** Causes of an abnormal plasma urea to creatinine ratio. * Causes of decreased creatinine synthesis; other conditions primarily affect urea concentration.

intake and sometimes in patients with liver disease. Plasma urea concentration rises during dehydration as a consequence of increased passive tubular reabsorption even when renal function is normal.

Factors affecting the ratio of plasma urea to creatinine are summarized in *Fig. 4.4*. Changes in plasma urea are a feature of renal impairment but it is important to consider possible extra-renal influences on urea concentrations before ascribing any changes to an alteration in renal function.

Urea diffuses readily across dialysis membranes and during renal dialysis a fall in plasma urea concentration is a poor guide to the efficacy of the process in removing other toxic substances from the blood.

### Plasma β₂-microglobulin

$\beta_2$-microglobulin is a small peptide (molecular weight 11,800 daltons), which forms part of the class I antigens of the major histocompatibility complex. It is present on the surface of most cells and in low concentrations in the plasma. It is completely filtered by the glomeruli and is reabsorbed and catabolized by proximal tubular cells.

The plasma concentration of $\beta_2$-microglobulin is a good index of GFR in normal people, being unaffected by diet or muscle mass. However, it is increased in certain malignancies and inflammatory diseases. Since it is normally reabsorbed and catabolized in the tubules, measurement of $\beta_2$-microglobulin excretion by radioimmunoassay is a sensitive, though expensive, method of assessing tubular integrity.

### Assessment of glomerular integrity

Impairment of glomerular integrity results in the filtration of large molecules which are normally retained and is manifest as proteinuria. Proteinuria can, however, occur for other reasons (*see page 65*).

With severe glomerular damage, red blood cells are detectable in the urine (haematuria). Whilst haematuria can occur as a result of lesions anywhere in the urinary tract, the red cells often have an abnormal morphology in glomerular disease. The presence of red cell casts (cells embedded in a proteinaceous matrix) in urinary sediment is strongly suggestive of glomerular dysfunction.

### Tests of renal tubular function

Formal tests of renal tubular function are performed less frequently than tests of glomerular function. The presence of glycosuria in a subject with a normal blood glucose concentration implies proximal tubular malfunction which may be either isolated (renal glycosuria) or part of a generalized tubular defect (Fanconi syndrome). Amino aciduria can occur with tubular defects and can be investigated by amino acid chromatography. Tests of proximal tubular bicarbonate reabsorption may be required in the assessment of proximal renal tubular acidosis.

The only tests of distal tubular function in widespread use are the water deprivation test, to assess renal concentrating ability (*see page 117*) and tests of urinary acidification, to diagnose distal renal tubular acidosis (*see page 69*).

### RENAL DISORDERS

Failure of renal function may occur rapidly, producing the syndrome of acute renal failure. This is potentially reversible since, if the patient survives the acute illness, normal renal function can be regained. However, chronic renal failure develops insidiously, often over many years, and is irreversible, leading eventually to end-stage renal failure. Patients with end-stage renal failure require either long-term renal replacement treatment (i.e., dialysis) or a successful renal transplant in order to survive.

The term 'glomerulonephritis' encompasses a group of renal diseases which are characterized by pathological changes in the glomeruli with an immunological basis, such as immune complex deposition. Glomerulonephritis may present in many ways: for example, as an acute nephritic syndrome with haematuria, hypertension and oedema: as acute or chronic renal failure, or as proteinuria leading to the nephrotic syndrome (proteinuria, hypoproteinaemia and oedema).

Many disorders primarily affect renal tubular function, but most are rare. Their metabolic and clinical consequences range from the trivial, such as isolated renal glycosuria, to the severe, for example, cystinuria.

## Acute renal failure

Acute renal failure is characterized by a rapid loss of renal function, with retention of urea, creatinine, hydrogen ions and other metabolic products and, usually but not always, oliguria (< 400 mL urine/24 h). Although potentially reversible, the consequences to homoeostatic mechanisms are so profound that this condition continues to be associated with a high mortality. Furthermore, acute renal failure often develops in patients who are already severely ill.

Acute renal failure is conventionally divided into three categories, according to whether renal functional impairment is related to a decrease in renal blood flow (prerenal), to intrinsic damage to the kidneys (intrarenal) or to urinary tract obstruction (postrenal). Should any of these occur in a patient whose renal function is already impaired, the consequences are likely to be more serious. Some clues to the presence of chronic disease in a patient with acute renal failure ('acute on chronic' renal failure) are discussed in *Case History 4.3*.

The term 'uraemia' (meaning 'urine in the blood') is often used as a synonym for renal failure (both acute and chronic). 'Azotaemia' is used in similar context and refers to an increase in the blood concentration of nitrogenous compounds.

### Prerenal acute renal failure

This is caused by circulatory insufficiency, as may occur with severe haemorrhage, burns, fluid loss, cardiac failure or hypotension and leads to renal hypoperfusion and a decrease in GFR. Renal hypoperfusion induces intense renal vasoconstriction; there is a redistribution of renal blood flow which results in a decrease in the GFR with preservation of tubular function. If left untreated, prerenal uraemia may progress to intrinsic failure (acute tubular necrosis). This may be prevented, however, if renal perfusion can be restored before structural damage has occurred.

### CASE HISTORY 4.1

A young man sustained multiple injuries in a motorcycle accident. He received blood transfusions and underwent surgery; 24 hours after admission he had only passed 500 mL of urine. He was clinically dehydrated and his blood pressure was 90/50 mmHg.

**Investigations**

| serum: | potassium | 5.6 mmol/L |
| | urea | 21.0 mmol/L |
| | creatinine | 140 µmol/L |
| urine: | sodium | 5 mmol/L |
| | urea | 480 mmol/L |

**Comment**
The diagnosis is prerenal uraemia. The urine contains little sodium and the urea has been concentrated by a factor of 22. These are normal physiological responses, implying that intrinsic renal function is intact and that the ability of the kidneys to function normally is constrained only by hypoperfusion. Osmolality was not measured, but in prerenal uraemia the urine to plasma osmolality ratio is characteristically greater than 1.5:1.

The distinguishing features of prerenal as opposed to intrinsic renal failure are listed in *Fig. 4.5*. These figures are not absolutely reliable. They are all invalidated if the patient has been given diuretics, and osmolalities are invalidated by the use of X-ray contrast media. In practice it may not be possible to distinguish between prerenal and intrinsic renal failure using biochemical tests; furthermore, if untreated, prerenal failure progresses to intrinsic renal failure. A concentrated, sodium-poor urine is a more reliable indicator of prerenal uraemia than a dilute sodium-containing urine is of intrinsic renal failure, since the latter is appropriate for a well hydrated healthy person. However, oliguria, although usually present, is not a constant feature of renal failure.

The increase in serum urea concentration in this patient is greater than the increase in creatinine. This is due in part both to passive reabsorption of urea and to increased synthesis from amino acids released as a result of tissue damage. The patient was given extra fluid intravenously and this resulted in a diuresis. The elicitation of this response is the only certain way of distinguishing prerenal from intrinsic renal failure. His serum urea and creatinine were normal 48 hours later.

| | Prerenal failure | Intrinsic failure |
|---|---|---|
| **Urine sodium concentration** | <20 mmol/L | >40 mmol/L |
| **Urine plasma urea concentration** | >10:1 | <3:1 |
| **Urine: plasma osmolality** | >1.5:1 | <1.1:1 |

**Fig. 4.5** Biochemical values in oliguria due to prerenal and intrinsic renal failure. Intermediate values occur in incipient intrinsic renal failure.

Prerenal uraemia is essentially the result of a normal physiological response to hypovolaemia or a fall in blood pressure. Stimulation of the renin–angiotensin–aldosterone system and vasopressin secretion results in the production of a small volume of highly concentrated urine with a low sodium concentration. Renal tubular function is normal, but the decreased GFR results in the retention of substances normally excreted by filtration, such as urea and creatinine. The decreased delivery of sodium to the distal tubule impairs hydrogen ion and potassium excretion; acidosis and hyperkalaemia are characteristic features of acute renal failure.

### Intrinsic acute renal failure

A wide variety of conditions can cause intrinsic acute renal failure (*Fig. 4.6*). Most cases are due to either nephrotoxins, including several drugs such as aminoglycosides and some cephalosporins, or renal ischaemia, both of which lead to renal tubular necrosis. Less common causes of acute renal failure include specific renal diseases and systemic conditions in which renal involvement is a prominent feature. The pathogenesis of this condition is incompletely understood and in any individual case several factors may be important.

Although glomerular damage is uncommon in acute tubular necrosis, the GFR falls due to glomerular hypoperfusion, itself a result of afferent arteriolar vasoconstriction. Failure of the GFR to recover after correction of the circulatory deficit is common. The reasons are not clear but contributing factors may include intrarenal release of vasoactive substances and tubular luminal obstruction by tubular debris or due to interstitial oedema.

There are typically three phases to the course of acute tubular necrosis: (i) initial oliguric phase; (ii) diuretic phase, in which urine output increases as the GFR increases but functional abnormalities persist, and (iii) recovery phase during which normal function returns.

In acute renal failure there is often a history of severe trauma, bleeding in relation to surgery, sepsis or the use of potentially nephrotoxic drugs. Although in prerenal uraemia the urine is concentrated, after the development of tubular damage the ability of the tubules to concentrate urine is lost and the ionic composition of the urine tends to resemble that of plasma. Proteinuria is always present and the urine is often dark due to the presence of haem pigments from the blood.

The characteristic biochemical changes in the plasma in acute renal failure are summarized in *Fig. 4.7*. Hyponatraemia is common; contributory factors include increased water formation from oxidative metabolism, continued intake of water

| Intrinsic acute renal failure | |
|---|---|
| **Causes** | **Examples** |
| specific renal diseases and systemic disease affecting kidneys | rapidly progressive glomerulonephritis systemic lupus erythematosus |
| nephrotoxins | aminoglycosides cephalosporins cis-platinum many other drugs and toxins |
| renal hypoperfusion | hypotension haemorrhage septicaemia low cardiac output burns crush injuries |
| intrarenal obstruction | Bence Jones protein |

**Fig. 4.6** Causes of acute renal failure.

| Biochemical changes in plasma in acute renal failure | |
|---|---|
| **Increased** | **Decreased** |
| potassium | sodium |
| urea | bicarbonate |
| creatinine | calcium |
| phosphate | |
| magnesium | |
| hydrogen ion | |
| urate | |

**Fig. 4.7** Biochemical changes in plasma in acute renal failure.

or injudicious fluid administration, decreased excretion and, possibly, loss of intracellular solute. Hyperkalaemia occurs as a result of decreased excretion of potassium together with both a loss of intracellular potassium to the ECF (due to tissue breakdown) and intracellular buffering of retained hydrogen ions. Decreased hydrogen ion excretion causes a non-respiratory acidosis.

Retention of phosphate and leakage of intracellular phosphate into the interstitial fluid leads to hyperphosphataemia which inhibits the $1\alpha$-hydroxylation of 25-hydroxycholecalciferol to calcitriol (*see page 187*). The resulting decreased plasma concentration of calcitriol causes skeletal resistance to the actions of parathyroid hormone, and there is a tendency to hypocalcaemia. Hypermagnesaemia is also often present as a result of decreased magnesium excretion.

If patients survive the acute illness, the urine output usually begins to increase after a period of time, which may be only a few days but can be several weeks (mean 10–11 days), and indicates the onset of the diuretic phase. This is due to an increase in GFR and initially there is often little improvement in tubular function. The composition of the urine is similar to that of protein-free plasma. During this phase, urine volume may exceed five litres per day and, because of its high ionic concentration, there is a considerable risk of dehydration and depletion of sodium and potassium.

Although the onset of the diuretic phase often heralds clinical improvement, plasma concentrations of urea and creatinine do not fall immediately since the GFR is still low and, therefore, insufficient to allow excretion of the surplus. The persisting high urea concentration in the blood, and hence in the glomerular filtrate, contributes to the diuresis by an osmotic effect. The acidosis also persists until tubular

function is restored. Plasma calcium concentration may rise during this phase, particularly after crush injuries, due to the release of calcium from damaged muscle. Temporary persistence of any elevation in the plasma concentration of parathyroid hormone will stimulate calcitriol synthesis and this may also cause hypercalcaemia.

Gradually, in the recovery phase, as the tubular cells regenerate and tubular function is restored, the diuresis subsides and the various abnormalities of renal function resolve. Patients who survive the acute illness usually recover completely. Some residual impairment of renal function is often demonstrable but it is not usually of clinical significance and may not be apparent from simple tests.

In very severe cases of acute renal failure, renal cortical necrosis may occur and there is no recovery of renal function.

---

**CASE HISTORY 4.2**

A young man was admitted to hospital with severe abdominal injuries after being knocked down by a car. On examination, he was severely shocked with a swollen, tender abdomen. He was given intravenous fluids and blood, and was taken to the operating theatre. At laparotomy, his spleen was found to be ruptured; splenectomy was performed. There was also mesenteric damage and a tear in the duodenum; the damaged gut was resected.

Three days later he became hypotensive and pyrexial and was taken back to theatre. Free fluid was present in the peritoneal cavity and a leak was found in a segment of gangrenous small intestine. Appropriate surgical procedures were performed. Following this, the patient became oliguric despite adequate hydration.

**Investigations**

| | | |
|---|---|---|
| serum: | sodium | 128 mmol/L |
| | potassium | 5.9 mmol/L |
| | bicarbonate | 16 mmol/L |
| | urea | 22.0 mmol/L |
| | creatinine | 225 µmol/L |
| | calcium | 1.72 mmol/L |
| | phosphate | 2.96 mmol/L |
| | albumin | 28 g/L |
| urine: | urea | 50 mmol/L |
| | sodium | 80 mmol/L |

### Comment

These findings are typical of acute renal failure in a septic, catabolic patient (see *Fig. 4.7*). He was treated with regular haemodialysis and parenteral nutrition; antibiotics were continued and his pyrexia settled. Eight days after the accident, the patient's urine output began to increase as shown in *Fig. 4.8*. The biochemical changes that occurred before and after the diuretic phase, until recovery of normal renal function, are also shown in *Fig. 4.8*.

### Postrenal renal failure

Obstruction to the flow of urine leads to an increase in hydrostatic pressure which acts in opposition to glomerular filtration and, if prolonged, leads to secondary renal tubular damage. Causes of obstruction include renal calculi, prostatic enlargement (hypertrophic or neoplastic), other neoplasms of the urinary tract and retroperitoneal fibrosis. Obstruction which occurs above the level of the vesicourethral junction must be bilateral to have a major effect on urine flow. Complete anuria is rare with acute renal failure from other causes and so is strongly indicative of the presence of obstruction. More often, however, obstruction is either intermittent or incomplete and urine production may even be normal in obstruction with overflow. The degree of reversibility of renal damage in obstructive renal failure depends to some extent on how longstanding it has been. It is more likely to be reversible if the obstruction is acute.

### *Management of acute renal failure*

Obstruction should always be excluded in a patient with renal failure, for example, by ultrasound examination. If present, obstruction should either be relieved or, if this is not immediately possible, urinary drainage should be established by an appropriate procedure.

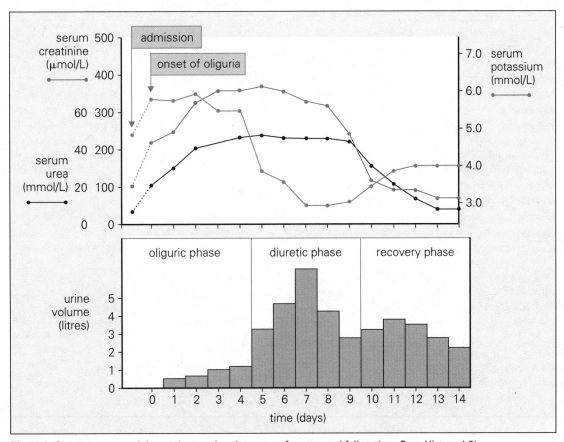

**Fig. 4.8** Serum urea, creatinine and potassium in a case of acute renal failure (see Case History 4.2)

Many cases of intrinsic renal failure are preventable and, if a patient is judged to be in the prerenal phase, it is important to attempt to halt the progression to acute tubular necrosis by measures to expand the ECF volume and improve renal perfusion. Volume repletion should be monitored by measurements of central venous pressure. Additional measures that can be employed include: the judicious use of mannitol, an osmotic diuretic; frusemide, a loop diuretic (both of these are also renal vasodilators), and dopamine, at a dose appropriate to promote renal vasodilatation.

If oliguria persists and acute tubular necrosis is diagnosed, it becomes necessary to minimize the severe adverse consequences of renal failure. The general principles of treatment include: strict control of sodium and water intake, to prevent overload; nutritional support, with some limitation of protein but adequate carbohydrate to minimize endogenous protein breakdown; prevention of metabolic complications, such as hyperkalaemia and acidosis, and prevention of infection. Care should be taken to avoid the use of potentially nephrotoxic drugs.

When renal failure is short-lived, conservative measures alone may suffice. However, the majority of patients will require renal replacement treatment, e.g., haemodialysis or haemofiltration. Specific indications for such treatment include: a dangerously high plasma potassium concentration, fluid overload, severe acidosis, a rapidly rising plasma urea or creatinine concentration, or a general deterioration in the patient's condition.

Dialysis or haemofiltration may have to be continued into the early part of the diuretic phase until the GFR has recovered sufficiently for the plasma concentration of creatinine to start falling. The main problem during the diuretic phase is to supply sufficient water and electrolytes to compensate for the excessive losses. Fluid replacement should not automatically be isovolaemic since the diuresis is partly due to

mobilization and excretion of excess ECF. From the onset of acute renal failure until its resolution, it is essential to monitor the patient's plasma creatinine, sodium, potassium, bicarbonate, calcium and phosphate concentrations, urinary volume and sodium and potassium excretion.

The general principles of management are similar whatever the cause of acute renal failure. In addition, specific measures may be indicated for certain diseases, for example, the control of infection or hypertension and the use of immunosuppressive drugs in immunologically mediated renal disease.

## Chronic renal failure

Many disease processes can lead to progressive, irreversible impairment of renal function. Effectively, all lead to a decrease in the number of functioning nephrons. Patients may remain asymptomatic until the GFR falls below 15 mL/min or lower. The natural history is of progression to end-stage renal failure, the state when conservative measures are no longer sufficient and dialysis or transplantation becomes necessary to save the patient's life. The time between presentation and end-stage renal failure is very variable; it may be a matter of weeks or as long as several years. The major pathological and clinical features are similar in all patients with chronic renal failure, whatever the cause.

### Consequences

The important metabolic features of end-stage renal failure are summarized in *Fig. 4.9*. Although there is impairment of urinary concentration, polyuria is never gross (not more than four litres per day) because the GFR is so low. The urine tends to be of a fixed specific gravity. The lack of urinary concentration is particularly noticed by the patient at night and nocturia is a common complaint. The ability to dilute the urine may be lost late in the course of renal failure and patients become very sensitive to the effects of either fluid loss or overload.

| End-stage renal disease | | |
|---|---|---|
| **Metabolic features** | **Biochemical changes in plasma** | |
| impairment of urinary concentration and dilution<br>impairment of electrolyte and hydrogen ion<br>  homoeostasis<br>retention of waste products of metabolism<br>impaired vitamin D metabolism<br>decreased erythropoietin synthesis | **Increased**<br>potassium<br>urea<br>creatinine<br>hydrogen ion<br>phosphate<br>magnesium | **Decreased**<br>sodium<br>bicarbonate<br>calcium |

**Fig 4.9** Metabolic and biochemical consequences of end-stage renal disease.

Sodium balance is usually maintained until the GFR falls below 20 mL/min. The majority of patients tend to retain sodium but severe renal sodium wasting is occasionally seen. This syndrome of 'salt-losing nephritis' occurs most often in patients whose renal disease particularly affects the tubules; for example, analgesic nephropathy, polycystic disease and chronic pyelonephritis.

Hyperkalaemia is a late feature of chronic renal failure; it may be precipitated by a sudden deterioration in renal function or by the injudicious use of potassium-sparing diuretics.

Patients with chronic renal failure tend to be acidotic. The urinary buffering capacity is impaired as a result of decreased phosphate excretion and ammonia synthesis. The ability of individual nephrons to reabsorb filtered bicarbonate is often impaired, probably, in part, as an effect of the raised blood level of parathyroid hormone. However, although plasma hydrogen ion concentration is increased and bicarbonate is decreased, these changes progress only slowly, due to buffering of excess hydrogen ions in bone.

Most patients with chronic renal failure become hypocalcaemic and, in time, many develop renal osteodystrophy.

The pathogenesis of this bone disease is complex (*Fig. 4.10*). Retention of phosphate causes a tendency to hyperphosphataemia, inhibiting calcitriol synthesis and leading to hypocalcaemia. This causes increased parathyroid hormone secretion (secondary hyperparathyroidism), which decreases the reabsorption of phosphate from each nephron, but eventually the falling GFR becomes the limiting factor in phosphate excretion and persistent hyperphosphataemia ensues. If the concentration of phosphate becomes so high that the solubility product of calcium and phosphate ($[Ca^{2+}] \times [Pi]$) is exceeded, metastatic calcification may occur. This is seen particularly in blood vessels and also in bone, where it causes sclerotic deposits. With advanced renal failure, the decrease in functioning renal tissue may also contribute to the decrease in calcitriol production. Another factor of importance is buffering of hydrogen ions by bone, which leads to demineralization.

Aluminium can cause osteomalacia. In the past the presence of aluminium in softened water used to prepare dialysis fluid has caused problems, as has the absorption of aluminium from orally administered salts given to bind phosphate in the gut and prevent hyperphosphataemia.

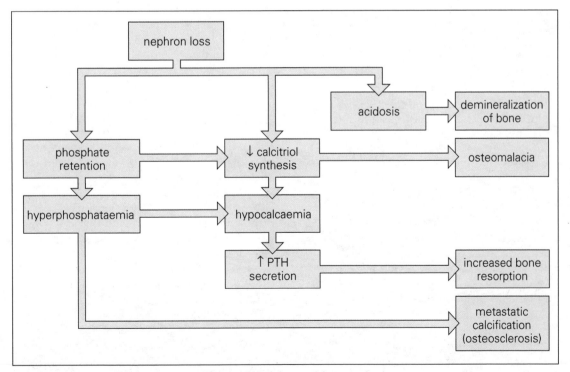

**Fig. 4.10** Pathogenesis of renal osteodystrophy. Aluminium toxicity may also be an important factor in patients on dialysis or those treated with oral aluminium salts.

In addition to the effect on calcitriol synthesis, other endocrine consequences of chronic renal failure include: decreased testosterone and oestrogen synthesis; abnormalities of thyroid function tests (seldom, however, associated with clinical thyroid disease), and abnormal glucose tolerance with hyperinsulinaemia due to insulin resistance. However, insulin-dependent diabetic patients who develop renal disease, often have decreased insulin requirements since insulin is metabolized in the kidney.

A normochromic normocytic anaemia is usual in end-stage renal failure, due to depression of bone marrow function by retained toxins and a decrease in the renal production of erythropoietin. A bleeding tendency may also be present and bleeding may exacerbate the anaemia.

The kidneys are small in most cases of chronic renal failure (unless due to amyloid or polycystic disease) and the demonstration of small kidneys by radiography or ultrasonography in a patient with renal disease is another indicator of chronicity. So, too, is the presence of hypertension.

Many other clinical features may be present in patients with end-stage renal disease (*Fig. 4.11*). The causes of many of these features are unknown, but they are presumably related to the retention of toxins which cannot be excreted. These 'uraemic toxins' include phenolic acids, polypeptides, polyamines and many other substances.

---

## CASE HISTORY 4.3

A 56-year-old man presented to his family doctor with weight loss, generalized weakness and lethargy of six months' duration. During this time, he had been passing more urine than usual, particularly at night. He had become impotent. On examination, the patient was found to be slightly anaemic and had a blood pressure of 180/110 mmHg. His urine contained protein but no glucose. A blood sample was taken for analysis.

### Investigations

| serum: | | |
|---|---|---|
| | sodium | 130 mmol/L |
| | potassium | 5.2 mmol/L |
| | bicarbonate | 16 mmol/L |
| | urea | 43.0 mmol/L |
| | creatinine | 640 µmol/L |
| | glucose (random) | 6.4 mmol/L |
| | calcium | 1.92 mmol/L |
| | phosphate | 2.42 mmol/L |
| | alkaline phosphatase | 205 IU/L |
| | haemoglobin | 9.1 g/dL |

### Comment

The doctor's first thought was that this patient had diabetes mellitus, but the absence of glycosuria militated against this and the results are typical of chronic renal failure. The history suggests slowly progressive, rather than acute, renal failure. The presence of anaemia and the raised alkaline phosphatase (due to renal osteodystrophy) are consistent with this diagnosis, although they are not specific findings.

## Management of chronic renal failure

Identification and subsequent treatment of the cause of chronic renal failure may prevent, or at least delay, further deterioration. In most cases, however, the cause is either unknown or untreatable and patients eventually require either maintenance dialysis or renal transplantation. Before dialysis or transplantation becomes necessary, considerable amelioration of symptoms and biochemical abnormalities can be obtained by conservative measures.

Since the kidneys become unable to control the water and sodium balance, it is essential that intake is matched to obligatory losses. Diuretics are often used to promote sodium excretion since adequate dietary salt restriction may be unacceptable to the patient. Bicarbonate can be given orally to control acidosis. Hyperkalaemia is usually of less significance in chronic than in acute renal failure, because it develops more slowly. It can usually be controlled with oral ion-exchange resins given in their sodium or calcium forms.

Hyperphosphataemia can be controlled by giving aluminium or magnesium salts by mouth. Osteodystrophy can be prevented, or treated if it does develop, by giving calcitriol or other 1α-hydroxylated derivatives of vitamin D, but care is necessary to avoid provoking hypercalcaemia.

Some limitation of dietary protein is beneficial to reduce the formation of nitrogenous waste products, but the limtation should not usually be so severe as to cause negative nitrogen balance. In patients who are not candidates for maintenance dialysis or transplantation, however, a very low protein intake can cause considerable symptomatic improvement in the terminal stage of renal failure, and may even slow the rate of decline in renal function. It is important to maintain an adequate intake of carbohydrate and fat.

Conservative measures must be continued in patients on maintenance dialysis. Patients having a successful renal transplant are freed of such constraints, although they require immunosuppressive therapy to prevent graft rejection.

Patients who have undergone transplantation require careful clinical and biochemical monitoring to assess graft function and to provide early warning of incipient graft rejection. Features of graft rejection include oliguria and pyrexia but these may not be present and a rise in plasma creatinine concentration may be the first sign. However, an increase in creatinine can also occur with nephrotoxicity due to cyclosporin, a frequently used immunosuppressive drug. Indicators of tubular damage, for example the urinary activity of the tubular enzyme N-acetyl-glucosaminidase, have been studied as possible indicators of early rejection, but none is specific to the process and they are not widely used.

## Proteinuria and the nephrotic syndrome

The glomeruli normally filter 7–10 g of protein per 24 hours, but almost all is reabsorbed by endocytosis and subsequently catabolized in the proximal tubules. Normal urinary protein excretion is less than 150 mg/24h. Approximately half of this is Tamm–Horsfall protein, a glycoprotein secreted by tubular cells; less than 35 mg is albumin.

The presence or absence of proteinuria is usually assessed using a reagent-impregnated strip (dip-stick) which is dipped into the urine. This reliably detects albumin at concentrations greater than 200 mg/L but is less sensitive to other proteins. False positive results are obtained with urine that is alkaline, contaminated by various antiseptics or contains X-ray contrast media. It should be appreciated that a particular concentration of protein will be more significant if a large volume of urine is being produced, since it will represent a greater total excretion than if urine volume is low.

The mechanisms of proteinuria are summarized in *Fig. 4.12*. Glomerular proteinuria may be sufficiently gross to cause hypoproteinaemia and oedema (the nephrotic syndrome).

| Clinical features of chronic renal failure |
|---|
| **Neurological** |
| lethargy |
| peripheral neuropathy |
| |
| **Musculoskeletal** |
| growth failure |
| bone pain |
| myopathy |
| |
| **Gastrointestinal** |
| anorexia |
| hiccough |
| nausea and vomiting |
| g.i. bleeding |
| |
| **Cardiovascular** |
| anaemia |
| hypertension |
| pericarditis |
| |
| **Dermal** |
| pruritis |
| pallor |
| purpura |
| |
| **Genitourinary** |
| nocturia |
| impotence |

**Fig. 4.11** Clinical features of chronic renal failure.

| Mechanisms of proteinuria |
|---|
| **Overflow** |
| due to presence in plasma |
| of a high concentration of a |
| low molecular weight protein, |
| which is filtered in a quantity |
| exceeding tubular reabsorptive |
| capacity, e.g., Bence Jones protein |
| |
| **Glomerular** |
| due to increased glomerular |
| permeability, e.g., albumin |
| |
| **Tubular** |
| due to impaired or saturated |
| reabsorption of protein filtered by |
| normal glomeruli, e.g., $\beta_2$-microglobulin |
| |
| **Secreted** |
| due to secretion by kidneys or |
| epithelium of urinary tract, |
| e.g., Tamm-Horsfall protein |

**Fig. 4.12** Mechanisms of proteinuria.

### Investigation of proteinuria

If a patient's urine gives a positive reaction for protein using a dip-stick, the presence of protein should be confirmed by an independent test in the laboratory. If Bence Jones proteinuria is suspected, a specific test must be used since this protein is not detectable by dip-stick. Before investigating renal function, incidental extrarenal causes of proteinuria such as fever, strenuous exercise and burns, should be excluded; such proteinuria is usually not of long-term significance.

When the presence of proteinuria has been confirmed, urinary protein excretion should be measured and simple tests of renal function performed. If these test results are normal and protein excretion is less than 500 mg/24h, the patient need not be subjected to further investigation but should be followed-up. With protein excretion in excess of this, or with abnormal test results, further investigation such as ultrasound examination, contrast radiography or biopsy, is necessary to determine the cause.

Orthostatic proteinuria is a benign condition in which proteinuria is present only when subjects are upright. It occurs in approximately 5% of young adults and can be induced in many more if they adopt a lordotic posture. The prevalence decreases with increasing age. Orthostatic proteinuria arises as a result of an increase in the hydrostatic pressure in the renal veins, itself a result of pressure of the liver on the inferior vena cava. It is of no clinical significance and can confidently be diagnosed if a sample of urine collected immediately on rising in the morning is protein-free.

Electrophoresis of a concentrated specimen of urine may help to distinguish between the various types of proteinuria. In tubular proteinuria, for example, the predominant proteins are of low molecular weight, being filtered proteins which are not reabsorbed. In glomerular proteinuria, higher molecular weight proteins are present. Electrophoresis of concentrated urine is the best technique for the detection of Bence Jones proteinuria.

In minimal change glomerulonephritis, the most frequent cause of nephrotic syndrome in children, the proteinuria is typically highly selective – that is, higher molecular weight proteins tend to be retained – while in most other causes of the condition, both high and low molecular weight proteins are excreted (low selectivity). Minimal change glomerulonephritis usually responds to steroids.

Measurement of selectivity, by comparing the clearances of IgG and albumin or transferrin, used to be used to indicate whether nephrotic syndrome was caused by minimal change glomerulonephritis, and to avoid the need for biopsy to make the diagnosis. However, the relationship is not constant, and most renal physicians now routinely treat nephrotic syndrome in children with steroids in the first instance, and reserve biopsy for non-responders. Minimal change disease is less common as a cause of nephrotic syndrome in adults, and biopsy is usually considered essential.

### The nephrotic syndrome

Hypoproteinaemia with oedema may develop if large amounts of protein are excreted in the urine. For this to occur, proteinuria must usually exceed 5 g/24h. Although the ability of the liver to synthesize protein is greater than this, much of the filtered protein is catabolized after endocytosis by renal tubular cells and is thus lost from the circulation, although it is not excreted in the urine. Conditions in which the nephrotic syndrome may occur are shown in *Fig. 4.13*.

The amount of proteinuria is not necessarily a useful guide to the severity of renal disease; for example, in minimal change glomerulonephritis, which has a good prognosis, the proteinuria may exceed that seen in patients with more aggressive glomerular lesions.

---

**CASE HISTORY 4.4**

An eight-year-old girl was admitted to hospital with generalized oedema. Her urine had become frothy and the family doctor had found proteinuria.

**Investigations**

| serum: | | |
|---|---|---|
| sodium | 130 mmol/L | |
| potassium | 3.6 mmol/L | |
| bicarbonate | 32 mmol/L | |
| urea | 2.0 mmol/L | |
| creatinine | 45 µmol/L | |
| calcium | 1.70 mmol/L | |
| total protein | 35 g/L | |
| albumin | 15 g/L | |
| triglyceride | 16 mmol/L | |
| cholesterol | 12 mmol/L | |

24 h urine protein excretion       12 g
The serum was grossly lipaemic.

**Comment**

The presence of proteinuria, hypoproteinaemia and oedema constitutes the nephrotic syndrome. The oedema is, in part, a result of redistribution of ECF

| The nephrotic syndrome | | |
|---|---|---|
| **Causes** | **Clinical and biochemical features** | |
| | **Feature** | **Mechanism** |
| minimal change glomerulonephritis | proteinuria | glomerular damage |
| membranous glomerulonephritis: | | |
| idiopathic | oedema | low plasma albumin secondary hyperaldosteronism |
| associated with carcinoma, drugs or infection; e.g., malaria, hepatitis B | increased susceptibility to infection | low plasma immunoglobulins and complement |
| systemic lupus erythematosus | thrombotic tendency | hyperfibrinogenaemia and low antithrombin III |
| diabetic nephropathy | | |
| other forms of glomerulonephritis | hyperlipidaemia | increased apolipoprotein synthesis |

**Fig. 4.13** The nephrotic syndrome: causes and clinical and biochemical features.

between the vascular and interstitial compartments; secondary aldosteronism, with evidence of potassium depletion, is often present as a consequence.

Loss of protein is not confined to albumin. Plasma concentrations of hormone-binding proteins, transferrin and antithrombin III are also reduced. On the other hand, there is usually an increase in the concentrations of high molecular weight proteins such as $\alpha_2$-macroglobulin, coagulation factors (fibrinogen, factor VIII, etc.) and the apolipoproteins. The increase in apolipoproteins causes secondary hypercholesterolaemia and hypertriglyceridaemia and these may in turn cause spurious hyponatraemia. In adults with persistent nephrotic syndrome, accelerated atherosclerosis may develop. Changes in the concentrations of coagulation factors can predispose to venous thrombosis, particularly in the renal veins. The hypocalcaemia is related in part to decreased protein binding and in part to renal excretion of vitamin D metabolites bound to vitamin D-binding globulin. Loss of immunoglobulins and complement components renders patients with nephrotic syndrome very susceptible to infection.

The GFR may be low, normal or raised in patients with the nephrotic syndrome. In minimal change glomerulonephritis, it is often raised and the low urea and creatinine concentrations in this patient reflect this. The quantity of protein excreted must be judged in relation to the GFR. A decrease in excretion is usually due to a decrease in glomerular permeability but it may occur because of a decrease in GFR. This may be due to the underlying disease or to the fall in plasma volume.

The clinical and biochemical features of the nephrotic syndrome are summarized in *Fig. 4.13*. There are two aspects to management: treatment of the underlying disorder, where the disorder can be identified and treatment is possible, and treatment of the consequences of protein loss. Minimal change glomerulonephritis often responds to corticosteroids or immunosuppressive drugs, but other types of glomerulonephritis are generally much less responsive to treatment.

General measures to counteract the consequences of protein loss include a high protein, low salt diet, although decreased appetite and impaired absorption of nutrients due to oedema of the gut may be limiting factors. A high protein intake must be introduced with caution when there is concurrent renal failure. It is important not to cause too rapid a diuresis since this could lead to hypovolaemia and thus impair renal function; potassium depletion must also be avoided. Spironolactone is the diuretic of the first choice but thiazides or frusemide may be necessary in addition. Prevention of infection is vital and antibiotics are often administered prophylactically. The risk of thrombosis, especially renal vein thrombosis which may cause a rapid increase in proteinuria, may warrant the prophylactic use of anticoagulants.

## Renal tubular disorders

Renal tubular disorders can be congenital or acquired; they can involve single or multiple aspects of tubular function. The congenital conditions are all rare; their clinical sequelae relate to the consequences of loss of substances which are normally completely or partially reabsorbed by the tubules.

### The Fanconi syndrome

This is a generalized disorder of tubular function characterized by glycosuria, amino aciduria, phosphaturia and acidosis. It can occur secondarily to a variety of conditions (*Fig. 4.14*). One of these is cystinosis, or Lignac–Fanconi disease, a rare inherited disease (only 1 in 40,000 live births in the United Kingdom) in which there is a defect in the transport of cystine out of lysosomes. This leads to cystine accumulation and the deposition of cystine crystals in many body tissues, including the kidney. Affected infants fail to thrive, develop rickets and polyuria with dehydration and eventually progress to renal failure. There is no specific treatment. Cystinosis should not be confused with cystinuria, a disorder of tubular transport.

Primary Fanconi syndrome can also develop in young adults; it is inherited, but the nature of the defect is not known.

### Renal tubular acidosis (RTA)

Proximal (type 2) RTA, which arises as a result of impaired bicarbonate reabsorption, is a component of the Fanconi syndrome but can also occur as an isolated phenomenon. A transient form can occur in infants. Bicarbonate can be completely reabsorbed if the plasma bicarbonate concentration is low, and thus patients may excrete normal amounts of acid but at the expense of systemic acidosis. Treatment consists in administering large amounts of bicarbonate, for example, 10 mmol/kg body weight/24 h. Distal (type 1 or classical) RTA occurs more frequently. It can be either inherited or acquired, for example, secondarily to hypercalcaemia or autoimmune diseases. There is a defect in hydrogen ion excretion and the urine cannot be acidified. Consequences include osteomalacia, hypercalciuria, nephrocalcinosis, renal calculi and often hypokalaemia. In general, hyperkalaemia is more usual in acidotic states, but in these types of RTA the impaired ability of the kidneys to excrete hydrogen ions necessitates increased potassium excretion when sodium is reabsorbed in the distal tubules, and this may cause potassium depletion and hypokalaemia. Treatment involves the administration of bicarbonate in sufficient quantities to buffer normal hydrogen ion production (1–3 mg/kg body weight/24 h) and potassium supplements.

The most frequently encountered type of RTA is type 4. It is associated with hypoaldosteronism, either secondary to adrenal disease, or to renal disease in which there is decreased renin secretion (hyporeninaemic hypoaldosteronism, e.g., diabetic nephropathy) or resistance to aldosterone (e.g., obstructive nephropathy). In contrast to the other types of RTA, there is hyperkalaemia. The urine can be maximally acidified, but only at the expense of a systemic acidosis. The clinical features are primarily those of the underlying cause. Management is directed at the underlying cause and correction of the hyperkalaemia.

The diagnosis of RTA requires a high index of suspicion. Typically, there is hyperchloraemia and a normal anion gap. Other causes of this combination, e.g., loss of alkaline fluid from the gut and treatment with carbonic anhydrase inhibitors, must be eliminated. Measurement of urine pH and plasma potassium concentration will usually indicate

---

| Causes of Fanconi syndrome |
| --- |
| idiopathic inherited metabolic disease:<br>  cystinosis (Lignac–Fanconi disease)<br>  galactosaemia<br>  fructose intolerance<br>  glycogen storage diseases<br>  tyrosinaemia<br>  Wilson's disease<br>nephrotoxins:<br>  heavy metals<br>  drugs<br>paraproteinaemia<br>amyloid |

**Fig. 4.14** Causes of the Fanconi syndrome.

the correct diagnosis. Confirmation of the diagnosis of type 1 RTA may require a formal urinary acidification test (*see Fig. 4.15*). Diagnosis of type 2 RTA may occasionally require determination of the renal threshold for bicarbonate.

### Defects of urinary concentration

Impairment of urinary concentration is a feature of nephrogenic diabetes insipidus, a primary tubular disorder. It is also a feature of cranial diabetes insipidus and chronic renal failure and can occur with hypercalcaemia, hypokalaemia and certain drugs, notably lithium. In nephrogenic diabetes insipidus, vasopressin secretion is normal but there is a defect involving either its receptors or one of the post receptor-binding events required for its normal action. Hypercalcaemia and hypokalaemia also interfere with this cAMP-mediated pathway.

### Glycosuria

Benign renal glycosuria is discussed on *page 174*. Renal glycosuria can also occur in association with other tubular abnormalities, for example, as part of the Fanconi syndrome.

### Amino aciduria

Renal amino aciduria may occur in combination with normal plasma levels of amino acids as a result of defective tubular reabsorption, for example, Hartnup disease and cystinuria. Overflow amino aciduria occurs secondarily to elevated plasma levels when the tubular transport mechanism is saturated, as in, for instance, phenylketonuria.

Cystinuria has an incidence of about one in 7,000 live births. Defective tubular reabsorption of cystine, ornithine, arginine and lysine leads to their excretion in the urine. The loss of these amino acids would alone be of little consequence, but cystine is relatively insoluble and cystinuria predisposes the patient to renal calculus formation. The management of cystinuria is discussed on *page 250*.

### Hypophosphataemic rickets

This condition, also known as vitamin D-resistant rickets, has a dominant X-linked pattern of inheritance. A defect in tubular phosphate reabsorption leads to severe rickets. This does not respond to treatment with vitamin D alone, even if administered in massive doses, but can be treated effectively with a combination of oral phosphate supplements and vitamin D, usually given as a $1\alpha$-hydroxylated derivative.

Hypophosphataemic rickets should not be confused with vitamin D-dependent rickets which is inherited as an autosomal recessive condition. The defect is in the $1\alpha$-hydroxylation of 25-hydroxycholecalciferol. This condition can be treated with $1\alpha$-hydroxylated derivatives of vitamin D alone.

## Urinary calculi

### Pathogenesis

Stones or calculi can form in urine when it is supersaturated with the crystalloid components of the calculus. Factors predisposing to this, and the commoner types of calculus that occur clinically, are shown in *Fig. 4.16*.

| Urinary acidification test | |
|---|---|
| **Procedure** | **Results** |
| take blood for bicarbonate measurements after overnight fast | normal response: urine pH < 5.2 in at least one sample if this pH is not obtained, serum bicarbonate should be measured. Test should be repeated if serum bicarbonate is not below the lower limit of normal |
| measure pH of freshly passed urine: if serum bicarbonate < 16 mmol/L and urine pH < 5.5, test unnecessary | |
| administer ammonium chloride (100 mg/kg body weight) orally | type 1 RTA: urine pH ≥6.5 |
| measure pH of freshly passed urine hourly for 8 h | |

**Fig. 4.15** Urinary acidification test. This test should not be performed in patients with liver disease.

---

| Urinary calculi |
|---|
| **Factors predisposing to formation** |
| dehydration |
| urinary tract infection |
| persistently alkaline urine |
| hypercalciuria |
| hyperuricosuria |
| hyperoxaluria |
| urinary stagnation (due to obstruction) |
| lack of urinary inhibitors of crystallization |
| |
| **Composition** |
| calcium oxalate (± phosphate) |
| calcium phosphate |
| magnesium ammonium phosphate ('triple phosphate') |
| uric acid |
| cystine |
| |
| **Biochemical investigations** |
| analysis of calculus (if available) |
| plasma: |
|     calcium |
|     urate |
|     phosphate |
| urine: |
|     pH |
|     qualitative test for cystine |
|     24 h excretion of calcium, oxalate and urate |
|     urinary acidification test |

**Fig. 4.16** Renal calculi: composition, factors predisposing to their formation and biochemical investigations.

Hypercalciuria is present in up to 25% of patients with calcium oxalate/phosphate stones. It may be associated with hypercalcaemia, for example, due to primary hyperparathyroidism. However, many patients with calcium-containing stones are normocalcaemic and in the majority the primary abnormality is an increase in intestinal calcium absorption.

Hyperoxaluria predisposes to renal calculus formation. Primary hyperoxaluria is a rare inherited metabolic disorder. Two types have been described; increased hepatic oxalate synthesis is common to both. In type 1 there is increased urinary excretion of oxalic and glycolic acids; renal failure develops in the majority of cases. Type 2 is a more benign condition in which there is increased urinary excretion of oxalic and glyceric acids; renal failure does not occur. Hyperoxaluria is usually caused by increased intestinal

absorption of dietary oxalate, with or without increased oxalate ingestion. This may be seen in patients with a variety of gastrointestinal disorders, in particular, with inflammatory bowel diseases and conditions associated with malabsorption. In these circumstances, non-absorbed free fatty acids bind to calcium. This limits the amount of calcium available to combine with oxalate to form calcium oxalate, an insoluble substance which is normally excreted in the faeces. As a result, an increased amount of oxalate remains in solution and can be absorbed into the bloodstream.

### Investigation

The history and examination may suggest an underlying cause for urinary calculi, such as inadequate fluid intake. Biochemical tests that should be performed on plasma and urine are shown in *Fig. 4.16*. The single most useful test is to analyse a stone, if available. The urine must be examined for evidence of infection in all patients presenting with urinary calculi. The radiographic appearance of a retained stone may be characteristic: for example, 'staghorn' calculi contain mixed phosphates and are related to chronic infection; pure uric acid stones (not containing calcium) are radiolucent as are cystine stones. An intravenous urogram may show a predisposing anatomical abnormality. Most calculi can be detected by ultrasound.

### Management

Small calculi are often passed spontaneously. Larger calculi may require surgical removal or disintegration by ultrasound. Any urinary tract infection should be treated. The identification of the cause of urinary calculus formation should make it possible to design an effective regimen to prevent further stone formation. This is particularly important in patients who form stones recurrently.

The management of cystinuria is considered on *page 250*. Hyperuricaemia should be treated with allopurinol (*see page 266*). Alkalinization of the urine increases the solubility of both cystine and uric acid but may be difficult to achieve. A high fluid intake is appropriate in all patients with a tendency to form urinary calculi.

If patients who form calcium stones are hypercalcaemic, the underlying cause should be treated. In the normocalcaemic majority, dietary manipulation to correct excessive intake of calcium or oxalate is appropriate. However, calcium restriction below maintenance levels is inadvisable since oxalate absorption may be increased and there may be adverse effects on the skeleton. In patients who do not respond to such measures, thiazide diuretics (which decrease urinary calcium excretion) are often very effective at preventing recurrence.

## SUMMARY

The kidneys are essential for the control of extracellular fluid volume and composition, hydrogen ion homoeostasis, the excretion of waste products of metabolism and as endocrine organs, particularly in relation to calcium homoeostasis, erythropoiesis and the control of blood pressure. The best simple test of overall renal function is the plasma creatinine concentration, while the presence of proteinuria is a sensitive, although not specific, indicator of kidney damage.

Acute renal failure is a life-threatening condition in which there is a deterioration in renal function which is potentially reversible. It is most frequently caused by either renal hypoperfusion or exposure to nephrotoxins. When hypoperfusion is responsible, it may be possible to prevent the development of intrinsic renal damage by restoration of normal perfusion. The biochemical features of acute renal failure include increases in plasma urea and creatinine concentrations, hyperkalaemia, hyperphosphataemia, acidosis and fluid retention. Patients are usually oliguric and require dialysis or haemofiltration until renal function recovers. The onset of recovery is heralded by an increase in urine production and a diuretic phase follows before normal renal function returns. During the diuretic phase there may be considerable losses of fluid and ions from the body.

In chronic renal failure, renal function is irreversibly lost and patients will eventually require transplantation or long-term dialysis. This condition usually develops slowly and because the kidneys have considerable functional reserves, patients tend to present late in the course of the illness. Retention of urea, creatinine and other waste products, and disturbance of sodium and water homoeostasis are characteristic but severe acidosis and hyperkalaemia are only late features of the condition. Bone disease, with hypocalcaemia and hyperphosphataemia, and anaemia result from impairment of renal endocrine function.

The nephrotic syndrome comprises proteinuria, hypoproteinaemia and oedema and can be a result of a variety of diseases affecting the glomeruli. The clinical and biochemical features stem from the loss of protein from the body. In addition to albumin, the loss of which is responsible for the oedema, the loss of other proteins leads to increased susceptibility to infection and hypercoagulability. Uraemia may or may not be present, depending on the nature of the underlying glomerular damage.

The formation of urinary calculi is essentially the result of supersaturation of the urine. Factors predisposing to calculus formation include the excretion of high solute loads, for example, of calcium, oxalate or urate, inadequate water intake and infection.

Conditions affecting the renal tubules alone are in general uncommon. They can be either congenital or acquired and can affect either single or multiple tubular functions. There may be either excessive loss of substances which are normally reabsorbed by the tubules, for example, phosphate, glucose and amino acids, or inadequate excretion of substances normally secreted by the tubules, for example, hydrogen ions, thus producing renal tubular acidosis.

## FURTHER READING

de Wardener HE (1985) *The Kidney*. 5th edition. Edinburgh: Churchill Livingstone.

Farrington K & Sweny P (1993) Nephrology, dialysis and transplantation. *Postgraduate Medical Journal*, **69**, 516–546.

Mandal AK & Herbert LA (eds.) (1990) Renal Disease. *The Medical Clinics of North America*, **74**, 859–1083.

Massry SG & Glassock RJ (eds.) (1989) *Textbook of Nephrology*. 2nd edition. Baltimore: Williams & Wilkins.

Smith L (ed.) (1990) Renal Stones. *Endocrinology and Metabolism Clinics of North America*, **19**, 767–965.

# 5. The Liver

## INTRODUCTION

The liver is of vital importance in intermediary metabolism and in the detoxification and elimination of toxic substances (*Fig. 5.1*). Damage to the organ may not obviously affect its activity since the liver has considerable functional reserve and, as a consequence, simple tests of liver function (e.g., plasma bilirubin and albumin concentrations) are insensitive indicators of liver disease. Tests reflecting liver cell damage (particularly the measurement of the activities of hepatic enzymes in plasma) are often superior in this respect. The categorization of such tests as 'liver function tests' is clearly a misnomer, but seems likely to endure. True tests of liver function, designed to provide a quantitative assessment of functional hepatic cell activity, exist (*see p. 76*) but are as yet infrequently used in routine clinical practice.

The results of biochemical tests rarely provide a precise diagnosis on their own since they reflect the basic pathological processes common to many conditions. However, biochemical tests are cheap, non-invasive and widely available, and are of value in directing the use of other diagnostic tests, notably imaging and liver biopsy. They are also useful in detecting the presence of liver disease and in following its progress.

The metabolic activity of the liver takes place within the parenchymal cells, which constitute 80% of the organ mass; the liver also contains Kupffer cells of the reticuloendothelial system. Parenchymal cells are contiguous with the venous sinusoids, which carry blood from the portal vein and hepatic artery, and with the biliary canaliculi, the smallest ramifications of the biliary system (*Fig. 5.2*). Substances destined for excretion in the bile are secreted from hepatocytes into the canaliculi, pass through the intrahepatic ducts and reach the duodenum via the common bile duct.

The most common disease processes affecting the liver are:
- Hepatitis, with damage to liver cells.
- Cirrhosis, in which increased fibrous tissue formation leads to shrinkage of the liver, decreased hepatocellular function and obstruction of bile flow.
- Tumours, most frequently secondary; for example, metastases from cancers of the large bowel, stomach and bronchus.

Patients with liver disease often present with characteristic symptoms and signs, but the clinical features may be non-specific and in some patients, liver disease is discovered

incidentally. Because of the intimate relationship between the liver and biliary system, extrahepatic biliary disease may present with clinical features suggestive of liver disease or may have secondary effects on the liver; for instance, obstruction to the common bile duct may cause jaundice and, if prolonged, a form of cirrhosis.

## BILIRUBIN METABOLISM

Bilirubin is derived mainly from the haem moiety of the haemoglobin molecules and is liberated when effete red cells are removed from the circulation by the reticulo-

| Major functions of the liver |
|---|
| **Carbohydrate metabolism**<br>gluconeogenesis<br>glycogen synthesis and breakdown |
| **Fat metabolism**<br>fatty acid synthesis<br>cholesterol synthesis and excretion<br>lipoprotein synthesis<br>ketogenesis<br>bile acid synthesis<br>25-hydroxylation of vitamin D |
| **Protein metabolism**<br>synthesis of plasma proteins (including some coagulation factors but not immunoglobulins)<br>urea synthesis |
| **Hormone metabolism**<br>metabolism and excretion of steroid hormones<br>metabolism of polypeptide hormones |
| **Drugs and foreign compounds**<br>metabolism and excretion |
| **Storage**<br>glycogen<br>vitamin A<br>vitamin $B_{12}$<br>iron |
| **Metabolism and excretion of bilirubin** |

**Fig. 5.1** Major functions of the liver.

endothelial system (*Fig. 5.3*); the iron in haem is reutilized but the tetrapyrrole ring is degraded to bilirubin. Other sources of bilirubin include myoglobin and the cytochromes.

Unconjugated bilirubin is not water-soluble; it is transported in the blood stream bound to albumin. In the liver, it is taken up by hepatocytes in a process involving specific

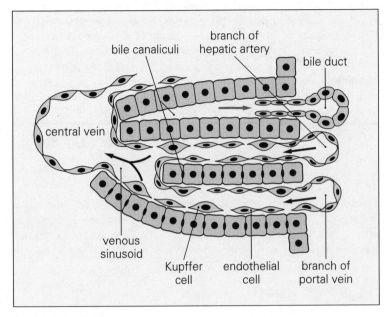

**Fig. 5.2** Microstructure of the liver. The liver consists of acini in which sheets of hepatocytes, one cell thick, are permeated by sinusoids carrying blood from the portal venules and hepatic arterioles to the central vein. Bile is secreted from the hepatocytes into canaliculi, which drain into the bile ducts.

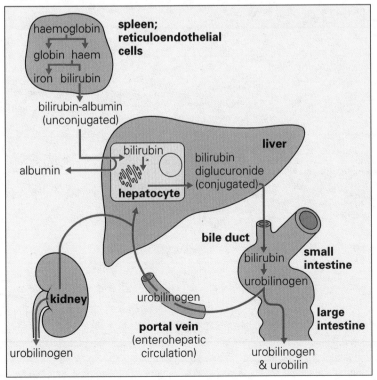

**Fig. 5.3** Excretion of bilirubin by the liver. Bilirubin, bound to albumin, is taken up into hepatocytes, conjugated in the smooth endoplasmic reticulum and excreted via the bile ducts into the gut, where it is converted to urobilinogen. Most of the urobilinogen is oxidized to urobilin in the colon and excreted in the stool. Some urobilinogen is absorbed from the small intestine and enters the enterohepatic circulation; while most is excreted in the bile, some reaches the systemic circulation and is excreted in the urine.

carrier proteins. Bililrubin is then transported to the smooth endoplasmic reticulum where it undergoes conjugation, principally with glucuronic acid to form a diglucuronide; this process is catalyzed by the enzyme bilirubin-uridyl diphosphate (UDP) glucuronyl transferase. Conjugated bilirubin is water-soluble and is secreted into the biliary canaliculi, eventually reaching the small intestine via the ducts of the biliary system. Secretion into the biliary canaliculi is the rate-limiting step in bilirubin metabolism. In the gut, bilirubin is converted by bacterial action into urobilinogen, a colourless compound. Some urobilinogen is absorbed from the gut into the portal blood; hepatic uptake of this is incomplete, and a small quantity reaches the systemic circulation and is excreted in the urine. Most of the urobilinogen in the gut is oxidized in the colon to a brown pigment, urobilin, which is excreted in the stool.

Some 300 mg of bilirubin is produced daily but the healthy liver can metabolize and excrete ten times this amount. The measurement of plasma bilirubin concentration is thus an insensitive test of liver function.

The bilirubin normally present in the plasma is mainly (approximately 95%) unconjugated; since it is protein bound, it is not filtered by the renal glomeruli and, in health, bilirubin is not detectable in the urine. Bilirubinuria reflects an increase in the plasma concentration of conjugated bilirubin, and is always pathological.

Jaundice, the yellow discoloration of tissues due to bilirubin deposition, is a frequent feature of liver disease. Clinical jaundice may not be discernible unless the plasma bilirubin concentration is more than two and half times the upper limit of normal, that is, more than 50 μmol/L. Hyperbilirubinaemia can be caused by increased production of bilirubin, impaired metabolism, decreased excretion or a combination of these. Causes of jaundice are listed in *Fig. 5.4*.

## BIOCHEMICAL ASSESSMENT OF LIVER FUNCTION

### Bilirubin

Hyperbilirubinaemia is not always present in patients with liver disease nor is it exclusively associated with liver disease. For example, it is not usually present in patients with well-compensated cirrhosis but it is a common feature of advanced pancreatic carcinoma.

| Major causes of jaundice | |
|---|---|
| **Pre-hepatic** | **Post-hepatic** |
| haemolysis<br>ineffective erythropoiesis | gallstones<br>biliary stricture<br>carcinoma of pancreas or biliary tree<br>cholangitis |
| **Hepatic** | |
| pre-microsomal:<br>    drugs, e.g., rifampicin, which interfere<br>      with bilirubin uptake<br>microsomal:<br>    prematurity<br>    hepatitis, e.g., viral or drug-induced<br>    Gilbert's syndrome<br>    Crigler–Najjar syndrome | post-microsomal:<br>    impaired excretion:<br>      hepatitis<br>      drugs, e.g., methyltestosterone, rifampicin<br>      Dubin–Johnson syndrome<br>intrahepatic obstruction:<br>    hepatitis<br>    cirrhosis<br>    infiltrations, e.g., lymphoma, amyloid<br>    biliary atresia<br>    tumours<br>    extra-hepatic sepsis |

**Fig. 5.4** Classification and major causes of jaundice. In hepatitis, bilirubin metabolism may be affected at at various steps. The jaundice is usually due to conjugated bilirubin.

## Unconjugated hyperbilirubinaemia

When an excess of bilirubin is unconjugated, the concentration in adults rarely exceeds 100 µmol/L. In the absence of liver disease, unconjugated hyperbilirubinaemia is most often due either to haemolysis or to Gilbert's syndrome, an inherited abnormality of bilirubin metabolism.

In haemolysis, hyperbilirubinaemia is due to increased production of bilirubin, which exceeds the capacity of the liver to remove and conjugate the pigment. Nevertheless, more bilirubin is excreted in the bile, the amount of urobilinogen entering the enterohepatic circulation is increased and urinary urobilinogen is increased. The laboratory findings in haemolytic (pre-hepatic) jaundice are summarized in *Fig. 5.5*.

Activity of the hepatic conjugating enzymes is usually low at birth but increases rapidly thereafter; the transient 'physiological' jaundice of the newborn reflects this. With excessive haemolysis, as in Rhesus incompatibility, or a lack of enzyme activity, as occurs in prematurity and in the Crigler–Najjar syndrome, there may be a massive rise in the plasma concentration of unconjugated bilirubin. If bilirubin levels exceed approximately 340 µmol/L, its uptake into the brain may cause severe brain damage (kernicterus).

## Conjugated hyperbilirubinaemia

This condition is due to leakage of bilirubin from either hepatocytes or the biliary system into the bloodstream when its normal route of excretion is blocked. The water-soluble conjugated bilirubin entering the systemic circulation is excreted in the urine, giving it a deep orange–brown colour.

In complete biliary obstruction, no bilirubin reaches the gut, no urobilin is formed and the stools are pale in colour. The differential diagnosis of jaundice due to conjugated bilirubin is considered on *pp 81–82*.

Hyperbilirubinaemia can be due to an excess of both conjugated and unconjugated bilirubin. The separate measurement of conjugated and unconjugated bilirubin concentration is useful in the diagnosis of neonatal jaundice where there may be some doubt as to the relative contribution of defective conjugation and other causes; it is less often required in adults. If the plasma bilirubin concentration is less than 100 µmol/L and other tests of liver function are normal, it can be inferred that the raised levels are due to the unconjugated form of the pigment. The urine can be tested to confirm this, since with unconjugated hyperbilirubinaemia there is no bilirubin in the urine.

A third fraction of bilirubin, consisting of conjugated bilirubin bound covalently to albumin, is found in the plasma of patients with long-standing conjugated hyperbilirubinaemia. This pigment has a half-life similar to that of albumin. Its persistence in the plasma during the resolution of liver disease or after the relief of obstruction explains the persistence of jaundice in the absence of bilirubinuria that can occur in these circumstances.

## Plasma enzymes

Enzymes used in the assessment of hepatic function include aspartate and alanine transaminases (also called aminotransferases; abbreviated AST and ALT, respectively), alkaline phosphatase (ALP) and γ-glutamyl transferase (GGT),

| Laboratory findings in haemolytic jaundice | |
|---|---|
| plasma bilirubin | unconjugated<br>rarely >100 µmol/L except in neonates |
| plasma enzymes | aspartate transaminase and hydroxybutyrate<br>  dehydrogenase slightly increased |
| plasma haptoglobins | decreased |
| urine urobilinogen | increased |
| peripheral blood | increased reticulocytes<br>decreased haemoglobin<br>possible evidence of haemolysis on blood film |

**Fig. 5.5** Laboratory findings in haemolytic jaundice.

as discussed in detail in Chapter 15. In general, these enzymes are not specific indicators of liver dysfunction. The hepatic isoenzyme of ALP is an exception, and ALT is more specific to the liver than AST.

Increased transaminase activities reflect cell damage; plasma levels may be 20 times the upper limit of normal (ULN) in patients with hepatitis. In cholestasis, plasma ALP activity is increased. This is a result of enzyme induction, itself a consequence of cholestasis, although the mechanism involved is not known. In severe obstructive jaundice, the plasma ALP activity may be up to ten times the ULN.

In practice, however, increases in the plasma activities of both enzymes are often present in patients with liver disease, although one may predominate. Thus, in primarily cholestatic disease there may be secondary hepatocellular damage and increased plasma transaminase activities, while cholestasis frequently occurs in hepatocellular disease. Increased GGT activity is found in both cholestasis and hepatocellular damage; this enzyme is a very sensitive indicator of liver disease but is non-specific. Thus, although certain patterns of plasma enzyme activities are frequently observed in various types of liver disease, they are not reliably diagnostic.

Plasma enzyme activities are very useful in following the progress of liver disease once the diagnosis has been made. Falling transaminase activity suggests a decrease in hepatocellular damage and falling ALP activity suggests a resolution of cholestasis. However, in fulminant hepatic failure, a decrease in transaminase activity may misleadingly suggest an improvement when it is actually due to almost complete destruction of parenchymal cells.

## Plasma proteins

Albumin is synthesized in the liver and its concentration in the plasma is in part a reflection of the functional capacity of the organ. Plasma albumin concentration is decreased in chronic liver disease, but tends to be normal in the early stages of acute hepatitis due to its long half-life (approximately 20 days). There are many other causes of hypoalbuminaemia, as discussed on *pp 203-204*, but a normal plasma albumin concentration in a patient with chronic liver disease does imply adequate synthetic function.

The prothrombin time is a test of plasma clotting activity and reflects the activity of vitamin K-dependent clotting factors synthesized by the liver, of which factor VII has the shortest half-life (4–6 hours). An increase in the prothrombin time is often an early feature of acute liver disease, but a prolonged prothrombin time may also reflect vitamin K deficiency. The cause can be determined by administering the vitamin parenterally; in the absence of liver disease, the prothrombin time should return to normal within 18 hours.

A polyclonal increase in immunoglobulins is frequently associated with cirrhosis, particularly when the disease is autoimmune in origin, and may cause the total plasma protein to be normal, or even increased, in spite of a low albumin concentration.

Serum protein electrophoresis is of little value in the diagnosis of liver disease; typical patterns may be seen in certain hepatic disorders, such as fusion of the β and γ bands due to an increase in IgA in alcoholic cirrhosis, but they are neither specific nor invariably present.

The measurement of individual immunoglobulins is also of little diagnostic value, although increases in specific autoantibodies may point to a diagnosis; for example, anti-smooth muscle antibody levels are increased in more than 70% of patients with chronic active hepatitis. Diagnostically useful changes in the concentration of other plasma proteins in liver disease are listed in *Fig. 5.6*.

## Other tests of liver function

Given the imperfections of the simple tests of liver function that have been discussed above, it is not surprising that many tests have been devised with a view to providing greater diagnostic sensitivity and specificity. Various dynamic tests, which give an indication of functional hepatic cell mass, are available, but are infrequently used. They may be considered as analogous to the use of clearance measurements for renal function, in that, utilizing marker substances that are excreted or metabolized by the liver, they measure either the rate of their removal from the blood or the rate of formation of a metabolite. Such tests include the bromsulphthalein and indocyanine green excretion tests and the galactose tolerance test. Newer dynamic tests include the $^{14}C$-aminopyrine demethylation breath test and the caffeine clearance test, both of which assess microsomal enzyme activity. They appear more sensitive than conventional tests but are more time-consuming and their use is likely to be confined to special situations, e.g., the monitoring of response to novel treatments.

Plasma bile acid concentrations are increased in liver disease but while this is a highly specific finding, bile acid measurements are no more sensitive than conventional tests. Measurements of bilirubin conjugates in plasma show considerable promise as sensitive tests of hepatic function but are technically demanding. So, too, is measurement of plasma glutathione-S-transferase activity, which appears to be a more sensitive and organ-specific indicator of liver damage than the transaminases.

| Plasma proteins of diagnostic value in liver disease | | |
|---|---|---|
| **Protein** | **Condition** | **Change in concentration** |
| albumin | chronic liver disease | ↓ |
| γ-globulins | cirrhosis, especially autoimmune | ↑ |
| $\alpha_1$-antitrypsin | cirrhosis due to $\alpha_1$-antitrypsin deficiency | ↓ |
| caeruloplasmin | Wilson's disease | ↓ |
| α-fetoprotein | primary hepatocellular carcinoma | greatly ↑ |
| transferrin | haemochromatosis | normal but 100% saturated with iron |

**Fig. 5.6** Plasma proteins of diagnostic value in liver disease.

# LIVER DISEASE

## Hepatitis

Acute hepatitis is most frequently caused by infectious agents, particularly viruses, and toxins. Patients may present with jaundice but this is often not apparent early in the course of the disease.

Early in the course of acute hepatitis, bilirubin and urobilinogen are usually readily detectable in the urine by a simple dip-stick technique. For as long as the plasma bilirubin is raised, bilirubin continues to be excreted in the urine. Urobilinogen may disappear from the urine at the height of the jaundice when there may be complete cholestasis, because no bilirubin reaches the gut, but it reappears as the hepatitis resolves and biliary excretion returns to normal. These changes (*Fig. 5.7*) are of no practical value in the management of hepatitis, but the detection of bilirubin in the urine is a simple and valuable diagnostic pointer to hepatitis in the pre-icteric stage of the illness.

The viruses primarily associated with hepatitis are hepatitis A, B and 'non-A, non-B' (principally hepatitis C virus but also D, which can complicate hepatitis B, and E), but many others, such as the Epstein–Barr virus and cytomegalovirus, can cause the disease. Many toxins and drugs can also cause acute hepatitis, including alcohol, paracetamol and carbon tetrachloride.

| Biochemical changes during acute hepatitis | | |
|---|---|---|
| | **Pre-icteric** | **Icteric** |
| plasma bilirubin | slight ↑ | large ↑ |
| plasma transaminases | large ↑ | ↑ |
| plasma ALP | normal | slight ↑ |
| urinary bilirubin | ↑ | ↑ |
| urinary urobilinogen | ↑ | absent |

**Fig. 5.7** Biochemical changes during acute hepatitis.

Most cases of viral hepatitis resolve completely. In severe cases, hepatic failure may develop, but most patients who survive the acute illness eventually recover completely, transaminase activities falling to normal in ten to twelve weeks. In some cases of infection with hepatitis B and C viruses, transaminase activities remain elevated; antigenaemia persists and chronic liver disease ensues. Infection with hepatitis A never leads to chronic disease.

---

**CASE HISTORY 5.1**

A 20-year-old student developed a flu-like illness with loss of appetite, nausea and pain in the right hypochondrium. On examination the liver was just palpable and was tender. Two days later he developed jaundice, his urine became darker in colour and his stools became pale.

**Investigations**

|  | on presentation | one week later |
|---|---|---|
| serum: |  |  |
| bilirubin | 38 μmol/L | 230 μmol/L |
| albumin | 40 g/L | 38 g/L |
| AST | 450 IU/L | 365 IU/L |
| ALP | 70 IU/L | 150 IU/L |
| GGT | 60 IU/L | 135 IU/L |
| urine: |  |  |
| bilirubin | positive | positive |
| urobilinogen | positive | negative |

**Comment**

The first set of results is characteristic of early hepatitis, with a raised transaminase reflecting cell damage. This usually precedes the rise in bilirubin and the development of jaundice. Impairment of the hepatic secretion of conjugated bilirubin and of urobilinogen uptake from the portal blood causes both these substances to be excreted in the urine.

The second set of results shows the expected high serum bilirubin but with a fall in AST as the phase of maximum cellular damage has passed. An increase in ALP, usually of not more than three times the ULN, is common at this stage. In hepatitis, the bilirubin in plasma is both conjugated and unconjugated, with the former predominating. Conjugated bilirubin is excreted in the urine and the pale stool reflects the decreased biliary excretion. The serum albumin has remained normal in this acute illness.

## Chronic hepatitis

Chronic hepatitis is defined as hepatic inflammation persisting without improvement for six months. Causes include autoimmune liver damage, chronic infection with hepatitis B or C, alcohol and drugs. There are various histological types and the prognosis varies between them. Chronic persistent hepatitis has a good prognosis; chronic active hepatitis may respond to treatment with immunosuppressive or antiviral agents, according to its aetiology, but the natural history is of progression to cirrhosis, which may be present at the time of diagnosis. Plasma transaminase activities are elevated in all types, reflecting the continuing hepatocellular damage. ALP activity is usually normal; indices of synthetic function (albumin, prothrombin time) are often abnormal in chronic active hepatitis but not in chronic persistent hepatitis.

## Cirrhosis

Causes of cirrhosis include chronic excessive alcohol intake, autoimmune disease, persistence of hepatitis B or C virus and various inherited metabolic diseases, such as Wilson's disease, haemochromatosis and $\alpha_1$-antitrypsin deficiency.

Due to the great functional capacity of the liver, metabolic and clinical abnormalities may not become apparent until late in the course of the disease; until this time, the cirrhosis is said to be 'compensated'. There are no reliable, simple biochemical tests to diagnose subclinical disease; dynamic tests of hepatic function (see p. 76) have the potential to do this but are time consuming and are not in routine clinical use.

Measurements of procollagen type III peptide in plasma are useful in monitoring fibrosis, one of the underlying pathological processes in cirrhosis, particularly when it is of alcoholic origin. This peptide is produced during collagen synthesis but its concentration in plasma can also be increased by inflammation and necrosis.

---

**CASE HISTORY 5.2**

A middle-aged female publican was admitted to hospital following a haematemesis. Endoscopy revealed the presence of oesophageal varices. The only biochemical abnormality was an elevated GGT (245 IU/L). Her varices were treated by sclerotherapy and no further bleeding occurred. The patient was told to abstain from alcohol. She was readmitted one year later, jaundiced, drowsy and with clinical signs of chronic liver disease.

### Investigations

serum:
| | |
|---|---|
| albumin | 25 g/L |
| bilirubin | 260 µmol/L |
| ALP | 315 IU/L |
| AST | 134 IU/L |
| GGT | 360 IU/L |

### Comment

The patient had continued to drink and the resulting liver damage eventually affected hepatic function. The serum albumin is decreased, serum bilirubin elevated and enzyme changes are consistent with cirrhosis and active liver cell damage; the prothrombin time was also prolonged.

Hepatic decompensation may be precipitated in chronic liver disease by sepsis, bleeding into the gut, for example, from varices, erosions and ulcers, and by various drugs, including diuretics. Diuretics may be given to treat ascites, a common feature of chronic liver disease, but must be used with great caution. Several factors probably contribute to the development of ascites, including hypoalbuminaemia, increased portal venous pressure, hepatic venous obstruction and increased hepatic lymph production.

Encephalopathy, characterized by a decrease in consciousness and impairment of higher functions, is often present in decompensated cirrhosis and may also be a feature of severe acute hepatitis. Substances implicated in encephalopathy include ammonia, which accumulates when urea synthesis is impaired, and false neurotransmitters, such as octopamine and β-phenylethanolamine. These false neurotransmitters are derived from the amino acids tyrosine and phenylalanine respectively, by bacterial decarboxylation in the gut, and are normally detoxified in the liver.

Treatment of hepatic encephalopathy involves: appropriate management of any precipitating factors such as gastrointestinal haemorrhage; restriction of dietary protein intake, and the provision of enemas or laxatives, for example, lactulose, to empty the bowels of nitrogen-containing material. Neomycin, a non-absorbable antibiotic, is used to sterilize the gut in order to reduce the production of toxins by bacteria. An adequate calorie intake is essential and fluid and electrolyte balance must be maintained. If ascites is present, sodium restriction is essential.

Alcohol is a common cause of liver disease. There are three main categories. Fat accumulation in the liver occurs frequently in people who abuse alcohol; it may also give rise to asymptomatic hepatomegaly with modest increases in plasma transaminases, a more marked increase in GGT activity, but a normal bilirubin concentration. Frank alcoholic hepatitis often develops after a bout of heavy drinking in patients with a history of excessive alcohol ingestion. Thirdly, chronic alcohol ingestion is a common cause of cirrhosis. The most important aspect of management, apart from general supportive measures and treatment of any complications, is to persuade the patient to abstain totally from alcohol. If this can be achieved, the prognosis in alcoholic cirrhosis is better than in cirrhosis due to other causes.

Renal failure is a recognized complication of chronic liver disease, particularly end-stage alcoholic cirrhosis. It may take the form of acute tubular necrosis, due for example to haemorrhage or infection, but more frequently is functional in nature. That is, the kidneys are histologically normal and tubular function is intact, the urine being concentrated and having a low sodium concentration. There is, however, no sustained benefit from extracellular fluid volume expansion. This 'hepato-renal syndrome' may arise spontaneously or be precipitated by fluid loss (diarrhoea, inappropriate use of diuretics). Response to treatment is generally poor and there is progressive azotaemia, fluid retention and severe hypotension although death is usually from liver rather than renal failure. The pathogenesis is incompletely understood; there is an increase in preglomerular vascular resistance, leading to decreased cortical blood flow, but the cause of this is uncertain.

Disturbance of endocrine function is common in patients with chronic liver disease. The most obvious is the feminization of males, with gynaecomastia, impotence, decreased body hair, testicular atrophy, etc. Both altered metabolism of androgens and oestrogens, and an increase in the plasma concentration of sex hormone binding globulin (see p.152) may be responsible.

### CASE HISTORY 5.3

A 40-year-old woman presented with jaundice.

There was no history of contact with hepatitis, recent foreign travel, injections or transfusions. She did not drink alcohol. She had been well in the past but had suffered from increasingly intense pruritus during the previous 18 months.

## Investigations

| serum: | total protein | 85 g/L |
| | albumin | 28 g/L |
| | bilirubin | 340 µmol/L |
| | ALP | 522 IU/L |
| | AST | 98 IU/L |
| | GGT | 242 IU/L |

### Comment

The very high alkaline phosphatase indicates a cholestatic jaundice; the low albumin is consistent with chronic liver disease. The clue to the diagnosis is the high total protein, implying a serum globulin level of 57 g/L. This is often seen in autoimmune liver disease. Further investigations revealed a high titre of antimitochondrial antibodies, characteristic of primary biliary cirrhosis. This diagnosis was confirmed by histological examination of tissue obtained by percutaneous liver biopsy.

Pruritus in chronic liver disease is due to the accumulation of bile salts. Measurement of plasma bile salts has been suggested as a sensitive test of hepatocellular function but has not been adopted routinely.

Once established, hepatic cirrhosis is irreversible. If possible, any underlying cause should be treated appropriately. Specific complications, including ascites, bleeding, for example from oesophageal varices resulting from portal hypertension, and malabsorption, may also be amenable to treatment. Causes of death include hepatic encephalopathy, uncontrollable bleeding and septicaemia.

The development of liver transplantation as treatment for cirrhosis has brought about a need for accurate prognostic tests. Several prognostic indices have been developed, based upon a combination of clinical features and the results of biochemical tests such as the plasma albumin and bilirubin concentrations. Surgery should not be undertaken while the short-term prognosis for the patient is still good, nor delayed until he is moribund.

## Tumours and infiltrations

The liver is a common site for tumour metastasis. Primary liver tumours are rare in the Western World but occur frequently in other geographical areas. Primary tumours are associated with cirrhosis, persistence of serological markers for hepatitis B and C, and various carcinogens, including aflatoxins. Plasma α-fetoprotein is elevated at diagnosis in approximately 70% of patients with primary hepatocellular carcinomas and is a valuable marker for this tumour although it can also be increased, usually to a lesser extent, in acute and chronic hepatitis and in cirrhosis. Infiltrative conditions which can affect the liver include lymphomas and amyloidosis. Patients with such conditions, and with intrahepatic tumours, are often not jaundiced. The only biochemical abnormality may be an increase in plasma ALP activity.

### CASE HISTORY 5.4

An elderly woman consulted her general practitioner because of weight loss and constipation. She had lost approximately 8 kg in weight in two months and had lost her appetite. She had previously opened her bowels daily but had recently had intervals of several days between movements and had passed only small amounts of stool on each occasion. On examination she was anaemic and had obviously lost weight. The liver was enlarged and had an irregular edge; a mass was palpable in the right iliac fossa.

### Investigations

| serum: | albumin | 30 g/L |
| | ALP | 314 IU/L |
| | bilirubin, AST and GGT | normal |
| stool occult blood | | positive |

A barium enema revealed a carcinoma of the caecum; an isotopic liver scan showed multiple filling defects characteristic of tumour deposits.

### Comment

An increase in serum ALP in a patient with carcinoma could be due to metastases in bone or liver. When the source of the enzyme is not obvious clinically, it can usually be inferred from isoenzyme studies. With hepatic metastases there is often no increase in plasma bilirubin concentrations unless lymph nodes at the porta hepatis are involved and obstruct the major bile ducts. Although tumour deposits within the liver can cause obstruction of small bile ducts, which is reflected by the increase in ALP, bilirubin leaking into the blood stream can be taken up and excreted by parts of the liver not affected by tumour. Thus, there is little or no increase in the plasma bilirubin concentration.

Hypoalbuminaemia is common in malignant disease and is usually multifactorial. Poor nutrition, increased catabolism (cancer cachexia) and replacement of normal hepatic tissue by tumour are all possible contributory causes in this case.

Carcinoma of the caecum is often clinically silent and may not present until extensive secondary spread has occurred.

## Cholestasis and jaundice

In a patient presenting with jaundice due to conjugated bilirubin, the possible diagnoses include intrinsic hepatocellular diseases and both intra- and extrahepatic cholestasis, that is, a failure of normal amounts of bile to reach the duodenum (*see Fig. 5.4*). Valuable diagnostic information may be provided by the history and examination. Biochemical tests can also give valuable information; for example, a high plasma transaminase activity suggests the presence of hepatocellular damage while a very ALP activity suggests cholestasis.

It is rarely possible to distinguish reliably between intra- and extrahepatic cholestasis from the results of biochemical tests alone. Other useful diagnostic techniques for the investigation of patients with cholestasis include ultrasound scanning, isotopic imaging, histological examination of tissue obtained by percutaneous biopsy and specialized radiological investigations such as either percutaneous or retrograde cholangiography (*Fig. 5.8*).

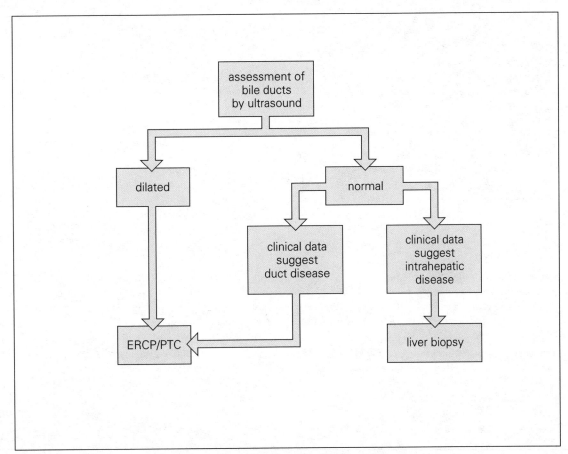

**Fig. 5.8** Procedures for the investigation of cholestatic jaundice. ERCP = endoscopic retrograde cholangiopancreatography; PTC = percutaneous transhepatic cholangiography (second choice procedure).

## CASE HISTORY 5.5

A retired publican presented to his family practitioner with a three-month history of epigastric pain radiating into the back and not related to meals. He was given antacids but returned one month later with more severe pain and weight loss. Over the past week his urine had become dark in colour and his stools pale. He had also become jaundiced. On examination, apart from the jaundice and signs of recent weight loss, no abnormality was found.

### Investigations

serum:
| | | |
|---|---|---|
| total protein | 72 g/L |
| albumin | 40 g/L |
| bilirubin | 380 μmol/L |
| ALP | 510 IU/L |
| AST | 80 IU/L |
| GGT | 115 IU/L |

Ultrasound examination demonstrated the presence of dilated bile ducts.

A barium meal and follow-through revealed indentation of the second part of the duodenum by an extrinsic mass, thought to be a carcinoma of the head of the pancreas.

A computerized tomogram of the abdomen also suggested the presence of tumour within the pancreas and this was confirmed at laparotomy.

### Comment

The results of the biochemical tests suggest that the jaundice is due to biliary obstruction and militate against, although do not exclude, the presence of liver disease. The clinical features are very suggestive of a carcinoma of the head of the pancreas obstructing the common bile duct as it enters the duodenum. However, the biochemical results, although compatible with this diagnosis, could also be caused by either a calculus obstructing the common bile duct, a metastatic tumour involving lymph nodes at the hilum of the liver or intrahepatic cholestasis.

Pancreatic carcinoma often presents with pain and cholestatic jaundice; there are, as yet, no reliable biochemical tests to aid in the diagnosis of this tumour.

## CASE HISTORY 5.6

An elderly man was admitted to hospital with acute abdominal pain. Clinically, he had generalized peritonitis and radiography suggested a perforated viscus. At laparotomy, he was found to have a ruptured diverticulum of the sigmoid colon. Peritoneal lavage was carried out and a defunctioning colostomy was constructed. Seventy-two hours later he was still very ill; he was hypotensive despite adequate fluid replacement and treatment with inotropic drugs; faeculent material was leaking from his wound, and he was slightly jaundiced.

### Investigations

Serum:
| | |
|---|---|
| bilirubin | 84 μmol/L |
| AST | 124 IU/L |
| ALP | 152 IU/L |

### Comment

Post-operative jaundice is a common clinical problem causes include:

- Increased bilirubin formation, e.g., due to haemolysis of transfused stored blood or resorption of haematomas.
- Hepatocellular damage, e.g., due to drugs, shock, transfusion-transmitted or coincidental hepatitis.
- Intrahepatic cholestasis, e.g., due to sepsis, hypotension, drugs or parenteral nutrition.
- Extrahepatic obstruction, e.g., due to calculi or perioperative damage to the bile ducts.

Post-operative jaundice is often multifactorial, as in this patient who was both hypotensive and septic. The elevated ALP is consistent with cholestasis but the elevated transaminase could be due to damage to other tissues besides the liver. The cause of cholestasis in septic patients is uncertain; impaired hepatic secretory capacity, obstruction due to swelling of Kupffer cells and changes in the composition of bile may all play a part.

| Inherited disorders of bilirubin metabolism | | |
|---|---|---|
| **Syndrome** | **Defect** | **Clinical features** |
| Gilbert's | decreased conjugation of bilirubin and decreased uptake in some cases (autosomal dominant?) | mild, fluctuant unconjugated hyperbilirubinaemia which increases on fasting<br>normal biopsy<br>normal lifespan |
| Crigler–Najjar | Type 1 (autosomal recessive) absence of conjugating enzyme<br><br>Type 2 (autosomal dominant) partial defect of conjugating enzyme | severe unconjugated hyperbilirubinaemia<br>early death due to kernicterus<br>partial response to phototherapy, none to phenobarbitone<br>severe unconjugated hyperbilirubinaemia, but good response to phenobarbitone and phototherapy<br>often survive to adulthood |
| Dubin–Johnson | decreased hepatic excretion of bilirubin (autosomal recessive) | mild, fluctuant conjugated hyperbilirubinaemia<br>hepatic pigment disposition (melanin)<br>increased coproporphyrin I/III ratio in urine<br>bilirubinuria<br>normal lifespan |
| Rotor | unknown (autosomal recessive) | similar to Dubin–Johnson but no hepatic pigmentation |

**Fig. 5.9** Inherited disorders of bilirubin metabolism. The precise nature of the metabolic defect in Dubin–Johnson syndrome is not known.

## Inherited abnormalities of bilirubin metabolism

There are four conditions in which jaundice is caused by an inherited abnormality of bilirubin metabolism: Gilbert's, Crigler–Najjar, Dubin–Johnson and Rotor syndromes. Their characteristics are summarized in *Fig. 5.9*. Gilbert's syndrome affects two to five per cent of the population but the others are rare.

**CASE HISTORY 5.7**

A medical student recovering from an attack of influenza was noticed to be slightly jaundiced. Worried that he might have hepatitis, the student had some blood taken for biochemical tests.

## Investigations

| serum: | bilirubin | 60 µmol/L |
|--------|-----------|-----------|
| | ALP | 7.4 IU/L |
| | AST | 35 IU/L |
| | haemoglobin | 16 g/dL |
| | reticulocytes | 1% |
| urine | bilirubin | negative |

### Comment

The negative urine bilirubin indicates that the excess bilirubin in the serum is unconjugated. There is no evidence of hepatocellular damage and the normal haemoglobin and reticulocyte count indicate that haemolysis cannot be the cause of the raised bilirubin. By elimination, the diagnosis is Gilbert's syndrome.

In this condition, there is reduced activity of UDP-glucuronyl transferase (the enzyme responsible for the conjugation of bilirubin) and often defective uptake of bilirubin into the liver cells. In cases where there is a family history, the pattern of inheritance is characteristic of an autosomal dominant, single gene defect.

The jaundice of Gilbert's syndrome is typically mild and present only intermittently. It is often noticed after an infection or a period of decreased food intake, possibly because fasting decreases hepatic UDP-glucuronic acid content or because free fatty acids compete with bilirubin for transport by albumin and uptake into liver cells. There may be mild malaise and hepatic tenderness but there are no other abnormal physical signs. The liver is histologically normal and there are no sequelae.

When suspected, the diagnosis should be confirmed and documented to avoid unnecessary investigations in the future. An increase in plasma bilirubin concentration of 20 µmol/L in response to either a 400 kcal food intake over 48 hours or an infusion of nicotinic acid (50 mg intravenously over 30 seconds, with blood samples taken every half hour for two hours, then hourly for three hours) is characteristic.

## Uncommon liver diseases

Wilson's disease is an inherited abnormality (autosomal recessive) of copper metabolism, characterized by decreased biliary excretion of copper and decreased incorporation of copper into caeruloplasmin, a plasma protein. Copper is deposited in the liver, the basal ganglia of the brain and the cornea of the eye. Patients with Wilson's disease may present either in childhood with a fulminating hepatitis, accompanied in many cases by haemolysis and a renal tubular defect, or as young adults with cirrhosis or manifestations of disease of the basal ganglia, e.g., dysarthria, tremor, and choreiform movements.

The biochemical features of Wilson's disease are a reduced plasma caeruloplasmin concentration, low–normal or low plasma copper (with increased binding to albumin) and increased urinary copper excretion. The decrease in caeruloplasmin is not unique to Wilson's disease, but is also seen in chronic hepatitis and malnutrition. The definitive diagnostic test is the demonstration of a high copper content in liver tissue obtained by biopsy; increased hepatic copper deposition is also seen to a lesser extent in primary biliary cirrhosis and in neonatal biliary atresia but these conditions have other distinguishing features.

Wilson's disease is treated with penicillamine which chelates copper and increases its urinary excretion; in chronic cases this often halts the progress of the disease. When patients present with fulminant hepatitis the prognosis is poor, but some cases have been treated successfully by liver transplantion; since the genetic defect is expressed in the liver, transplantation effectively cures the disease.

Haemochromatosis (see p. 259), an inherited disorder characterized by excessive iron uptake from the gut and iron deposition in the tissues, can affect many organs including the liver.

$\alpha_1$-Antitrypsin deficiency (see p. 204), an inherited condition characterized either by the absence of this protein from the plasma or by the presence of an abnormal protein, is another rare cause of cirrhosis.

## Fulminant hepatic failure

This clinical syndrome develops when there is massive liver cell necrosis. Such severe destruction of liver tissue is fortunately rare, but it is particularly associated with viral hepatitis and paracetamol poisoning. The underlying hepatic lesion is usually potentially reversible since the liver has a considerable capacity for regeneration, but the metabolic disturbance is profound and the prognosis poor; fulminant hepatic failure is often accompanied by renal failure.

Metabolic features of fulminant hepatic failure include severe hyponatraemia, hypocalcaemia and hypoglycaemia. Hydrogen ion homoeostasis is also disturbed. Lactic acidosis may develop as a result of the failure of hepatic gluconeogenesis from lactate, but may be masked by a respiratory alkalosis caused by toxic stimulation of the respiratory centre. Generalized depression of the brain stem may lead to respiratory arrest. In some cases, a metabolic alkalosis predominates; this is in part related to excessive urinary potassium loss, due to intracellular potassium depletion and secondary aldosteronism, and in part to the accumulation of basic substances, such as ammonia, in the blood.

Despite the fact that renal failure may also be present, the plasma urea concentration is often low, reflecting decreased hepatic synthesis. The plasma creatinine concentration is a more reliable guide both to renal function and to whether the patient should be haemodialyzed. The prothrombin time is greatly prolonged as a result of impaired hepatic synthesis of clotting factors and bleeding is a common clinical problem.

### Management

Management involves support of vital functions and correction of the metabolic imbalances. Respiratory failure may necessitate artificial ventilation and haemodialysis may be necessary if renal failure occurs. Close cooperation between the laboratory and clinical staff is vital in the management of fulminant hepatic failure. Artificial hepatic support has little to offer and hepatic transplantation should be considered in the most severely ill.

As with cirrhosis, the advent of liver transplantation as treatment for fulminant hepatic failure has highlighted a need for good prognostic tests. The prothrombin time, and the ratio of the concentration of factor V (which decreases) to that of factor VIII (which increases) are valuable in this respect.

## Liver transplantation

Liver transplantation is now increasingly used for the treatment of irreversible, severe liver disease. Donor organs are scarce and careful patient selection is vital. Following surgery, the major complications are immediate non-function, infection and rejection. The results of measurements of plasma transaminases and other liver function tests may suggest the development of complications, but diagnosis usually rests on imaging techniques or biopsy. The monitoring of immunosuppressive treatment with cyclosporin is discussed in *Chapter 20*.

## Gallstones

Gallstones are composed primarily of cholesterol with varying amounts of bilirubin and calcium salts. Cholesterol is maintained in solution in bile by virtue of the surface-active properties of bile salts and lecithin, but while a change in the proportion of these components may predispose to stone formation, other factors are also involved. Stones consisting primarily of bilirubin diglucuronide may develop in patients with chronic haemolytic anaemias.

Gallstones may be clinically silent. They can, however, cause biliary colic and obstruction and predispose to cholecystitis, cholangitis and pancreatitis. Biochemical tests may be of value in the management of these conditions, but the analysis of biliary calculi is of no importance in the routine diagnosis or surgical management of patients with gallstones.

## Drugs and the liver

The liver plays a central role in the metabolism of many drugs, converting them to polar, water-soluble metabolites which can be excreted in bile and urine. The enzymes involved are located in the smooth endoplasmic reticulum of the hepatocytes. Metabolism usually involves two types of reaction: phase 1 metabolism, for example, oxidation or demethylation by cytochrome P450-linked enzymes; and phase 2 metabolism in which phase 1 metabolites are conjugated with polar molecules, for example, glucuronic acid or glutathione.

Drug-induced liver damage may be predictable, arising when a toxic metabolite is produced by a phase 1 reaction at a rate which exceeds the detoxicating capacity of the phase 2 reaction as occurs, for example, in a paracetamol overdose. However, many drugs may have toxic effects when used in therapeutic doses (*Fig. 5.10*); this response (idiosyncratic hepatotoxicity) is unpredictable and is independent of the dose of the drug administered. Some idiosyncratic reactions to drugs, such as halothane-induced liver damage, have an immunological basis; the binding of a metabolite to a liver cell protein alters its antigenicity and provokes an immune response.

Some drugs are associated with the development of cholestasis; this may be an idiosyncratic response, as is the case with chlorpromazine, and additionally there is often evidence of liver cell damage. Other drugs, for instance 17α-alkyl-substituted steroids, including some anabolic steroids, predictably cause cholestasis without hepatocellular damage when administered in high doses.

Minor degrees of hepatic dysfunction occur relatively frequently as results of idiosyncratic responses, but overt hepatotoxicity is fortunately rare. The simple tests of liver function and damage are important for the detection of hepatotoxicity during trials of new drugs.

| Some drugs causing liver disease |
|---|
| **Dose-dependent hepatotoxicity**<br>paracetamol (in overdose)<br>salicylates (high doses only)<br>tetracyclines (high doses only)<br>azathioprine<br>methotrexate |
| **Idiosyncratic hepatotoxicity**<br>isoniazid*<br>halothane<br>methyldopa*<br>rifampicin<br>dantrolene*<br>nitrofurantoin* |
| **Dose-dependent cholestasis**<br>methyltestosterone |
| **Idiosyncratic cholestatic hepatitis**<br>chlorpromazine<br>erythromycin estolate<br>chlorpropamide<br>tolbutamide |
| * Signifies that chronic hepatitis can occur. |

**Fig. 5.10** Some drugs causing liver disease. Rifampicin also impairs bilirubin uptake and excretion, and induces hepatic enzymes involved in drug metabolism.

## SUMMARY

The liver has a central role in intermediary metabolism and is also responsible for: detoxification of many foreign compounds; deamination of amino acids and synthesis of urea; synthesis and excretion of bile; metabolism of some hormones; synthesis of plasma proteins; and storage of certain vitamins.

Because of its considerable functional reserve, biochemical tests tend to be insensitive indicators of hepatic function, although they can be highly sensitive indicators of damage to the liver. The results of biochemical tests often indicate the nature of a liver disease (*Fig. 5.11*), but less often indicate a specific diagnosis.

The most frequently performed biochemical tests are the measurement of plasma bilirubin and albumin concentrations and the measurement of the activities of transaminases, alkaline phosphatase (ALP) and γ-glutamyl transferase (GGT) in the plasma.

A raised plasma bilirubin concentration is a frequent but not invariable finding in patients with liver disease. However, conjugated hyperbilirubinaemia can result from extrahepatic biliary obstruction and a mild, unconjugated hyperbilirubinaemia is often a result of haemolysis. Greatly increased plasma transaminase activities are characteristic of hepatocellular damage; greatly increased ALP activity is characteristic of biliary obstruction. However, transaminases may be increased irrespective of either the nature or cause

| Test \ Condition | Acute hepatitis | Chronic active hepatitis | Chronic persistent hepatitis | Cirrhosis | Cholestasis | Malignancy and infiltrations |
|---|---|---|---|---|---|---|
| **Bilirubin** | N to ↑↑ | N to ↑ | N | N to ↑ | ↑ to ↑↑↑ | N |
| **Transaminases** | ↑↑↑ | ↑↑ | ↑ | N to ↑ | N to ↑ | N to ↑ |
| **Alkaline phosphatase** | N to ↑ | N§ | N | N to ↑↑ | ↑↑↑ | ↑↑ |
| **Albumin** | N | N to ↓ | N | N to ↓ | N | N to ↓ |
| **γ-Globulins** | N | ↑ | ↑ | ↑ | N | N |
| **Prothrombin time** | N to ↑* | N to ↑ | N | N to ↑* | N to ↑† | N |

**Fig. 5.11** Patterns of abnormalities of simple liver function tests in various liver diseases. The severity of the abnormalities is dependent on the degree of liver damage and its effect on liver function.
* Not corrected by parenteral vitamin K.  † Corrected by parenteral vitamin K.  § May be increased if cirrhosis is present.

of hepatocellular damage and ALP may be increased with both intra- and extrahepatic obstruction. In many patients with liver disease, moderate increases in both enzymes are observed. Further, changes in neither of these enzymes are specific to liver disease.

Plasma GGT activity is frequently increased in liver disease but an isolated increase may indicate excessive alcohol consumption; the finding of an increase in GGT in a patient with an increased plasma ALP activity implies a hepatic origin for the latter. Albumin is synthesized by the liver but because of its long plasma half-life, plasma albumin concentration tends to be decreased only in chronic liver disease. Many other factors can also affect albumin concentration. Blood clotting factors are synthesized in the liver and the prothrombin time provides a sensitive and rapidly responsive index of hepatic synthetic capacity.

Serum protein electrophoresis has no role in the investigation of liver disease; plasma immunoglobulins are of limited value but serological tests for specific autoantibodies are valuable in the differential diagnosis of chronic liver disease. Other tests which may be useful in specific liver diseases include the measurement of $\alpha$-fetoprotein (liver cancer), $\alpha_1$-antitrypsin ($\alpha_1$-antitrypsin deficiency) and copper and caeruloplasmin (Wilson's disease).

Biochemical tests which reflect liver damage and function are in general cheap and simple to perform but they often do not provide a precise diagnosis. They are, however, invaluable in monitoring the course of liver disease and the response of patients to treatment.

## FURTHER READING

Johnson P J (1989) Role of the standard 'liver function tests' in clinical practice. *Annals of Clinical Biochemistry*, **26**, 463–471.

Johnson P J & McFarlane I G (1989) *The Laboratory Investigation of Liver Disease*. London: Bailliere Tindall.

Lake J R (ed.) (1993) Advances in liver transplantation. *Gastroenterology Clinics of North America*, **22**, 213–481.

Laker M F (1990) Liver function tests. *British Medical Journal*, **301**, 250–251.

Rustgi V K (ed.) (1989) Hepatic Disease. *The Medical Clinics of North America,* **73**, 753–1053.

Sherlock S & Dooley J (1992) *Diseases of the Liver and Biliary System*. 9th edition. Oxford: Blackwell Scientific.

# 6. The Gastrointestinal Tract

## INTRODUCTION

The digestion and absorption of food is a complex process which depends upon the integrated activity of the organs of the alimentary tract. Food is mixed with the various digestive fluids, which contain enzymes and cofactors, and is broken down into small molecules which are absorbed by the intestinal epithelium. Complex carbohydrates such as starch are converted to mono- and disaccharides, the latter undergoing further hydrolysis by intestinal brush border disaccharidases (e.g., lactase) to allow absorption of the constituent monosaccharides. Proteins are broken down by proteases (secreted as inactive precursors) and peptidases to oligopeptides and amino acids. The absorption of fat is a complex process. Mechanical mixing and the action of bile salts create an emulsion of triglycerides which acts as a substrate for pancreatic lipase. This enzyme converts triglycerides to free fatty acids and monoglycerides. These are then incorporated with bile salts into mixed micelles and are absorbed from these into intestinal epithelial cells where they are re-esterified.

All these processes require the intimate mixing of enzymes, cofactors and substrates, and the maintenance of the optimum pH for enzyme activity. Disorders of the stomach, pancreas, liver and small intestine can result in the malabsorption of nutrients.

## THE STOMACH

In the stomach, food mixes with acidic gastric juice, which contains the proenzyme of pepsin, and intrinsic factor, essential for the absorption of vitamin $B_{12}$. Secretion of gastric juice is under the combined control of the vagus nerve and the hormone, gastrin.

Gastrin is secreted by G-cells in the antrum of the stomach itself and has several physiological functions (*Fig. 6.1*). It is a polypeptide hormone, present in the blood stream mainly in two forms: G-17 and G-34, containing 17 and 34 amino acids respectively. Other gastrin molecules have been identified in the blood, but the physiological significance of this heterogeneity is not known. All the variants have an identical C-terminal amino acid sequence.

### Disorders and investigation of gastric function

Biochemical tests are of limited use in the diagnosis of gastric disorders; the stomach can be directly inspected by endoscopy, and contrast radiography can also provide valuable information. Biochemical tests are used principally to investigate conditions in which gastric acid secretion is either excessive or inadequate.

Excessive gastric acid secretion is an important factor in the pathogenesis of duodenal, though not of gastric, ulcers.

| Gastrin | |
|---|---|
| **Functions** | **Control of secretion** |
| stimulation of: <br>    gastric acid secretion <br>    pepsin secretion <br>    gastric motility <br>    growth of gastric mucosa | stimulated by: <br>    increased vagal discharge <br>    gastric distension <br>    food, particularly amino <br>        acids and peptides, in <br>        stomach <br>    calcium in blood <br><br> inhibited by: <br>    gastric acidity <br>    gastrointestinal hormones, <br>        e.g., secretin |

**Fig. 6.1** Gastrin: functions and control of secretion.

| Pentagastrin test | |
|---|---|
| **Procedure** | **Results** |
| fast patient overnight | resting juice: normally <50 mL with a low acid content; large volume suggests gastric stasis |
| pass nasogastric tube under fluoroscopic control into stomach | basal acid secretion: normally <5 mmol/h; rates >15 mmol/h are characteristic of the Zollinger–Ellison syndrome |
| position tip in antrum | |
| aspirate gastric juice (resting juice) | stimulated acid secretion: normally <45 mmol/h in males and <35 mmol/h in females; pH does not fall below 7.0 in achlorhydria |
| aspirate stomach every 15 min, or continuously, for 1 h (basal secretion), | |
| combine samples for analysis | |
| give pentagastrin 6 µg/kg body weight i.m. | |
| aspirate stomach every 15 min, or continuously, for 1 h (stimulated secretion) | |
| analyze samples separately | |
| measure pH of all samples | |
| if acidic, titrate with sodium hydroxide and calculate acid secretion | |

**Fig. 6.2** Pentagastrin test.

The management of both types of peptic ulceration has changed radically since the introduction of $H_2$-blockers (antagonists of $H_2$-histamine receptors) and inhibitors of $H^+$, $K^+$-ATPase. These drugs inhibit gastric acid secretion and, as a result of their use, surgical procedures are now required far less frequently.

Maximal gastric acid secretion can be measured by the pentagastrin test (*Fig. 6.2*); pentagastrin is a synthetic analogue of gastrin. Acid secretion tends to be higher than normal in patients with duodenal ulceration and low in patients with gastric ulceration, but these findings are inconsistent and of no diagnostic use.

In achlorhydria, basal gastric acid secretion is low or completely undetectable and there is no response to pentagastrin. This condition is most frequently seen in patients with atrophic gastritis, but is also present in pernicious anaemia and in association with gastric carcinoma.

Tests of gastric acid secretion are now performed only infrequently. They may be useful to exclude achlorhydria

as a cause of hypergastrinaemia when this has been found in a patient with duodenal ulceration. Gastric acid secretion is also stimulated by stress, this response being mediated via the vagus nerve. The secretion of acid in response to stress induced by hypoglycaemia is still occasionally used to assess the completeness of a vagotomy, for example, if a patient thus treated develops recurrent ulceration.

Measurement of plasma gastrin concentration is now the first-line biochemical test for the investigation of atypical peptic ulceration, for example, duodenal ulcers resistant to medical treatment, recurrent duodenal ulcers after surgery, multiple duodenal ulcers and jejunal ulcers. A further indication is the presence of excessive gastric secretion detected endoscopically or radiologically. As gastrin is very labile, the blood must be mixed with aprotinin, a protease inhibitor, immediately after venesection to prevent degradation. Treatment with inhibitors of gastric acid secretion stimulates gastrin secretion and such drugs must be stopped before gastrin is measured.

| Causes of hypergastrinaemia | | | |
|---|---|---|---|
| **Disorder** | **Gastric acid secretion** | **Gastrin response to:** secretin | protein meal |
| Zollinger–Ellison syndrome | greatly ↑ | ↑ | normal |
| hypersecretion of gastrin by antral G-cells | greatly ↑ | none or ↓ | greatly ↑ |
| pernicious anaemia | ↓ | ↓ | ↑ |
| post vagotomy | ↓ | ↓ | ↑ |
| chronic renal failure | variable | ↓ | normal |

**Fig. 6.3** Some causes of hypergastrinaemia.

Atypical peptic ulceration is a feature of Zollinger–Ellison syndrome, a rare condition in which hypergastrinaemia is caused by a tumour (gastrinoma) of the pancreas, duodenum or, less frequently, the G-cells of the stomach. Approximately 60% of gastrinomas are malignant and in approximately 20% of cases they occur as part of a syndrome of multiple endocrine neoplasia (MEN). Plasma gastrin concentrations typically exceed 200 ng/L (normal <50). Patients usually present with recurrent or atypical peptic ulceration and sometimes have steatorrhoea due to inhibition of pancreatic lipase by the excessive gastric acid.

Zollinger–Ellison syndrome is treated by surgical removal of the tumour, where possible. Vagotomy and long-term treatment with inhibitors of gastric acid secretion may also be necessary and may be the only possible treatment if the tumour cannot be resected.

Other causes of hypergastrinaemia are described in *Fig. 6.3*. The response to an intravenous bolus of secretin (1–2 U/kg body weight) or to a protein-rich meal may be useful in distinguishing between some of them and this is also shown in *Fig. 6.3*.

## THE PANCREAS

The pancreas is an essential endocrine organ producing insulin, glucagon, pancreatic polypeptide and other hormones; its endocrine functions are discussed *in Chapter 11*. The exocrine secretion of the pancreas is an alkaline, bicarbonate-rich juice containing various enzymes essential for normal digestion: the proenzyme forms of the proteases,

trypsin, chymotrypsin and carboxypeptidase; the lipolytic enzyme, lipase, co-lipase and amylase.

The secretion of pancreatic juice is primarily under the control of two hormones secreted by the small intestine: secretin, a 27 amino acid polypeptide, which stimulates the secretion of an alkaline fluid, and cholecystokinin (CCK), which stimulates the secretion of pancreatic enzymes. Like gastrin, CCK is a heterogeneous hormone; the predominant form in the gut is a 33 amino acid polypeptide, but an eight amino acid form is present in some parts of the central nervous system and may function as a neurotransmitter. Both secretin and CCK are secreted in response to the presence of acid in the duodenum.

## Investigation of exocrine pancreatic function

Tests of pancreatic function fall into two groups: direct and indirect, according to whether or not it is necessary to intubate the patient to obtain a sample of pancreatic juice. Tests involving intubation are unpleasant for the patient and the procedure itself requires considerable skill and time. Many tests have been developed and one example is described for each group.

### Direct tests
SECRETIN–CHOLECYSTOKININ TEST
In this test (*Fig. 6.4*) a double-lumen tube is used, with one orifice in the stomach and the other in the duodenum near the opening of the pancreatic duct; this allows separate removal of gastric and duodenal juices and prevents the gastric juice from contaminating the juice in the duodenum.

The volume of juice, the bicarbonate output, and amylase or tryptic activity are measured.

A decrease in bicarbonate secretion is characteristic of chronic pancreatic insufficiency; enzyme activity is usually also reduced. Abnormal results are seen in some cases of pancreatic cancer, particularly when the tumour is in the head of the pancreas; enzyme secretion tends to be affected to a greater extent than bicarbonate. The range of normal responses is very wide; *Fig. 6.4* gives typical lower limits of normal. The sensitivity of this test for the diagnosis of exocrine pancreatic insufficiency is approximately 85%, and the specificity, approximately 90%.

OTHER DIRECT TESTS

In the Lundh test of pancreatic function, pancreatic secretion is stimulated physiologically by giving a test meal containing corn oil, skimmed milk powder and dextrose. A single-lumen tube is used and duodenal juice is aspirated over a period of two hours and analyzed for tryptic activity. This is decreased in chronic pancreatic insufficiency. If properly performed, the test has similar sensitivity to the secretin–cholecystokinin test for the detection of pancreatic insufficiency, although the specificity is somewhat lower.

Pure pancreatic juice can be collected by endoscopic cannulation of the pancreatic duct, but the measurement of enzymes and bicarbonate in this fluid does not appear to offer any advantage over the other tests described. The concentration of lactoferrin, an iron-containing glycoprotein, appears to be increased in patients with chronic pancreatitis; similar results are obtained if the protein is measured in duodenal juice.

### Indirect tests

FLUORESCEIN DILAURATE TEST

This test (*Fig. 6.5*) is based on the principle that fluorescein dilaurate, administered orally, is hydrolyzed in the gut by pancreatic esterase. The fluorescein released is absorbed from the gut, conjugated in the liver to fluorescein glucuronide and excreted in the urine where it can be measured. However, since pancreatic esterase is dependent on bile salts for its activity, the test effectively assesses combined pancreatico–biliary function; results may wrongly suggest pancreatic insufficiency if bile salt secretion is defective.

The possibility of any defect in intestinal absorption, hepatic conjugation or renal excretion affecting the result is controlled by comparing fluorescein excretion after giving

| Secretin-cholecystokinin test | | |
|---|---|---|
| **Procedure** | **Results** | |
| fast patient overnight | lower limits of normal: | |
| intubate with a double-lumen tube | volume of aspirate in 60 min | 150 mL |
| aspirate throughout test but discard all gastric juice | peak bicarbonate concentration | 90 mmol/L |
| keep all samples on ice | | |
| 0 min: discard resting duodenal juice give secretin i.v. collect duodenal juice for three 10 min periods over 30 min | peak tryptic activity | 30 IU/mL |
| | peak amylase activity | 270 IU/mL |
| 30 min: give CCK i.v. collect duodenal juice as before | | |
| analyze samples immediately for bicarbonate, amylase and tryptic activity and measure volume of juice | | |

**Fig. 6.4** Secretin–cholecystokinin test. The doses of secretin and CCK depend upon the brand of hormone used. The values for enzyme activity are guides only; they are method-dependent and should ideally be determined by individual laboratories.

| Fluorescein dilaurate test | |
|---|---|
| **Procedure** | **Results** |
| day 1 (test):<br>    give 0.5 mmol fluorescein dilaurate orally<br>    ensure adequate fluid intake<br>    collect urine for 10 h<br>    measure amount of fluorescein excreted<br><br>day 2 (control):<br>    give 0.5 mmol fluorescein orally<br>    follow same procedure as day 1 | $\dfrac{\text{fluorescein excreted on day 1}}{\text{fluorescein excreted on day 2}} \times 100 = \dfrac{\text{test}}{\text{control}}$ index<br><br>normal pancreatic function: $\dfrac{\text{test}}{\text{control}}$ index > 30%<br><br>pancreatic insufficiency: $\dfrac{\text{test}}{\text{control}}$ index < 20% |

**Fig. 6.5** Fluorescein dilaurate test.

the ester with that after giving an equivalent amount of free fluorescein on the following day. Although less specific than the direct tests, this is a sensitive, simple and cheap test for assessing pancreatic function.

OTHER INDIRECT TESTS

The principle of the $^{14}$C-PABA test is similar to that of the fluorescein dilaurate test, although a different enzyme is involved; the synthetic peptide, N-benzoyl-L-tyrosyl-p-aminobenzoic acid (BT-PABA) is hydrolyzed to p-aminobenzoic acid (PABA) by chymotrypsin. PABA is absorbed from the gut and excreted unchanged in the urine. To eliminate extrapancreatic factors, the BT-PABA is given with a tracer quantity of $^{14}$C-labelled PABA and the amounts of PABA and $^{14}$C excreted are measured and expressed as a ratio of the doses given.

This test is both sensitive and specific (both up to 90%) for detecting pancreatic insufficiency, but has the disadvantage that facilities for counting β-emission are required. It is not suitable for use in pregnancy or in renal failure and some drugs, including paracetamol and sulphonamides, interfere with the measurement of PABA.

The use of breath tests is described later in the section on tests of intestinal function. The measurement of serum amylase activity, valuable in the diagnosis of acute pancreatitis, is of no value in the assessment of pancreatic function.

## Disorders of pancreatic function

Disorders of the exocrine pancreas include acute and chronic pancreatitis, pancreatic carcinoma and cystic fibrosis. Clinical evidence of impaired exocrine function is usually only seen in advanced disease. Endocrine function tends to be well-preserved in all these conditions, although glucose intolerance may develop in severe or advanced disease. Diabetes mellitus and other conditions affecting only the endocrine pancreas are discussed in *Chapter 11*.

Other gastrointestinal disorders may mimic the effects of pancreatic disease; for example, enzymes may be destroyed in Zollinger–Ellison syndrome or be rendered less effective by an insufficient concentration of bile salts, while the control of pancreatic exocrine secretion may be affected by previous gastric surgery.

### Acute pancreatitis

This condition presents as an acute abdomen with severe pain and a variable degree of shock. The most frequent known causes are excessive alcohol ingestion and gallstones; many cases are idiopathic. Less common causes include infection, hypertriglyceridaemia and hypercalcaemia. The pancreas becomes acutely inflamed and, in severe cases, haemorrhagic. The initial lesion in acute pancreatitis is uncertain; either overstimulation of leukocytes, in response to damage induced by oxygen free radicals, or intrapancreatic activation of enzyme precursors may be involved.

---

**CASE HISTORY 6.1**

A 53-year-old man, who admitted to a heavy alcohol intake over many years, developed severe abdominal pain which radiated through to the back. The pain had started quite suddenly, 18 hours before admission to hospital. He had no previous history of gastrointestinal disease. On examination, the patient was mildly shocked and his abdomen was tender in the epigastric region with slight guarding. There was no evidence of either intestinal obstruction or perforation of a viscus on radiographic examination. Blood was taken for urgent biochemical investigation.

## Investigations

serum:
| | | |
|---|---|---|
| urea | 10 mmol/L | |
| creatinine | 90 μmol/L | |
| calcium | 2.10 mmol/L | |
| albumin | 30 g/L | |
| glucose | 12 mmol/L | |
| amylase | 5000 IU/L | |

## Comment

The level of amylase in the serum cannot be used alone to diagnose pancreatitis (see Chapter 15) and it is necessary to consider all the available evidence. In this case, the history is suggestive of pancreatitis and the clinical findings, although non-specific, are consistent with this diagnosis. The radiological findings militate against, but do not exclude, intestinal obstruction and perforation, two important differential diagnoses.

The finding of a very high amylase activity strongly supports a diagnosis of acute pancreatitis. The slightly raised urea, with normal creatinine, can be explained by renal hypoperfusion due to shock. Loss of protein-rich exudate into the peritoneal cavity commonly causes a fall in plasma albumin concentration and contributes to the hypocalcaemia which is often present, especially in severe cases of acute pancreatitis. The formation of insoluble calcium salts of fatty acids, released within and around the inflamed pancreas by pancreatic lipase, may also contribute to hypocalcaemia, and hormonal disturbances, for example, glucagon-stimulated release of calcitonin, have also been implicated. Hyperglycaemia may occur, but is usually transient.

In severe pancreatitis, methaemalbumin may be detectable in the plasma, but this finding is not sufficiently consistent to be of diagnostic value. The plasma of patients with pancreatitis may be lipaemic and there may be a mild increase in bilirubin concentration and alkaline phosphatase activity. An early elevation in plasma aspartate transaminase activity is characteristic of pancreatitis caused by gallstones.

The management of acute pancreatitis is essentially conservative. The gut is 'rested' by nasogastric aspiration, and fluid, electrolyte and protein losses are replaced intravenously; parenteral nutrition may be required if the condition does not settle within a short period. Pain is controlled with appropriate analgesics; opiates may exacerbate the condition and should be avoided. Progress can be followed by serial measurements of amylase and C-reactive protein, and by imaging (ultrasound and CT scanning).

### Chronic pancreatitis

Chronic pancreatitis is an uncommon condition which usually presents with abdominal pain or malabsorption and occasionally with impaired glucose tolerance. The malabsorption is due to impaired digestion of foodstuffs, but there is considerable functional reserve and pancreatic lipase output must be reduced to only 10% of normal before steatorrhoea is produced. Such a reduction only occurs in extensive disease or if the main pancreatic duct is obstructed. Alcohol is an important aetiological factor and there may be a history of recurrent acute pancreatitis.

Tests of exocrine function are unhelpful in the investigation of pain thought to be of pancreatic origin, but are used to establish that pancreatic insufficiency is present in patients who present with malabsorption. Pancreatic calcification is frequently visible on plain abdominal X-ray of patients with advanced chronic pancreatitis. Ultrasound imaging will exclude gallstones or a dilated biliary system, and show the morphology of the pancreas. If abnormal, it should be followed by CT scanning. Endoscopic retrograde cholangiopancreatography (ERCP) is capable of revealing the characteristic anatomical changes of chronic pancreatitis long before the results of functional tests become abnormal.

The treatment of chronic pancreatitis involves treatment of the underlying cause, if known, and, since damage to the organ is irreversible, long-term treatment of its consequences by, for example, prevention of malabsorption by the addition of pancreatic extracts to food.

### Carcinoma of the pancreas

Pancreatic carcinoma may be difficult to diagnose (see Case History 5.5). Presentation often occurs as a result of metastases rather than as a direct effect of the primary tumour. Other presentations include obstructive jaundice, when a tumour in the head of the pancreas obstructs the common bile duct, and malabsorption. Biochemical tests of pancreatic function are rarely of any use in diagnosis, and other techniques, such as contrast radiography, are far more powerful diagnostic tools.

Pancreatic carcinoma is therefore usually diagnosed late, by which time metastases are often present and only palliative surgical procedures are feasible. However, even in advanced disease, the demonstration of a rise in serum amylase after administration of CCK suggests that surgical drainage of the pancreatic duct may be beneficial in relieving pain.

### Cystic fibrosis

This is an inherited condition in which increased viscosity of pancreatic exocrine secretions results in obstruction of the pancreatic ducts and eventual fibrosis of the gland. the resultant malabsorption can be prevented by adding pancreatic extract to the food. Cystic fibrosis also affects mucus secretion in the bronchi, predisposing to recurrent respiratory infections and bronchiectasis, and biliary secretion, leading in some cases to cirrhosis. The diagnosis of cystic fibrosis is considered in *Chapter 16*.

## THE SMALL INTESTINE

The small intestine is the site of absorption of all nutrients; most of this absorption takes place in the duodenum and jejunum, but vitamin $B_{12}$ and bile salts are absorbed in the terminal ileum. Approximately 8 L of fluid enter the gut every 24 h. This is derived from ingested food and water and from the digestive juices, including those secreted by the small intestine itself. Most of this fluid, and the salts it contains, is reabsorbed in the jejunum, ileum and large intestine.

## Investigation of intestinal function

### Tests of carbohydrate absorption

A variety of tests involving the ingestion of carbohydrates and the measurement of their plasma concentrations or urinary excretion have been developed for the investigation of small intestinal function. The best known is the xylose absorption test (*Fig. 6.6*). D-Xylose, a plant sugar, is absorbed from the jejunum without prior digestion. It is not metabolized in the body and is excreted unchanged in the urine where it can be measured. An accurately timed urine collection is essential.

Misleadingly low results are obtained if the glomerular filtration rate is decreased, as occurs in renal failure and many normal elderly people. Other factors which can produce misleading results include delayed gastric emptying, oedema and obesity. An alternative approach is to measure serum xylose concentration 60 minutes after administering the xylose.

This test is cheap and simple to perform. Although abnormal results are almost always found in severe coeliac disease and disorders of the proximal small intestine caus-

| Xylose absorption test | |
|---|---|
| **Procedure** | **Results** |
| fast patient overnight; bladder must be emptied before test | normal plasma xylose at 60 min >1.3 mmol/L |
| 0 min:<br>    give 5 g D-xylose in water<br>    collect all urine passed until end of test<br>    patient should drink at least 500 mL of<br>        water over the next 2 h | normal urine xylose excretion >7.0 mmol/5 h |
| 1 h:<br>    draw blood and determine xylose<br>        concentration | |
| 5 h:<br>    collect final urine<br>    analyze urine for xylose | |

**Fig. 6.6** Xylose absorption test. Urinary xylose excretion can be measured over two hours (normal excretion > 4.0 mmol) but this is less reliable.

ing malabsorption, xylose absorption may be normal in milder disease. It cannot therefore be used to screen for malabsorption but may be helpful in the differential diagnosis of steatorrhoea. Xylose absorption is usually normal in patients with pancreatic disease and small intestinal disease affecting only the terminal ileum. It may be decreased in patients with bacterial overgrowth of the small intestine, due to bacterial fermentation. This provides the basis of a test for bacterial overgrowth (see p. 97). The diagnostic performance of the xylose test is improved by giving the xylose together with 3-O-methyl-D-glucose (2.5 g) and comparing the absorption of the two sugars by measurement of their plasma concentrations. The normal molar [xylose]/[3-O-methyl-D-glucose] ratio is 1:3; it is reliably decreased in mucosal disease and a normal result effectively excludes untreated coeliac disease.

Some small intestinal conditions give rise to increased gut permeability; this can be assessed together with absorptive capacity by giving an oral mixture of D-xylose and 3-O-methyl-D-glucose together with L-rhamnose (1.0 g) and lactulose (5.0 g) and measuring their urinary excretions. The percent dose excreted is calculated; the normal lactulose/rhamnose excretion ratio is <0.06; it is increased in untreated coeliac disease and in active small intestinal Crohn's disease, in which gut permeability to lactulose is increased but the absorption of rhamnose is decreased.

Impaired absorption of glucose may produce a 'flat' response in a glucose tolerance test. However, the number of other factors involved in determining the response to a glucose load is such that this test is of no practical value in the diagnosis of malabsorption.

Intestinal disaccharidase deficiency can be diagnosed by administering the appropriate disaccharide orally and measuring the blood glucose response. To increase sensitivity, the test is performed with the disaccharide (50 g) and then with the equivalent quantities (25 g each) of the constituent monosaccharides. The commonest of these disorders is lactase deficiency, which may be congenital or acquired; it often occurs transiently when there is damage to gut mucosa, such as after gastroenteritis. Lactose itself cannot be absorbed and in lactase deficiency lactose reaches the colon and undergoes bacterial fermentation; hydrogen, a byproduct of this process, can be measured in expired air (Fig. 6.7). Breath hydrogen excretion is also high in patients with bacterial overgrowth in the small intestine. Less common disaccharidase deficiencies include sucrase-isomaltase and maltase deficiencies. The definitive test for disaccharidase deficiencies is measurement of the appropriate enzyme in a biopsy sample.

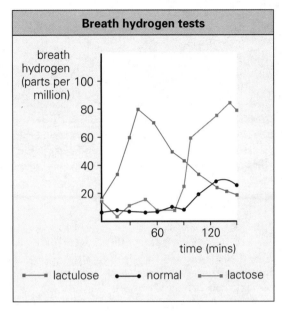

**Fig. 6.7** Breath hydrogen tests. Hydrogen is not produced by mammalian cells; its presence in expired air is due to bacterial fermentation of unabsorbed carbohydrate. Typical results are shown from the test performed in a patient with bacterial colonization of the small intestine when challenged with oral lactulose (10 g), where the lactulose acts as a substrate for bacterial metabolism, and in a patient with intestinal lactase deficiency when challenged with oral lactose (50 g). Hydrogen is generated by the fermentation of unabsorbed lactose in the colon with the result that the increase in breath hydrogen occurs later than with small intestinal bacterial overgrowth.

### Tests of amino acid absorption

Tests of amino acid absorption from the gut are only used as research procedures. Generalized malabsorption of amino acids occurs only with extensive small bowel disease. Malabsorption of specific amino acids occurs in certain inherited metabolic disorders; for example, deficiency of tryptophan may occur in Hartnup disease, an inherited disorder of the transport of neutral amino acids. In cystinuria there is impaired transport of the dibasic amino acids lysine, cystine, ornithine and arginine, but this condition is not associated with a deficiency syndrome.

Loss of protein from the gut in a protein-losing enteropathy can be assessed by measuring faecal radioactivity after parenteral administration of isotopically labelled proteins, e.g., [51]Cr-albumin, or polyvinylpyrrolidine. Such investigations are not commonly performed, however, since the cause of any hypoproteinaemia is usually obvious in such conditions.

### Tests of fat absorption

Because the absorption of fat is a complex process, the effects of fat malabsorption are often a prominent feature of generalized malabsorption. For this reason, and because fat malabsorption can occur with gastric, pancreatic, hepatic and intestinal disease, tests of fat absorption are frequently used in the diagnosis of the malabsorption syndrome (see p. 98).

FAECAL FAT TEST

Fat absorption has traditionally been assessed by measuring the excretion of fat in faeces. After digestion, dietary fat is normally absorbed completely in the small intestine; a small quantity of fat (<18 mmol/24 h) is excreted in faeces but this is derived from enterocytes.

With malabsorption of fat, its excretion in the faeces is increased. However, a major problem with its measurement is the need to obtain an accurately timed faecal collection. Collections should preferably be made for five consecutive days, although, for practical reasons, three day collections are often used.

Accuracy of timing can be improved by using a non-absorbable coloured marker such as carmine. This is administered orally and faecal collection is started when marker appears in the stool; a second marker is given 120 (or 72) hours after the first, and collection is terminated when this appears.

This test is unpleasant for all concerned and is only of value if carried out correctly. Dietetic guidance should be sought to ensure that the patient consumes 90–100 g fat per day for 48 hours before and during the period of collection; if less fat is ingested, minor degrees of malabsorption may be missed. In severe malabsorption with obvious steatorrhoea, quantifying the faecal fat excretion adds nothing to the diagnosis.

$^{14}$C-TRIOLEIN BREATH TEST

Due to the unpleasantness of the faecal fat test and its impracticality as an outpatient procedure, there has been considerable enthusiasm for the development of alternative tests. The $^{14}$C-triolein breath test is probably the most reliable alternative (Fig. 6.8). Facilities for counting β-radiation are required, but the test takes only a few hours and can be performed on a day ward. The test is based on the principle that when $^{14}$C-labelled triglyceride is taken orally, digested and absorbed, some of the label appears in the breath as $^{14}$C-labelled carbon dioxide. Since it is the specific activity of the expired carbon dioxide that is measured, a constant rate of production of carbon dioxide from all other sources must be assumed; patients must be fasting and must rest throughout the test.

The $^{14}$C-triolein breath test is not reliable in patients with diabetes, obesity, thyroid disease or chronic respiratory insufficiency and is not suitable for use in pregnancy. Properly performed, however, it is a sensitive test for fat malabsorption and results correlate well with those of faecal fat excretion. However, neither test differentiates between the different causes of fat malabsorption.

Modifications of the $^{14}$C-triolein test have been described, in which the respective absorptions of labelled triglyceride and labelled free fatty acids are compared, with the intention of distinguishing between pancreatic and intestinal causes of malabsorption. Such tests are not reliable. In practice, the $^{14}$C-triolein breath test is best used to diagnose fat malabsorption in doubtful cases. Specific tests, e.g., of pancreatic function, should be used to diagnose the cause.

### Tests for bacterial overgrowth

Bacterial overgrowth in the small intestine can occur in a number of conditions, particularly when there is stasis of gut contents, for example, due to a stricture or in jejunal diverticulosis. Bacterial deconjugation of bile acids leads to failure of mixed micelle formation and malabsorption of fat.

The most reliable diagnostic test for bacterial overgrowth is aspiration and culture of duodenal contents. However, this method has disadvantages: it is an invasive procedure and the cultures are sometimes negative when other evidence of bacterial overgrowth is overwhelming.

The measurement of urinary indicans (products of the bacterial metabolism of tryptophan) was formerly widely used to screen for bacterial overgrowth, but results correlate poorly with those of duodenal aspiration.

Bacterial overgrowth can be diagnosed with a breath test using $^{14}$C-labelled xylose given orally (Fig. 6.9). The principle is that the xylose is metabolized by bacteria in the lumen of the gut, producing $^{14}$C-labelled carbon dioxide which is measured in the expired air. This procedure is similar to that for the $^{14}$C-triolein test. This test appears to be more specific and sensitive than the $^{14}$C-glycocholic acid test, the principle of which is that bacteria deconjugate the glycocholic acid (a bile acid), releasing $^{14}$C-labelled glycine, which is absorbed in the proximal small gut and metabolized, producing $^{14}$C-labelled carbon dioxide. Intact bile acids are absorbed in the terminal ileum.

The disadvantages associated with the use of radioactive isotopes in these tests can be obviated by the use of the stable isotope, $^{13}C$. However, measurement of this isotope requires facilities for mass spectrometry and is more difficult than measurement of radioactivity.

### Tests of terminal ileal function

Terminal ileal function is tested in the Schilling test, a test used to assess the absorption of vitamin $B_{12}$, particularly in patients with suspected pernicious anaemia. Vitamin $B_{12}$ is absorbed in the terminal ileum. Abnormal results are seen in many patients with disease of the terminal ileum, but false negatives do occur and abnormal results may be seen in patients with bacterial overgrowth of the small intestine. The Schilling test is usually performed by a haematologist.

### Non-biochemical tests of intestinal function

The mucosa of the small intestine can be biopsied endoscopically or using a Crosby capsule; this is the definitive procedure for the diagnosis of coeliac disease (gluten-induced enteropathy, *see Case History 6.3*). The diagnosis of disaccharidase deficiencies can also be confirmed by measuring the enzyme in an intestinal biopsy.

Characteristic radiographical appearances are seen in patients with certain intestinal diseases, for example, Crohn's disease (see *Case History 6.4*). Biochemical tests, however, continue to be used for diagnosis of the malabsorption syndrome.

| $^{14}$C-triolein breath test |
|---|
| **Procedure** |
| fast patient overnight |
| collect basal sample of expired $CO_2$ (1 mmol) |
| give 10 μCi $^{14}$C-triolein in 60 g fat meal |
| collect 1 mmol samples of expired $CO_2$ hourly for 7 h |
| measure radioactivity of $CO_2$ samples |
| **Results** |
| combine radioactivities of samples and express as percentage of ingested radioactivity |

typical patterns of $^{14}CO_2$ excretion

**Fig. 6.8** $^{14}$C-triolein breath test. $CO_2$ samples are collected by bubbling expired air into vials containing 1mmol hyamine which reacts with the $CO_2$. An indicator is used which changes colour when the reaction is complete. Individual laboratories should determine their own lower limit of normal for $^{14}CO_2$ excretion.

| $^{14}$C-xylose breath test |
|---|
| **Procedure** |
| fast patient overnight |
| collect basal sample of expired $CO_2$ (1 mmol) |
| give 1 g xylose containing 10 μCi $^{14}$C-xylose |
| collect 1 mmol samples of expired $CO_2$ hourly for 7 h |
| measure radioactivity of $CO_2$ samples |
| **Results** |
| combine radioactivities of samples and express as percentage of ingested radioactivity |

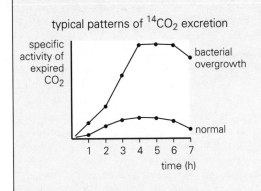

typical patterns of $^{14}CO_2$ excretion

**Fig. 6.9** $^{14}$C-xylose breath test for the diagnosis of intestinal bacterial overgrowth. $CO_2$ is collected as in the $^{14}$C-triolein test.

# DISORDERS OF INTESTINAL FUNCTION

## Malabsorption

The term malabsorption strictly refers to impaired absorption of the products of digestion, whilst maldigestion is failure of digestion which may be responsible for non-absorption of nutrients, for example, in pancreatic insufficiency. In practice, since the resultant clinical syndromes are basically the same, the term malabsorption is commonly used to encompass both disorders.

The clinical features of malabsorption are varied and stem from either deficiency of nutrients or retention of nutrients within the bowel lumen. The clinical features and common causes of malabsorption are shown in *Fig. 6.10*.

More than one mechanism can be responsible for malabsorption in individual cases. After gastric surgery, for example, impaired mixing of food with digestive juices, decreased stimuli to their secretion, rapid transit and bacterial colonization of a blind afferent loop may all contribute to malabsorption.

Investigations are required for two purposes: to diagnose malabsorption and to determine its cause. If the diagnosis is obvious clinically, e.g., if steatorrhoea is present, only tests to determine the cause are required. If the diagnosis is uncertain simple tests, for example, haemoglobin, red cell indices, prothrombin time, plasma albumin, calcium, phosphate and alkaline phosphatase, should be performed first; if the results of these are normal, malabsorption is unlikely and further expensive or invasive tests can often be avoided.

---

### CASE HISTORY 6.2

A middle-aged publican presented with flatulence and abdominal distention. On questioning, he admitted to weight loss and to passing frequent, bulky, foul-smelling bowel motions which were difficult to flush away.

**Investigations**

serum:
| | | |
|---|---|---|
| calcium | 2.10 mmol/L |
| phosphate | 0.70 mmol/L |
| glucose (fasting) | 12 mmol/L |
| alkaline phosphatase | 264 IU/L |
| albumin | 40 g/L |

A plain abdominal radiograph revealed pancreatic calcification.

**Comment**

The clinical features are characteristic of malabsorption (*Fig. 6.10*). The patient is hypocalcaemic and hypophosphataemic with a raised alkaline phosphatase due to vitamin D deficiency with secondary hyperparathyroidism. With gross steatorrhoea, further investigations to establish that the patient has malabsorption are not necessary, but the cause must be determined.

The presence of pancreatic calcification is very suggestive of alcohol-induced chronic pancreatitis. The raised fasting level of glucose, indicating glucose intolerance, is compatible with chronic pancreatitis and no further investigations of pancreatic function

---

| Malabsorption | |
|---|---|
| **Clinical features** | **Causes** |
| **Retention of non-absorbed nutrients**<br>diarrhoea, steatorrhoea<br>abdominal discomfort and distension<br>flatulence<br><br>**Decreased absorption of nutrients**<br>anaemia (iron, folate and vitamin $B_{12}$ deficiency)<br>osteomalacia and rickets (vitamin D deficiency)<br>oedema (hypoalbuminaemia)<br>bleeding tendency (vitamin K deficiency)<br>weight loss; growth failure in children | pancreatic enzyme deficiency, e.g., chronic pancreatitis and cystic fibrosis<br>bile salt deficiency, e.g., biliary obstruction and hepatic disease<br>intestinal, e.g., coeliac disease, tropical sprue, Crohn's disease and partial resection<br>bacterial overgrowth, e.g., gastric surgery, internal fistulae, strictures and jejunal diverticulosis |

**Fig. 6.10** Malabsorption: clinical features and common causes. There may be several reasons for the development of malabsorption in individual cases.

were performed. The patient was given pancreatic extract to add to his food and the symptoms regressed. This therapeutic response provides further confirmation of the diagnosis of pancreatic insufficiency.

## CASE HISTORY 6.3

A three-year-old boy was referred for the investigation of failure to thrive; he was below the third centile for height and the tenth for weight, although both parents were tall. The boy had frequent diarrhoea and did not appear to enjoy his food. On examination, he was anaemic and had abdominal distension; there was obvious wasting of the muscles of the limbs, buttocks and shoulder girdle.

### Investigations

Serum: albumin                           30 g/L
       xylose (1 h after 5 g orally)     0.5 mmol/L
haemoglobin                              9.7 g/dL

A jejunal biopsy showed total villous atrophy. A blood film showed hypochromic, microcytic red cells.

### Comment

There are many causes of growth failure. In this case, the history and findings on examination suggest a gastrointestinal disorder. Hypoproteinaemia and a hypochromic, microcytic anaemia, characteristic of iron deficiency, are common in patients with malabsorption. The grossly abnormal xylose absorption (*see Fig. 6.6*) indicates an intestinal lesion. The biopsy appearance is characteristic of coeliac disease, or gluten-induced enteropathy.

In this condition, damage to the small intestine occurs on exposure to gluten, a protein present in wheat and some other cereal flours; it varies considerably in severity. It may present either in infancy with severe failure to thrive and gross steatorrhoea, in later childhood or not until adult life. Growth failure is almost invariable in children. Complete withdrawal of gluten from the diet results in the regrowth of intestinal villi and resolution of symptoms. Secondary lactose intolerance is common and may persist for a period after treatment has been started

## CASE HISTORY 6.4

A 35-year-old woman was referred for the investigation of diarrhoea and abdominal pain. She had lost weight and was clinically anaemic. She had had two previous episodes of the same symptoms, lasting for several weeks on each occasion in the preceding two years, but had not sought medical advice.

### Investigations

serum: albumin             28 g/L
       haemoglobin         8.5g d/L
       red cell volume     110 fL

A $^{14}$C-triolein breath test was performed; the excretion of $^{14}$C-carbon dioxide was very low and for a few hours after having had a fat meal the woman experienced abdominal discomfort and distension. A barium meal and follow-through revealed narrowing and ulceration of the terminal ileum, with an ileo-ileal fistula.

### Comment

Weight loss is a common feature of gastrointestinal disease, even without malabsorption, and the breath test was used to screen for possible malabsorption.

The patient did not have steatorrhoea; this was ascribed to her habitual low fat diet, prescribed for familial hypercholesterolaemia some years before. The development of symptoms when she was challenged with fat suggests that her symptoms might have been more florid if she had had a normal fat intake. There was nothing in the history specifically to suggest a biliary or pancreatic disorder and the diagnosis was made radiologically.

The radiographical appearances are typical of Crohn's disease, an inflammatory disease of the gut in which ulceration and fibrosis occur and may lead to the formation of strictures and fistulae. Although the condition can affect any part of the gut, the ileum is most often involved. The course is often one of remission and exacerbations.

In the acute illness, sulphasalazine, steroids or azathioprine may be used and nutritional support is often necessary. Surgery may be required for intestinal obstruction or fistulae, or if medical treatment fails. Malabsorption in Crohn's disease may be due to either damage to the ileum or bacterial overgrowth of a stagnant loop, a possible consequence of internal fistula formation.

## The short bowel syndrome and intestinal failure

The short bowel syndrome encompasses the disorders that can occur following resection of part of the small intestine. When a large segment of bowel has to be removed, for example, following vascular occlusion, the result may be intestinal failure, in which the function of the gut is compromised to the extent that the patient's life is threatened. Other causes of intestinal failure include Crohn's disease, radiation enteritis, systemic sclerosis and desmoid tumours.

The gut has considerable reserve capacity, and the severity of dysfunction in short gut syndrome is related to the site of resection, the length of the segment resected and the extent to which adaptation (an increase in the absorptive capacity of the remaining gut) occurs. Thus less dysfunction follows resection of mid-jejunum than of proximal small intestine (essential for the absorption of most nutrients) or of ileum (essential for bile acid and vitamin $B_{12}$ absorption). Preservation of the ileocaecal valve reduces colonization of the small intestine by colonic bacteria and increases transit time. In practice, survival without long-term parenteral nutrition is unlikely if a patient is left with less than 60 cm of small intestine following bowel resection.

The major problem in the first few days following gut resection is fluid and mineral loss; accurate measurement and replacement of the losses is essential. This loss may decrease as adaptation occurs, or be controllable with drugs. Parenteral nutrition is usually required, at least initially, but adaptation is promoted by the presence of nutrients in the lumen of the gut, as well as by pancreatic and biliary secretions and certain gastrointestinal hormones, and so early enteral feeding is also desirable. If this is tolerated (e.g., without causing an increase in fluid loss), it can be gradually increased while parenteral support is decreased. Occasionally, when there has been massive resection, long-term parenteral nutrition is required.

Long-term complications of the short bowel syndrome include persistent diarrhoea, nutrient deficiencies, gallstones (due to bile salt wasting) and renal calculi (due to hyperoxaluria, see p. 70). Deficiencies of some nutrients are commoner than of others. Vitamin $B_{12}$ deficiency can complicate ileal resection; zinc deficiency is common with persistent diarrhoea, and malabsorption of vitamin D, calcium and magnesium, together with resistance to the action of vitamin D, the basis of which is poorly understood, can cause metabolic bone disease. Persisting lactase deficiency may limit milk intake, further compromising calcium absorption.

| Gastrointestinal hormones | | |
|---|---|---|
| **Hormone** | **Location** | **Function** |
| gastrin | gastric antrum | stimulates gastric acid secretion (see Fig. 6.1) |
| CCK | duodenum, jejunum | stimulates pancreatic enzyme secretion and gallbladder contraction |
| secretin | duodenum, jejunum | stimulates pancreatic bicarbonate secretion |
| pancreatic polypeptide (PP) | pancreas | inhibits exocrine pancreatic secretion |
| gastric inhibitory polypeptide (GIP) | duodenum, jejunum | releases insulin in response to glucose and inhibits gastric acid secretion |
| vasoactive intestinal polypeptide (VIP) | entire GI tract | ? neurotransmitter and regulates GI motility and secretion |
| motilin | duodenum, jejunum | stimulates GI motility |

**Fig. 6.11** Gastrointestinal hormones: locations and functions. ? = exact function unknown

## Other intestinal disorders

Given the amount of fluid that enters the gut each day, there is considerable potential for fluid and electrolyte depletion in situations of impaired reabsorption. Dehydration can complicate prolonged vomiting and diarrhoea, and enterocutaneous fistulae. Magnesium and potassium depletion are also frequently associated with excessive loss of fluid from the gastrointestinal tract.

In some cases, there is increased secretion of fluid into the gut; for example, in cholera, massive fluid loss can occur very rapidly. Secretory diarrhoea also occurs with villous adenomata of the rectum, tumours which secrete large volumes of potassium-rich mucus, and with tumours secreting vasoactive intestinal polypeptide (VIP) which cause profuse, watery diarrhoea, the Werner–Morrison syndrome.

## GASTROINTESTINAL HORMONES

The functions of gastrin, secretin, CCK, insulin and glucagon have been well understood for some time. In recent years, a number of other gastrointestinal polypeptide hormones have been discovered (*Fig. 6.11*). Although many of their properties are known, their exact physiological functions are incompletely understood.

At present, assays for these hormones are available only in specialized laboratories and the indication for measuring them for diagnostic purposes is largely confined to cases of suspected hormone-secreting tumours, for example, in the Werner–Morrison syndrome.

## SUMMARY

The gastrointestinal tract is responsible for the digestion and absorption of food. This process also depends upon normal hepatic and pancreatic function and is controlled by both neural and humoral mechanisms.

The malabsorption syndrome can be a result of intestinal, pancreatic or hepatic dysfunction. Significant malabsorption can readily be excluded by simple tests on blood or serum. If malabsorption is obvious clinically, for instance, because of weight loss and gross steatorrhoea, tests for malabsorption add nothing to the diagnosis. Such tests, for example, the $^{14}$C-triolein breath test, should be used only in doubtful cases. Once a diagnosis of malabsorption has been made, investigations are required to determine the cause if this is not obvious clinically. Biochemical, histological and radiological data may all be useful in this context.

Formal assessment of gastric acid secretion is now seldom required, but measurement of the hormone gastrin, which stimulates gastric acid secretion, is valuable in patients with atypical peptic ulceration, since this may be due to a gastrin-secreting tumour. Many other gut hormones have been described. The measurement of some of them may similarly be useful in the investigation of patients suspected of having a hormone-secreting tumour.

Chronic pancreatitis usually presents with malabsorption, but acute pancreatitis typically presents as an acute abdomen. Increased serum amylase activity is characteristic of, though not specific to, acute pancreatitis. In the acute condition, shock, renal failure, hypocalcaemia and hyperglycaemia may be complicating factors.

Approximately 8 L of fluid are secreted into the gut each day, the great majority of which is reabsorbed. The loss of fluid and salts from the gut because of vomiting, diarrhoea or a fistula can lead to severe salt and water depletion.

## FURTHER READING

Bouchier I A D, Allan R N, Hodgson H F J & Keighley M R B (eds.) (1993) *Textbook of Gastroenterology*. 2nd edition London: W.B. Saunders.

Lawson N & Chesner I (1994) Tests of exocrine pancreatic function. *Annals of Clinical Biochemistry*, **31**, 305–314.

Romano T J & Dobbins J W (1989) Evaluation of the Patient with Suspected Malabsorption. *Gastrointestinal Clinics of North America*, **18**, 467–484.

Sleisenger M H (ed.) (1983) Malabsorption and nutritional support. *Clinics in Gastroenterology*, **12**, 323–613.

Steinberg W M (ed.) (1990) Disorders of the Pancreas. *Gastrointestinal Clinics of North America*, **19**, 783–997.

# 7. The Hypothalamus and Pituitary Gland

## INTRODUCTION

The pituitary gland consists of two parts, the anterior pituitary, or adenohypophysis, and the posterior pituitary, or neurohypophysis. Though very closely related anatomically, they are embryologically and functionally quite distinct. The anterior pituitary comprises primarily glandular tissue, while the posterior pituitary is of neural origin. The pituitary gland is situated at the base of the brain, in close relation to the hypothalamus (*Fig. 7.1*) which has an essential role in the regulation of pituitary function.

## ANTERIOR PITUITARY HORMONES

The anterior pituitary secretes several hormones, some of which are trophic, that is, they stimulate the activity of other endocrine glands (*Fig. 7.2*). The secretion of hormones by the anterior pituitary is controlled by hormones secreted by the hypothalamus which reach the pituitary through a system of portal blood vessels. The secretion of hypothalamic hormones is influenced by higher centres in the brain and the secretion of both hypothalamic and pituitary hormones is regulated by feedback from the hormones whose production they stimulate in target organs.

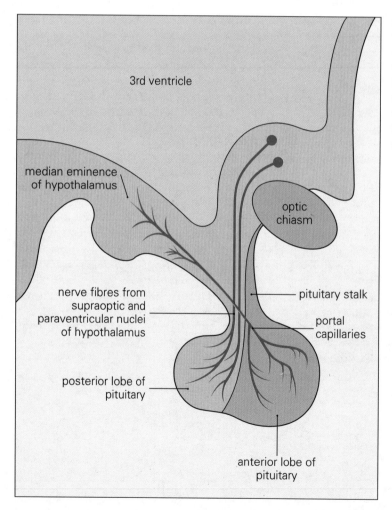

**Fig. 7.1** Anatomical relationship of the pituitary gland and hypothalamus. The portal blood vessels, through which hypothalamic hormones reach the anterior pituitary, and nerve fibres which transport hypothalamic hormones to the posterior pituitary are shown.

3rd ventricle

median eminence of hypothalamus

optic chiasm

nerve fibres from supraoptic and paraventricular nuclei of hypothalamus

pituitary stalk

portal capillaries

posterior lobe of pituitary

anterior lobe of pituitary

| Anterior pituitary hormones | | |
|---|---|---|
| **Hormone** | **Target organ** | **Action** |
| growth hormone (GH) | liver | somatomedin synthesis, hence growth stimulation |
| | others | metabolic regulation |
| prolactin | breast | lactation |
| thyroid-stimulating hormone (TSH) | thyroid | thyroid hormone synthesis and release |
| follicle-stimulating hormone (FSH) | ovary | oestrogen synthesis oogenesis |
| | testis | spermatogenesis |
| luteinizing hormone (LH) | ovary | ovulation corpus luteum, hence progesterone production |
| | testis | testosterone synthesis |
| adrenocorticotrophic hormone (ACTH) | adrenal cortex | glucocorticoid synthesis and release |
| | skin | pigmentation |
| β-lipotrophin | | precursor of endorphins |

**Fig. 7.2** Anterior pituitary hormones and their actions. All the actions shown are stimulatory; trophic hormones stimulate both synthesis and release of hormones by their target organs.

## Growth hormone

Growth hormone (GH) is a 191-amino acid polypeptide hormone. It is essential for normal growth, although in the main it acts indirectly by stimulating the liver to produce insulin-like growth factor-1 (IGF-1), also known as somatomedin-C. GH also has a number of metabolic effects which are summarized in *Fig. 7.3*. The release of GH is controlled by two hypothalamic hormones, growth hormone releasing hormone (GHRH) and growth hormone release inhibiting hormone (somatostatin). Somatomedin-C exerts negative feedback at the level of the pituitary, where it modulates the actions of GHRH, and at the level of the hypothalamus where, together with GH itself, it stimulates the release of somatostatin. The concentration of GH in the blood varies widely through the day and it may be undetectable (<1 mU/L) with present assays for long periods.

Physiological secretion occurs in sporadic bursts, lasting for one to two hours, mainly during sleep. Peak concentrations may be as high as 40 mU/L. Secretion can be stimulated by

| Metabolic actions of growth hormone |
|---|
| increases lipolysis (hence ketogenic) |
| increases hepatic glucose production and decreases tissue glucose uptake (hence diabetogenic) |
| increases protein synthesis (hence anabolic) |

**Fig. 7.3** Metabolic actions of growth hormone.

stress, exercise, a fall in blood glucose concentration, fasting and ingestion of certain amino acids. Such stimuli are employed in provocative tests for diagnosing GH deficiency, particularly in children. GH secretion is inhibited by a rise in blood glucose and this effect provides the rationale for the use of the oral glucose tolerance test in the diagnosis of excessive GH secretion. Excessive secretion due to a pituitary tumour causes gigantism in children and acromegaly in adults; deficiency causes growth retardation in children but is usually clinically silent in adults.

Somatostatin, the 14-amino acid hypothalamic peptide which inhibits GH secretion, has many other actions both within the hypothalamic–pituitary axis and elsewhere. For example, it inhibits the release of thyroid-stimulating hormone (TSH) in response to thyrotrophin releasing hormone (TRH) and it is present in the gut and pancreatic islets where it inhibits the secretion of many gastrointestinal hormones including gastrin, insulin and glucagon. The physiological significance of these actions is poorly understood. Rare somatostatin-secreting tumours of the pancreas have been described and somatostatin secretion may also occur from medullary carcinomas of thyroid and small cell carcinomas of the lung. Somatostatin analogues are used therapeutically to stop bleeding from the upper gastrointestinal tract, to inhibit hormone secretion by tumours, and to treat acromegaly.

## Prolactin

Prolactin is a 198-amino acid polypeptide hormone; its principal physiological action is to initiate and sustain lactation. Prolactin secretion is controlled by the hypothalamus through the release of dopamine, which inhibits the process. There is no known hypothalamic prolactin releasing hormone. Although both TRH and vasoactive intestinal polypeptide (VIP) stimulate prolactin secretion, it is not thought that this is physiologically important. Increased prolactin secretion occurs with prolactin-secreting tumours and is also frequently seen with other pituitary tumours, due to their obstruction of blood flow from the hypothalamus and thus the dopamine-dependent inhibition of prolactin secretion. In the absence of dopamine, prolactin secretion is autonomous.

The secretion of prolactin is pulsatile, increases during sleep and during stress, and in women is dependent upon oestrogen status, making it difficult to define a precise upper limit for plasma prolactin concentration in normal men and women, although 400 mU/L is often regarded as the upper reference limit. There is no defined lower reference limit for plasma prolactin concentration. Its secretion increases during pregnancy but levels fall to normal within approximately seven days after birth if a woman does not breast feed. With breast feeding, levels start to decline after about three months, even if breast feeding is continued beyond this time. The consequences of hyperprolactinaemia are discussed on p. 114. Prolactin deficiency is uncommon but does occur, for example, with pituitary infarction; its only manifestation is failure of lactation.

## Thyroid-stimulating hormone

Thyroid-stimulating hormone (TSH) is a glycoprotein (molecular weight 28,000 daltons) composed of an α- and βsubunit; the α-subunit is common to TSH and the gonadotrophins and is almost identical to that of human chorionic gonadotrophin (hCG), but the β-subunit is unique to TSH.

The normal plasma concentration of TSH is 0.1–4.0 mU/L. TSH binds to specific receptors on thyroid cells and this stimulates the synthesis and secretion of thyroid hormones. Secretion of TSH is stimulated by the hypothalamic tripeptide, thyrotrophin releasing hormone (TRH), and this effect, and probably the release of TRH itself, is inhibited by high circulating levels of thyroid hormones.

Thus thyroid hormone synthesis is regulated by a negative feedback system: if plasma concentrations of thyroid hormones decrease, TSH secretion increases, stimulating thyroid hormone synthesis; if thyroid hormone levels increase, TSH secretion is suppressed. In primary hypothyroidism, TSH secretion is increased; in hyperthyroidism it is decreased. TSH deficiency can cause hypothyroidism but hyperthyroidism due to a TSH-secreting tumour is very rare.

## Gonadotrophins

Follicle-stimulating hormone (FSH) and luteinizing hormone (LH) are both glycoproteins of molecular weight approximately 30,000 daltons consisting of two subunits: the β-subunits are unique to each hormone but the α-subunit is the same in each, is present also in TSH and is similar to that in hCG.

The synthesis and release of both hormones are stimulated by the hypothalamic decapeptide, gonadotrophin releasing hormone (GnRH), this effect being modulated by circulating gonadal steroids. GnRH is secreted episodically, resulting in pulsatile secretion of gonadotrophins with peaks in plasma concentration occurring at approximately 90-minute intervals. In males, LH stimulates testosterone secretion by Leydig cells and both testosterone and oestradiol, derived from the Leydig cells themselves and from the metabolism of testosterone, feed back to block the action of GnRH on LH secretion. FSH, in concert with high intratesticular testosterone concentrations, stimulates spermatogenesis and its secretion is inhibited by inhibin (*Fig. 7.4*), a hormone produced during spermatogenesis.

In the female, the relationships are more complex. Oestrogen (primarily oestradiol) secretion by the ovary is stimulated primarily by FSH in the first part of the menstrual cycle; both hormones are necessary for the development of Graafian follicles. As oestrogen concentrations in the blood rise, FSH secretion declines until oestrogens trigger a positive feedback mechanism, causing an explosive release of LH and, to a lesser extent, FSH. The increase in LH stimulates ovulation and development of the corpus luteum but rising levels of oestrogens and progesterone then inhibit FSH and LH secretion; inhibin from the ovaries also appears to inhibit FSH secretion. If conception does not occur, declining levels of oestrogens and progesterone from the regressing corpus luteum trigger menstruation and LH and FSH release, initiating the maturation of further follicles in a new cycle (*Fig. 7.5*). Before puberty, plasma levels of LH and FSH are very low and unresponsive to exogenous GnRH. With the approach of puberty, FSH secretion increases before that of LH.

Increased levels of gonadotrophins are seen in ovarian failure in women, whether pathological or after the natural menopause. High levels of FSH are seen in azoospermic men and LH is increased if testosterone secretion is decreased.

Gonadotrophin-secreting tumours of the pituitary are uncommon. They can secrete LH or FSH. Decreased gonadotrophin secretion, leading to secondary gonadal failure, is more common. It can either be an isolated phenomenon, due to hypothalamic dysfunction, or occur with generalized pituitary failure. A case of hypogonadotrophic hypogonadism is described in *Case History 10.1*.

## Adrenocorticotrophic hormone

Adrenocorticotrophic hormone (ACTH) is a polypeptide (molecular weight 4500 daltons), comprising a single chain of 39 amino acids. Its biological function, which is to stimulate adrenal glucocorticoid (but not mineralocorticoid) secretion, is dependent upon the N-terminal 24 amino acids. ACTH is a fragment of a much larger precursor, pro-opiomelanocortin (molecular weight 31,000 daltons) (*Fig. 7.6*) which is the precursor not only of ACTH but also of β-lipotrophin, itself the precursor of endogenous opioid peptides (endorphins). The control of the release of β-lipotrophin and the endorphins has not been fully elucidated, but ACTH release is controlled by a hypothalamic peptide, corticotrophin releasing hormone (CRH). ACTH secretion is pulsatile and also shows diurnal variation, the plasma concentration being highest at approximately 0800h and lowest at midnight. Secretion is greatly increased by stress and is inhibited by cortisol. Thus cortisol secretion by the adrenal cortex is controlled by negative feedback, but this and the circadian variation can be overcome by the effects of stress. The normal range for plasma ACTH concentration is 10–80 pg/mL.

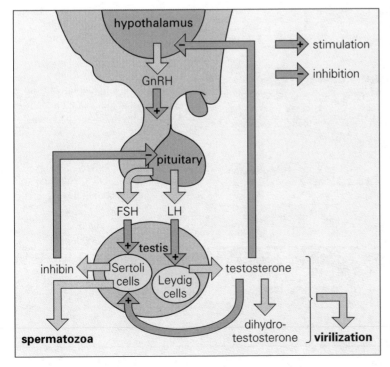

**Fig. 7.4** Control of testicular function by pituitary gonadotrophins.

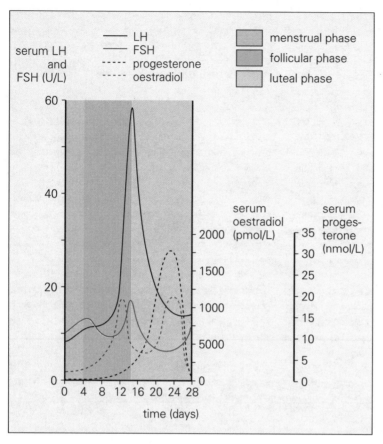

**Fig. 7.5** Changes in the plasma concentration of pituitary gonadotrophins during the menstrual cycle. The resultant changes in oestrogens (17β-oestradiol) and progesterone concentration are also shown.

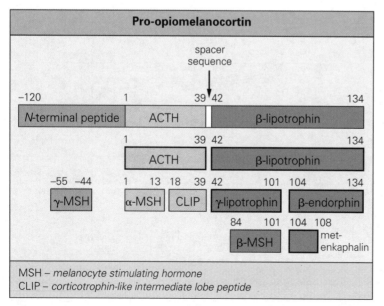

**Fig. 7.6** ACTH is derived by proteolysis of a precursor, pro-opiomelanocortin. β-lipotrophin is derived from the same precursor and is itself the precursor of endorphins and enkephalins (naturally occurring peptides with opioid-like activity). Melanocyte stimulating hormones are secreted in some species, but not man. (Those hormones which are secreted in man are shown in heavier outlines.)

Increased secretion of ACTH by the pituitary is seen with pituitary tumours (Cushing's disease) and in primary adrenal failure (Addison's disease). The hormone may also be secreted ectopically by non-pituitary tumours. Excessive ACTH synthesis is associated with increased pigmentation. This is due to the melanocyte-stimulating action of ACTH. Although a separate melanocyte-stimulating hormone (MSH) has been described in other animals it does not occur in man. Decreased secretion of ACTH may be an isolated phenomenon but is more commonly associated with generalized pituitary failure.

## MEASUREMENT OF ANTERIOR PITUITARY HORMONES

Hormones produced by the anterior pituitary can be measured in serum by immunoassay, although in some cases the sensitivity of the assays is insufficient to distinguish reliably between normal and reduced concentrations. The pulsatility of the secretion of some of these hormones makes it inappropriate to rely on single measurements for diagnostic purposes. Hence, when measuring trophic hormones, it is often useful to measure both the pituitary hormone and that produced by the target organ. For example, a low serum thyroxine concentration with an elevated serum TSH implies primary hypothyroidism, whereas a low TSH with a low thyroxine suggests decreased pituitary secretion of TSH causing secondary hypothyroidism.

Dynamic tests are important tools in the investigation of pituitary function and, indeed, the function of other endocrine organs. There are two types: stimulatory tests, used to investigate suspected hypofunction, and suppression tests, used to investigate suspected hyperfunction. Tests relating to individual hormones will be described in later sections of this chapter in the context of the clinical conditions in which they are used. The use of the clomiphene test in the investigation of hypogonadism due to isolated gonadotrophin deficiency is discussed in *Chapter 10*.

In assessing patients with suspected anterior pituitary dysfunction, it is often convenient to test the capacity of the gland to secrete GH, prolactin, ACTH, TSH and the gonadotrophins in a single procedure. The combined pituitary function test (triple bolus test) involves giving a single intravenous bolus of a mixture of TRH, GnRH and insulin. The insulin induces hypoglycaemia, the stress of which stimulates ACTH and GH release. The test is potentially hazardous because of the possible sequelae of hypoglycaemia. A doctor should always be present when the test is performed. It is contraindicated in patients with a history of fits or ischaemic heart disease and it should not be performed

in patients whose 0900 h serum cortisol concentration is low. 50 mL of 50% dextrose solution must be available for immediate administration should severe hypoglycaemia develop. Giving glucose because of severe symptomatic hypoglycaemia does not invalidate the results of the test. The stress need only be very brief to be effective. It is important that documented hypoglycaemia is obtained, since if it does not occur a failure of ACTH response might be due to the inadequacy of the stimulus rather than to pituitary failure. If hypoglycaemia does not develop, a further dose of insulin must be given. The protocol for this test and the normal responses are shown in *Fig. 7.7*.

It may be preferable to give the insulin by continuous intravenous infusion. The rate can be adjusted until hypoglycaemia develops, whereupon the infusion is stopped. This is a more certain and safer way of producing hypoglycaemia than giving a single bolus of insulin. When the induction of hypoglycaemia is contraindicated, glucagon can be used to stimulate cortisol and GH secretion instead of insulin.

Because the assay of ACTH is technically more demanding, it is usual to measure cortisol instead in these tests. Should an abnormal response be found, it is necessary to demonstrate that the adrenal gland is normally sensitive to ACTH by performing a Synacthen test if this has not been done already. Prolactin secretion is stimulated by both stress and TRH. However, the normal response is variable and since prolactin deficiency is rarely a clinical problem, plasma prolactin concentrations are often not measured in patients undergoing combined tests of pituitary function.

The validity of using the TRH and GnRH tests in the assessment of pituitary function has been criticized on the basis that they measure the ability of the gland to secrete pre-formed hormones as a short-term response to a pharmacological stimulus (albeit with a substance identical to a natural hormone); this may not reflect the ability of the pituitary to respond to normal physiological stimuli. This point is discussed further in *Chapters 9 and 10*.

## DISORDERS OF ANTERIOR PITUITARY FUNCTION

### Hypopituitarism

Destructive lesions of the pituitary tend to present with evidence of pituitary hypofunction. Partial hypopituitarism is seen more frequently than complete loss of pituitary function. The presenting features depend on several factors; age is particularly important. Decreased GH secretion is an early feature of pituitary failure (*see p. 111*), but whilst its effects can be dramatic in children, they are of less significance in adults. In general, GH and gonadotrophin secretion (LH

| Combined test of anterior pituitary function | | | | | |
|---|---|---|---|---|---|

### Procedure

1. fast patient overnight and weigh

2. insert and heparinize i.v. cannula

3. draw and discard 1 mL of blood before collecting each sample and heparinize cannula after each sample is drawn

4. after 30 min take basal blood sample and analyze for glucose, cortisol (or ACTH), FSH, LH, TSH, free thyroxine, GH and testosterone/oestradiol.

5. give 200 μg TRH, 100 μg GnRH and 0.15 U/kg body weight soluble insulin

6. take blood samples for analysis as follows:

| time (min) | assay | | | | |
|---|---|---|---|---|---|
| | glucose | cortisol | FSH, LH | TSH | GH |
| 0 | * | * | * | * | * |
| 15 | * | | | | |
| 20 | | | * | * | |
| 30 | * | * | | | * |
| 45 | * | | | | |
| 60 | * | * | * | * | * |
| 90 | * | * | | | * |
| 120 | * | * | | | * |

7. repeat insulin dose at 45 min if patient has not become clinically (sweating) or biochemically (blood glucose < 2.2 mmol/L) hypoglycaemic and extend sampling accordingly

### Normal response

| cortisol | increment<br>peak | >200 nmol/L<br>>500 nmol/L (the same criteria apply if glucagon is used) |
|---|---|---|
| GH | peak | >20 mU/L (after glucagon: 15 mU/L in males and 20 mU/L in females) |
| FSH | increment | >1.5 times basal level |
| LH | increment | >5 times basal level |
| TSH | increment | ≥ 2 mU/L (elderly)<br>≥ 5 mU/L (young adults) |

**Fig. 7.7** Combined test (triple bolus test) of anterior pituitary function. In patients thought to be very likely to be hypopituitary, the insulin dose should be 0.1 U/kg body weight; in patients with Cushing's disease or acromegaly, a dose of 0.30 U/kg may be used. When glucagon (1mg intramuscularly) is used instead of insulin, blood samples for cortisol and GH should be taken at 30 min intervals from 90 to 240 min after the injection (GH and cortisol responses occur later than when insulin is used).

before FSH) are affected before that of ACTH. It is very uncommon for hypothyroidism to be the presenting feature of pituitary failure. Isolated deficiency of some of the anterior pituitary hormones can occur but this is usually congenital. In most such cases, it is apparently due to failure of secretion of the relevant hypothalamic hormone. Haemorrhage into a pituitary tumour can cause 'pituitary apoplexy'. The onset is sudden, usually with headache, signs of meningism, visual deterioration and loss of consciousness. Immediate treatment with intravenous fluids and hydrocortisone is required, often followed by surgery.

In suspected pituitary hypofunction, stimulatory tests are used to assess the ability of the gland to produce hormones. With a suspected pituitary tumour, the possibility of both excessive hormone secretion by the tumour and decreases in the production of other hormones must be investigated. The underlying causes must be determined where possible and pituitary tumours should be carefully assessed, by examination of the visual fields, skull radiography and imaging techniques, e.g., computerized tomography (CT) or magnetic resonance imaging (MRI), to define their anatomical extent; this may determine the correct management. Some of the many causes and clinical features of hypopituitarism are indicated in *Fig. 7.8*.

Clinical evidence of posterior pituitary dysfunction (diabetes insipidus) must be sought and, if present, confirmed by appropriate tests (*see pp 117–119*). Diabetes insipidus is uncommon except with large pituitary tumours but can develop, often transiently, after surgery. Even in patients with impaired vasopressin (antidiuretic hormone, ADH) secretion, diabetes insipidus may not be apparent if ACTH secretion is also impaired, since cortisol, the secretion of which is dependent on ACTH, is necessary for normal water excretion.

## CASE HISTORY 7.1

A 50-year-old man tripped and fell as he was running for a bus. He hit his head against the kerb and was knocked out for a few seconds. An ambulance was called and he was taken to the local hospital.

There was no sign of physical injury on examination but a skull radiograph showed enlargement of the pituitary fossa. The casualty officer questioned the patient further. Over the preceding 12 months he had lost his libido and found it necessary to shave less frequently than before; he had also noticed some loss of axillary and pubic hair. He frequently felt dizzy when getting out of bed in the morning and despite

spending a lot of time in the sun had not acquired his usual summer tan.

### Investigations

serum:

| | | |
|---|---|---|
| cortisol (0900 h) | 300 nmol/L | |
| GH | < 2 mU/L | |
| free thyroxine | 12 pmol/L | |
| TSH | 2 mU/L | |
| testosterone | 4 nmol/L | |
| LH | <1.5 U/L | |
| FSH | <1.0 U/L | |
| prolactin | <50 mU/L | |

combined glucagon, TRH and GnRH stimulation test:

serum:

| | |
|---|---|
| cortisol (maximum) | 350 nmol/L at 180 min |
| LH, FSH | no increment over basal values |
| GH | no increment over basal value |
| TSH | 5 mU/L at 20 min; 3 mU/L at 60 min |

### Comment

The clinical features are typical of hypopituitarism (*Fig. 7.8*) and the test results confirm this diagnosis. GH, gonadotrophin and prolactin concentrations are all low; the cortisol concentration is in the lower part of the normal range. These hormones show little or no response to appropriate stimuli. The low testosterone is secondary to the lack of gonadotrophins. In view of the overwhelming evidence for the diagnosis, it was not considered necessary to perform a Synacthen test. The serum free thyroxine is near the lower end of the normal range; if this were related to incipient thyroid failure, a higher TSH concentration would be expected. There is a TSH response to TRH, but even this is towards the lower limit of normal.

Cortisol replacement therapy was started immediately and testosterone and thyroxine were also given. Within a few hours, the patient became polyuric and signs of water depletion developed. The serum sodium concentration, which was low on admission (128 mmol/L), rose to 149 mmol/L. Diabetes insipidus, due to impaired release of vasopressin, can be masked by simultaneous cortisol deficiency and revealed when replacement therapy is started, as in this case.

The patient was given synthetic vasopressin which controlled his polyuria. He subsequently underwent surgery and a chromophobe adenoma was successfully removed. On follow-up, there was no evidence of recovery of pituitary function and he remained on replacement therapy.

| Hypopituitarism | | |
|---|---|---|
| **Causes** | | |

**Tumours**
pituitary tumours:
 adenoma
 craniopharyngioma
cerebral tumours:
 primary
 secondary

**Miscellaneous**
sarcoidosis
histiocytosis X
haemochromatosis

**Hypothalamic disorders**
tumours
functional disturbances, e.g., anorexia
 nervosa and starvation, causing reversible
 hypogonadotrophic hypogonadism
isolated GH and gonadotrophin secretion due
 to impaired secretion of hypothalamic
 releasing hormones

**Vascular disease**
post-partum necrosis (Sheehan's syndrome)
infarction, especially of tumours
severe hypotension
cranial arteritis

**Trauma**

**Infection**
meningitis, especially tuberculous
syphilis

**Iatrogenic**
surgery
irradiation
prolonged treatment with glucocorticoids or
 thyroid hormones causing isolated ACTH
 and TSH suppression respectively

| Clinical features | |
|---|---|
| **Hormone** | **Features of deficiency** |
| growth hormone | children: growth retardation<br>adults: decreased muscle bulk<br>any tendency to hypoglycaemia may be accentuated |
| prolactin | failure of lactation |
| gonadotrophins | children: delayed puberty<br>females: oligomenorrhoea, infertility, atrophy of breasts<br> and genitalia |
| | males: impotence, azoospermia, testicular atrophy<br>both sexes: decreased libido, loss of body hair, fine<br> wrinkling of skin |
| ACTH | weight loss, weakness, hypotension, hypoglycaemia and<br> other features of glucocorticoid deficiency, usually of<br> insidious onset unless stressed; decreased skin pigmentation |
| TSH | weight gain, cold intolerance, fatigue, etc. |
| vasopressin | thirst, polyuria |

**Fig. 7.8** Main causes and clinical features of hypopituitarism.

| Assessment of growth hormone status | |
| --- | --- |
| **Procedure** | **Normal GH response** |
| arginine infusion test:<br>  give 0.5 g/kg body weight (maximum 30 g) i.v. over 30 min<br>  take blood samples at 30 min intervals for 2 h | peak >15 mU/L |
| Bovril (yeast extract) test:<br>  give 20 g/1.5 m$^2$ body surface area orally in water<br>  take blood samples at 30 min intervals for 2 h | peak >20 mU/L |
| exercise test:<br>  patient runs up and down stairs as fast as possible for 10 min | peak >20 mU/L |
| insulin/glucagon test: *see Fig 7.7* | |

**Fig. 7.9** Procedure for assessing GH status. Other secretagogues which may be used in provocative tests include clonidine, metoclopramide and GHRH. The insulin hypoglycaemia test is the most widely used.

### Anorexia nervosa

Anorexia nervosa, a disorder characterized by self-imposed starvation and a preoccupation with body size, may clinically resemble hypopituitarism. Amenorrhoea, due to decreased gonadotrophin secretion, is common to both conditions. However, pubic and axillary hair, which may be lost in hypopituitarism, is normal in anorexia nervosa and there may even be additional (lanugo) hair on the body. The weight loss of anorexia nervosa is usually severe in comparison with that which can occur in hypopituitarism. Plasma cortisol and GH concentrations tend to be elevated in anorexia nervosa.

### Growth hormone deficiency

GH deficiency is an uncommon but important cause of growth retardation. GH may be undetectable in plasma in normal children which means that, while a random level of greater than 20 mU/L excludes significant deficiency, a low concentration in a random blood sample is not diagnostic. GH status can be assessed by various stimulatory tests (*Fig. 7.9*). Although these provocative tests are widely used in the investigation of poor growth, their relevance to the physiological secretion of GH is questionable, and both false negative and false positive results occur. More reliable information may be provided by the measurement of GH secretion during sleep, by means of frequent blood sampling through an indwelling cannula.

**CASE HISTORY 7.2**

A ten-year-old boy was referred to hospital for investigation of short stature. He had always been small, but his parents became worried when his seven-year-old brother overtook him in height. He had been measured two years before and had only grown 3 cm since then. On examination, there was no abnormality apart from his short stature. The history and appropriate tests excluded many of the recognized causes of growth retardation (*see p. 309*).

**Investigations**

serum GH:  4 mU/L (after vigorous exercise)
        4 mU/L (during documented hypogly-
        caemia induced by insulin)

**Comment**

The diagnosis of GH deficiency depends upon the demonstration of subnormal growth velocity and subnormal plasma GH concentrations. Both features are present in this case. If plasma GH concentration is normal (>20 mU/L), either after exercise or in a sample obtained while the child is asleep, this obviates the need to perform the more invasive and hazardous insulin hypoglycaemia test. However, the exercise must be sufficient to make the patient breathless, for example, repeated running up and down stairs. In this case, the response was subnormal and to confirm GH deficiency the insulin hypoglycaemia test was performed; the response was again subnormal.

A fall in blood glucose concentration is sufficient to stimulate GH secretion in normal people, but it is advisable to achieve documented hypoglycaemia (blood glucose <2.2 mmol/L) to ensure an adequate stimulus. Sex steroids are important in determining the magnitude of the response. Equivocal responses in children with pubertal delay require that the test is repeated after priming with either testosterone in boys or oestrogen in girls.

There was no other evidence of pituitary hypofunction in this boy and no evidence of a destructive pituitary lesion. A diagnosis of idiopathic GH deficiency was made. He began treatment with GH and grew at a normal rate thereafter, although he was always shorter than his peers. Typically, the lost height is not completely restored when GH deficiency is treated.

Until the mid 1980s, the only source of GH for patients requiring replacement therapy was pituitary glands of human cadavers and supplies were very limited. However, human biosynthetic GH is now available, produced by bacteria into whose genome the DNA sequence encoding GH has been inserted. Since most cases of isolated GH deficiency are now known to be due to growth hormone releasing hormone (GHRH) deficiency, GHRH may have a therapeutic role in the future. In adults, decreased GH secretion is of uncertain significance and there is as yet no good evidence that replacement treatment is beneficial. The use of GH to promote anabolism in severely catabolic patients is under investigation. Its use to increase muscle mass, e.g., in weightlifters, is inadvisable since harmful side effects can result.

## Pituitary tumours

Pituitary tumours may be purely destructive but are often functional, producing excessive quantities of a hormone.

The order of frequency with which hormone secretion occurs in patients with pituitary tumours is prolactin (relatively common) > GH > ACTH > gonadotrophins > TSH (very rare). Any pituitary tumour may give rise to clinical features due to the destruction of normal pituitary tissue, that is hypopituitarism, and of intracranial space-occupying lesions such as headache, vomiting and papilloedema. Visual field defects may develop when an upward growing tumour impinges on the optic chiasm and occasionally a patient's sight may be threatened.

### Growth hormone excess: acromegaly and gigantism
Acromegaly and gigantism are usually (95% of cases) the result of excessive GH secretion by a pituitary tumour. As a result, there is increased growth of soft tissues and bone. If this occurs before the epiphyses have fused, growth of long bones occurs leading to gigantism. More commonly, GH-secreting tumours occur in adults, producing acromegaly, with increased growth of soft tissues, hands, feet, jaw and internal organs. The GH concentration in a random serum sample is usually raised, but because GH secretion is normally episodic, the clinical diagnosis should be confirmed biochemically by demonstrating a failure of GH suppression in response to an oral glucose tolerance test. In normal subjects, plasma GH concentration falls to less than 2 mU/L during this procedure. In acromegaly and gigantism, GH fails to suppress normally and there may even be an increase in concentration. The glucose response may indicate impaired glucose tolerance (approximately 25% of patients) or, less frequently (10%), diabetes mellitus.

In many patients with acromegaly, TRH causes an increase in GH secretion; the reason for, or relevance of this observation is unclear. Plasma somatomedin-C (IGF-1) concentrations are elevated in patients with acromegaly. Somatomedin-C measurements are helpful in the assessment of otherwise borderline cases, and are used to follow the response of patients to treatment.

The clinical features of excessive GH secretion are related both to the somatic and to the metabolic effects of the hormone (Fig. 7.10). In addition, features due directly to the presence of the pituitary tumour are often present. Hyperprolactinaemia, due either to interference with the normal inhibition of prolactin secretion or (less frequently) to its secretion by the tumour itself, occurs in 30% of patients with acromegaly but there may be impaired secretion of other pituitary hormones. Acromegaly is occasionally a feature of multiple endocrine neoplasia (MEN type I). Approximately 5% of cases are the result of either ectopic secretion of GHRH (e.g., by a bronchial carcinoid tumour) or of GH (by a pancreatic islet cell tumour).

| Clinical features of excessive growth hormone secretion | | |
|---|---|---|
| **Somatic** | **Metabolic** | **Local effects of tumour** |
| increased growth of:<br>    skin, subcutaneous tissues<br>    skull and jaw<br>    hands, feet<br>    long bones, if before fusion<br>        of epiphyses<br><br>excessive sweating, greasy<br>    skin, acne<br>goitre<br>cardiomegaly, hypertension | elevated, non-suppressible<br>    plasma GH concentration<br><br>glucose intolerance<br><br>clinical diabetes mellitus<br><br><br>hypercalcaemia,<br>    hyperphosphataemia | headache<br><br>visual field defects<br><br>hypopituitarism<br><br>diabetes insipidus |

**Fig. 7.10** Clinical features of excessive GH secretion.

**CASE HISTORY 7.3**

A 40-year-old man consulted his general practitioner because he had become impotent. He had also been embarrassed by excessive sweating in the absence of exertion. His wife thought that his facial features had become coarser, and he had recently had to buy a larger pair of shoes than normal because his old ones had become uncomfortable. The GP found mild hypertension and a trace of glycosuria and referred him to an endocrine clinic with a presumptive diagnosis of acromegaly.

**Investigations**

combined pituitary function test: (*see Fig. 7.11*)

oral glucose tolerance test:

| | | | |
|---|---|---|---|
| blood glucose | (initial) | 8.5 mmol/L |
| | (2 h) | 11.5 mmol/L |
| serum GH | (initial) | 22 mU/L |
| | (minimum) | 20 mU/L |

serum: prolactin (at 0 min)          800 mU/L
    testosterone      11 nmol/L
visual fields: partial bitemporal hemianopia

skull radiograph: enlarged pituitary fossa with erosion of anterior clinoid processes

pituitary CT scan: pituitary tumour with suprasellar extension

**Comment**

The clinical diagnosis is confirmed by the high basal GH level which is not suppressed by glucose. The glucose tolerance test gives a diabetic result; abnormal glucose tolerance is seen in about 25% of cases of acromegaly, but clinical diabetes mellitus is present in only about 10%.

The basal prolactin concentration is increased. Gonadotrophins are low and do not increase in response to GnRH. The serum testosterone concentration is at the low end of the normal range due to inadequate testicular stimulation by LH. The cortisol and TSH responses are normal.

The presence of a tumour is confirmed by the radiographic appearances; the optic chiasm lies immediately above the pituitary and compression of it can cause either visual field defects, characteristically a bitemporal hemi- or quadrantanopia, or threaten complete visual failure.

| Case History 7.3: combined pituitary function test | | | | | |
|---|---|---|---|---|---|
| Time (min) | Blood glucose (mmol/L) | Serum cortisol (nmol/L) | Serum LH (U/L) | Serum FSH (U/L) | Serum TSH (mU/L) |
| 0 | 7.6 | 400 | 2.0 | 1.5 | 0.8 |
| 15 | 3.4 | | | | |
| 20 | | | 2.2 | 1.7 | 9.7 |
| 30 | 2.0 | 700 | | | |
| 45 | 2.1 | | | | |
| 60 | 3.3 | 680 | 2.1 | 1.5 | 4.3 |
| 90 | 4.0 | 600 | | | |
| 120 | 4.5 | 550 | | | |

**Fig. 7.11** Results of a combined pituitary function test (see Case History 7.3).

Treatment of acromegaly and gigantism is aimed at reducing excessive GH secretion, preventing or treating deficiencies of other pituitary hormones and preventing damage to surrounding structures, particularly the optic nerves, by the tumour. In practice, it is often difficult to achieve all these goals. The main modes of treatment are surgery, external irradiation and medical therapy. Transphenoidal resection of the pituitary tumour is the treatment of choice in the majority of cases. Occasionally, with large tumours with suprasellar extension, transfrontal craniotomy is necessary. If there is continuing evidence of excessive GH secretion, external irradiation or, more frequently, medical therapy can be used. The most widely used drugs are octreotide, a long-acting analogue of somatostatin, and bromocriptine, a dopamine agonist which stimulates GH secretion in normal subjects but inhibits it in many patients with acromegaly.

When there is accompanying hypopituitarism, appropriate replacement treatment with cortisol, gonadal steroids or gonadotrophins, and thyroxine must be given. All patients with acromegaly and gigantism must be followed up and reassessed regularly for evidence of either recurrence or further loss of normal pituitary function.

### Hyperprolactinaemia

Hyperprolactinaemia is a common endocrine abnormality. It is an important cause of infertility in both males and females, impotence in males and menstrual irregularity in females. These effects are thought to be mediated through inhibition of the pulsatility of GnRH by prolactin. The causes and clinical features of hyperprolactinaemia are summarized in Fig. 7.12. There may also be features related to the cause of the hyperprolactinaemia. The causes include various drugs, which either block pituitary dopaminergic receptors or deplete the brain of dopamine, in addition to pituitary tumours (prolactinoma) and destructive pituitary lesions which interfere with the normal inhibition of prolactin secretion. Prolactinomas are often small (microadenomas, <10 mm diameter) but larger tumours (macroadenomas) do occur, which erode the pituitary fossa and extend outside its confines. Overall, prolactinomas occur more frequently in women but affected men are more likely to have a macroadenoma.

Prolactin is secreted in response to both stress and TRH, and plasma levels also depend on oestrogen status. It is therefore difficult to define an upper limit of normal for plasma prolactin concentration. Less than 400 mU/L is probably normal and more than 600 mU/L, abnormal. Slightly elevated concentrations of prolactin are less likely to be of significance in well-oestrogenized women. Patients with prolactin-secreting tumours usually have basal levels in excess of 2000 mU/L.

Numerous dynamic tests have been proposed to aid in the diagnosis of suspected prolactin-secreting tumours. The most widely used is the measurement of the prolactin response to TRH, which is diminished in most patients with prolactinomas. However, this is not a consistent, nor a specific finding and neither the TRH nor any other dynamic test is of established value in the diagnosis of prolactinomas. However, if a tumour is diagnosed, patients must be tested for deficient secretion of other anterior pituitary hormones. With small tumours, other pituitary functions are usually normal.

The majority of patients with small prolactin-secreting tumours are treated either with bromocriptine (or another dopamine agonist), or by transphenoidal resection. Surgery may be curative but recurrence is common. Bromocriptine treatment usually needs to be given chronically although in some patients, hyperprolactinaemia does not recur on withdrawal of the drug. With larger tumours, the chances of effecting a cure are lower, but shrinkage of the tumour and substantial reductions in prolactin concentration occur in approximately 75% of patients treated with bromocriptine. Such treatment can be used as a preliminary to surgery. External irradiation may be helpful in some cases.

### Cushing's disease

Cushing's disease, in which increased secretion of cortisol by the adrenal cortex is secondary to increased secretion of ACTH by the anterior pituitary, is discussed in *Chapter 8*. Patients who have been treated for Cushing's disease by adrenalectomy alone may later develop hyperpigmentation and the clinical features of a large pituitary tumour (Nelson's syndrome). The pigmentation is due to the melanocyte-stimulating activity of ACTH and its precursors. Nelson's syndrome is uncommon in patients in whom treatment for Cushing's disease has included pituitary surgery or irradiation in addition to adrenalectomy.

### Other conditions related to pituitary tumours

Tumours which secrete TSH or gonadotrophins are rare. Occasionally, TSH-secreting tumours develop in patients with long-standing untreated hypothyroidism but these regress when replacement treatment is given. Thirty per cent of pituitary tumours, usually chromophobe adenomas, are non-functioning. They can present with features of hypopituitarism or due to the physical presence of the tumour and are occasionally diagnosed incidentally from a skull radiograph taken for some other purpose.

| Hyperprolactinaemia |
|---|
| **Causes** |
| **Physiological** <br> stress, sleep, pregnancy, suckling |
| **Drugs** <br> dopaminergic receptor blockers, <br>    e.g., phenothiazines, haloperidol <br> dopamine-depleting agents, <br>    e.g., methyldopa, reserpine <br> others, <br>    e.g., oestrogens, TRH |
| **Pituitary disorders** <br> prolactin-secreting tumour (prolactinoma) <br> tumours blocking dopaminergic inhibition <br>    of prolactin secretion <br> pituitary stalk section and surgery |
| **Others** <br> hypothyroidism <br> ectopic secretion <br> chronic renal failure |
| **Clinical features** |
| **Females** <br> oligomenorrhoea and amenorrhoea <br> infertility <br> galactorrhoea |
| **Males** <br> impotence <br> infertility <br> gynaecomastia |

**Fig. 7.12** Causes and clinical features of hyperprolactinaemia.

Some non-functioning pituitary tumours are able to synthesize hormones but do not secrete them or secrete only the α-subunit. Measurement of plasma α-subunit concentration may be useful in assessing the success of treatment in such cases.

## POSTERIOR PITUITARY HORMONES

The posterior pituitary secretes two hormones, vasopressin (antidiuretic hormone, ADH) and oxytocin. These hormones are synthesized in the hypothalamus and pass down nerve axons into the posterior pituitary, from where they are released into the circulation. Oxytocin is involved in the control of uterine contractility and of milk release from the lactating breast. Disorders of its secretion are probably uncommon and are not clinically important. In contrast, vasopressin is essential to life and disorders of its secretion are well recognized.

## Vasopressin

Vasopressin has a vital role in the control of the tonicity of the extracellular fluid, and hence indirectly of the intracellular fluid, and of water balance. Excessive secretion results in dilutional hyponatraemia, with a risk of water intoxication, while decreased secretion results in diabetes insipidus, a condition in which there is uncontrolled excretion of water with a tendency to severe dehydration. The syndromes of excessive secretion of vasopressin are discussed *on p. 23*; they are frequently seen in conditions which do not affect the pituitary directly. Diabetes insipidus, on the other hand, is usually due to pituitary or hypothalamic disease (*Fig. 7.13*), although it can also be due to a failure of the kidneys to respond to the hormone (nephrogenic diabetes insipidus).

In diabetes insipidus, the lack of vasopressin results in polyuria and thirst. Unless the hypothalamic thirst centre is also damaged, thirst leads to increased fluid intake (polydipsia). The differential diagnosis includes other conditions causing polyuria and polydipsia, for example, diabetes mellitus, chronic renal failure, hypercalcaemia and hypokalaemia. Simple tests will eliminate these possibilities.

A compulsive desire to drink (psychogenic or primary polydipsia) also causes polyuria. However, in this case polyuria is secondary to increased fluid intake, while in diabetes insipidus the opposite applies, polydipsia being a response to polyuria. In both conditions, the urine is dilute, but in diabetes insipidus there is a tendency towards an increased plasma osmolality (>295 mmol/kg) and hypernatraemia, whereas with primary polydipsia, the tendency is to a decreased osmolality (<280 mmol/kg) and hyponatraemia. If a random urine osmolality is greater than 750 mmol/kg, diabetes insipidus is excluded.

If there is any doubt about the diagnosis, a fluid deprivation test should be performed (*Fig. 7.14*). This is effectively a biological assay for vasopressin which is difficult to measure in plasma. Patients with diabetes insipidus may become dangerously dehydrated if denied access to fluid; they may also exercise considerable ingenuity to obtain fluid. Close supervision is therefore required and the test must always be performed by day, not overnight.

| Causes of diabetes insipidus |
| --- |

**Cranial**
tumours:
   craniopharyngioma
   secondary tumours
   pituitary tumours with suprasellar extension
granulomatous disease
meningitis and encephalitis
vascular disorders
trauma
surgery (often transient)
idiopathic
familial

**Nephrogenic**
congenital
metabolic:
   hypokalaemia
   hypercalcaemia
drugs:
   lithium
   demeclocycline
post-obstructive uropathy
chronic renal disease:
   pyelonephritis
   polycystic disease
   amyloid
   sickle cell disease

**Fig. 7.13** Causes of diabetes insipidus.

In a normal subject, the urine becomes concentrated in response to fluid deprivation and plasma osmolality does not exceed 295 mmol/kg. In diabetes insipidus, the urine does not become concentrated and plasma osmolality rises. In patients who are water overloaded before the test is started, the urine may not become concentrated; plasma osmolality is usually low and may remain so since vasopressin secretion is only stimulated if it rises above 285 mmol/kg. Thus the urine becomes concentrated only if the plasma osmolality exceeds this level.

At the end of the eight-hour period, the patient is allowed to drink water and is given 1-desamino-D-argininevasopressin (desmopressin), a synthetic analogue of vasopressin. In cranial diabetes insipidus, the urine should become concentrated; in patients whose kidneys are insensitive to vasopressin (nephrogenic diabetes insipidus) it remains dilute. If the water deprivation test is to be carried out on a patient with anterior pituitary disease, adequate cortisol replacement must be provided.

| Fluid deprivation test |
| --- |
| **Procedure** |
| allow fluids overnight before test and give light breakfast with no fluid; no smoking permitted |
| weigh patient |
| allow no fluid for 8 h; patient must be under constant supervision during this time |
| every hour: <br> 1. weigh patient; stop test if body weight falls by >3% <br> 2. ask patient to empty bladder; measure volume and osmolality of urine |
| collect blood for measurement of plasma osmolality at 30 min and 3.5, 6.5 and 7.5 h; stop test if osmolality exceeds 300 mmol/kg |
| after 8 h allow patient to drink and give 20 µg desmopressin intranasally |
| collect urine hourly for a further 4 h |
| **Results** |
| diabetes insipidus diagnosed if: <br> weight loss >3% initial body weight <br> plasma osmolality exceeds 300 mmol/kg <br> urine : plasma osmolality ratio does not exceed 1.9, provided plasma osmolality exceeds 285 mmol/kg <br><br> nephrogenic diabetes insipidus diagnosed if urine does not become concentrated after 4 h of desmopressin |

**Fig. 7.14** Fluid deprivation test. The first eight hours test for the ability to concentrate the urine and hence differentiate between diabetes insipidus and primary polydipsia. The final hours, after the administration of desmopressin, test for the kidneys' ability to respond to vasopressin and therefore differentiate between cranial and nephrogenic diabetes insipidus. The results of this test may be equivocal, necessitating further investigation.

If the results of a fluid deprivation test are equivocal, the plasma vasopressin response to hypertonic saline infusion should be assessed. The response is normal in patients with nephrogenic diabetes insipidus or primary polydipsia, but decreased in patients with cranial diabetes insipidus (*Fig. 7.15*). The former two conditions can be distinguished by comparing plasma vasopressin concentration with urine osmolality after a period of fluid deprivation (*Fig. 7.16*). In nephrogenic diabetes insipidus, plasma vasopressin is much higher than normal. Alternatively, since vasopressin measurements are not widely available, a closely supervised therapeutic trial of desmopressin treatment can be used. This causes an improvement in cranial diabetes insipidus, has no effect in the nephrogenic type and causes increasing

hyponatraemia in primary polydipsia. An algorithm for the investigation of polyuria is given in *Fig. 7.17*.

**CASE HISTORY 7.4**

A middle-aged woman, who had undergone mastectomy and local radiotherapy for carcinoma of the breast two years previously, attended for her regular outpatient appointment. There was no sign of recurrence but she complained of increasing thirst over the previous months and that she was passing copious amounts of urine. The thirst became intolerable if she went without water for more than a few hours and her sleep was disturbed by the frequent need to pass urine and have a drink. There was no glycosuria; serum creatinine, potassium and calcium concentrations were all normal. She was admitted for investigation.

### Investigations

random plasma: osmolality      295 mmol/kg
             sodium        144 mmol/L
urine osmolality           90 mmol/kg

Fluid deprivation test: after six hours' water deprivation her weight had fallen from 60 kg to 57.6 kg; the test was therefore stopped.

at end of test:    plasma osmolality 307 mmol/kg
                urine osmolality    220 mmol/kg

She was then allowed to drink and was given a dose of desmopressin. Following this her urine osmolality rose to 610 mmol/kg.

### Comment

The history of intolerable thirst with a slightly raised plasma osmolality yet dilute urine is very suggestive of diabetes insipidus and this diagnosis is confirmed by the failure to conserve water and concentrate the urine during water deprivation. She responded to desmopressin, indicating that vasopressin deficiency, rather than renal insensitivity to the hormone, was the cause of her symptoms.

She was treated successfully with regular administration of desmopressin and her symptoms resolved. A skull radiograph was normal but CT scanning revealed a small lesion in the region of the hypothalamus. The patient died one year later, with extensive cerebral metastatic deposits from her breast carcinoma.

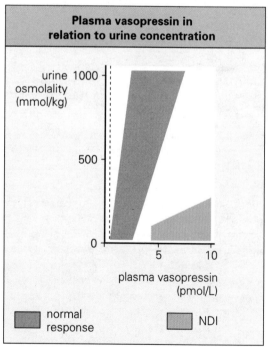

**Fig. 7.15** Hypertonic saline infusion.
Typical responses to the intravenous infusion of 5% saline are shown for patients with nephrogenic diabetes insipidus (NDI), cranial diabetes insipidus (CDI) and primary polydipsia (PP).

**Fig. 7.16** Plasma vasopressin in relation to urine concentration. In nephrogenic diabetes insipidus (NDI), vasopressin concentrations are inappropriately high in relation to urine osmolality.

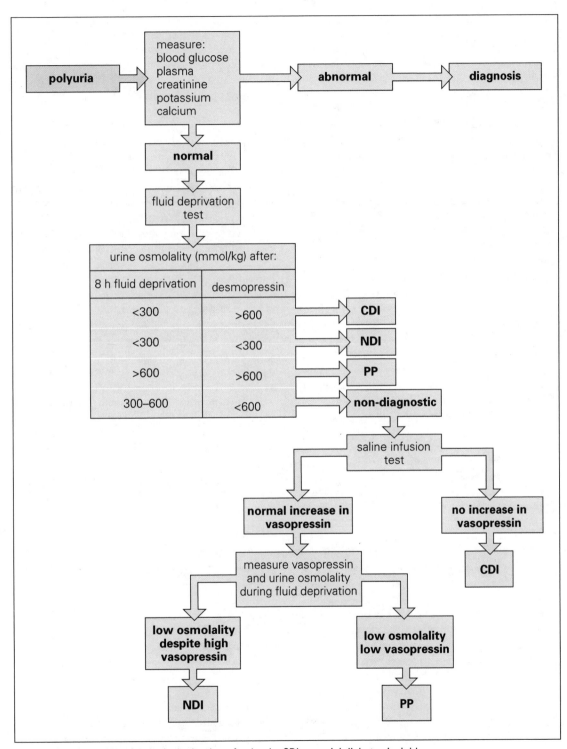

**Fig. 7.17** An algorithm for the investigation of polyuria. CDI = cranial diabetes insipidus, NDI = nephrogenic diabetes insipidus, PP = primary polydipsia.

In about one-third of cases of cranial diabetes insipidus there is no obvious underlying cause. Some of these cases have a familial incidence and the onset may then be very sudden. Urine output in diabetes insipidus may exceed 10 L/24 h although less than this is more usual. Patients with nephrogenic diabetes insipidus are insensitive to vasopressin, which is secreted in either normal or increased amounts in such patients. The congenital form is inherited as an X-linked recessive disorder; the defect is in the adenylate cyclase mechanism responsible for mediating the action of vasopressin after it has become bound to receptors.

### Management of diabetes insipidus

Patients must always have access to adequate fluid and whenever possible, the underlying disease should be treated. Cranial diabetes insipidus is usually treated with desmopressin, given as a nasal spray, although mild cases may successfully be treated with chlorpropamide, an oral hypoglycaemic agent which also increases renal sensitivity to vasopressin (hypoglycaemia is a possible side-effect). Patients must learn to monitor their fluid output and input in order to avoid water intoxication. This may be a particular problem if the sensation of thirst is blunted.

Patients with nephrogenic diabetes insipidus, because they do not respond to vasopressin, must maintain an adequate water intake to avoid dehydration. Hydronephrosis and hydroureter secondary to bladder distension may occur and lead to renal impairment. Thiazide diuretics, which induce a state of sodium depletion, increasing renal sodium and water retention, may reduce the polyuria. Potassium supplements or the concomitant use of a potassium-sparing diuretic may be necessary to prevent hypokalaemia.

## SUMMARY

The anterior pituitary gland secretes growth hormone and prolactin, and trophic hormones which control the activity of the gonads (luteinizing hormone and follicle-stimulating hormone), thyroid (thyroid-stimulating hormone) and the adrenal cortex (adrenocorticotrophic hormone). The secretion of all these hormones is regulated by hypothalamic hormones, which reach the pituitary through a portal system of blood vessels. The trophic hormones are in addition controlled by feedback mechanisms involving the hormones produced by the respective target organs.

Anterior pituitary hypofunction may result in the inadequate production of one or more hormones and the clinical manifestations depend upon the particular pattern of deficiency. It may either be the result of disease affecting the pituitary itself or be secondary to hypothalamic disease, with failure of production of hypothalamic hormones. Pituitary hypofunction (hypopituitarism) is investigated by tests designed to stimulate the production of pituitary hormones.

Pituitary tumours can cause hypopituitarism by destroying normal pituitary tissue, but may be functional and produce syndromes related to excessive hormone secretion. Pituitary tumours producing prolactin, growth hormone and adrenocorticotrophic hormone are well-recognized but secretion of gonadotrophins or thyroid-stimulating hormone is rare. In addition to their endocrine effects, both functional and non-functional tumours can give rise to clinical features characteristic of intracranial space occupying lesions.

The posterior pituitary gland secretes oxytocin and vasopressin. Both are synthesized in the hypothalamus and reach the posterior pituitary through nerve axons. Because of this, damage to the posterior pituitary may only cause temporary failure of hormone secretion. Oxytocin stimulates uterine contraction during labour but does not appear to be an essential hormone.

Vasopressin is essential as it controls water excretion by altering the permeability of the renal collecting tubules to water in response to changes in extracellular fluid osmolality. Excessive vasopressin secretion produces water retention with a dilutional hyponatraemia. Defective vasopressin secretion results in diabetes insipidus, with uncontrolled renal water loss. Diabetes insipidus can also be due to renal insensitivity to vasopressin; the two types can be distinguished from each other, and from psychogenic polydipsia, by a fluid deprivation test.

## FURTHER READING

Besser G M & Thorner M O (eds) (1994) *Clinical Endocrinology: An Illustrated Text*. 2nd edition. London: Wolfe.

Hall R & Besser M (eds) (1989) *Fundamentals of Clinical Endocrinology*. 4th edition. London: Churchill Livingstone.

Molitch M E (ed.) (1987) Pituitary Tumours: Diagnosis and Management. *Endocrinology and Metabolism Clinics of North America*, **16**, 475–828.

Wilson J D & Foster D W (eds) (1992) *Williams–Textbook of Endocrinology*. 8th edition. Philadelphia: WB Saunders Company.

# 8. The Adrenal Glands

## INTRODUCTION

The adrenal glands have two functionally distinct parts, the cortex and the medulla. The adrenal cortex is essential to life; it produces three classes of steroid hormone, glucocorticoids, mineralocorticoids and androgens. The medulla, which is functionally part of the sympathetic nervous system, is not essential to life and its pathological importance is related mainly to the occurrence of rare catecholamine-secreting tumours.

Glucocorticoids, of which the most important is cortisol, are secreted in response to adrenocorticotrophic hormone (ACTH), which is itself secreted by the pituitary in response to hypothalamic corticotrophin releasing hormone (CRH). Cortisol exerts negative feedback control on ACTH release. Glucocorticoids have many physiological functions (*Fig. 8.1*) and are particularly important in mediating the body's response to stress.

The most important mineralocorticoid is aldosterone. This is secreted in response to angiotensin II, produced as a result of the activation of the renin–angiotensin system by a decrease in renal blood flow and other indicators of decreased extracellular fluid volume (*Fig. 8.2*). Secretion of aldosterone is also directly stimulated by hyperkalaemia. The main action of aldosterone is to stimulate sodium reabsorption in the distal convoluted tubules in the kidney in exchange for potassium and hydrogen ions; it thus has a central role in the determination of the extracellular fluid (ECF) volume. ACTH does not have a major physiological role in aldosterone secretion. A single injection of ACTH

| Functions of glucocorticoids |
|---|
| increase protein catabolism |
| increase hepatic glycogen synthesis |
| increase hepatic gluconeogenesis |
| inhibit ACTH secretion (negative feedback mechanism) |
| sensitize arterioles to action of noradrenaline, hence involved in maintenance of blood pressure |
| permissive effect on water excretion; required for initiation of diuresis in response to water loading |

**Fig. 8.1** Principal physiological functions of glucocorticoids.

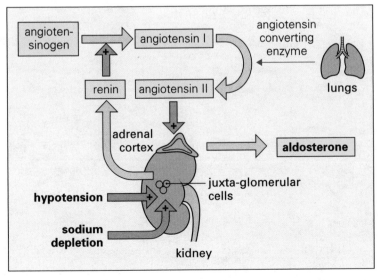

**Fig. 8.2** Stimulation of aldosterone secretion through activation of the renin–angiotensin system. Renin, released into the plasma from the juxtaglomerular cells of the kidney in response to various stimuli, catalyzes the formation of angiotensin I from angiotensinogen, an $\alpha_2$-globulin. Angiotensin I is metabolized to an octapeptide, angiotensin II, by angiotensin converting enzyme during its passage through the lungs. Angiotensin II stimulates the release of aldosterone from the adrenal cortex.

increases plasma aldosterone concentration, but ACTH infusion does not cause a sustained increase. Curiously, the secretion of aldosterone by adrenal tumours is affected by ACTH (*see p. 133*).

The adrenal cortex is also a source of androgens, including dehydroepiandrosterone (DHEA), DHEA-sulphate (DHEAS) and androstenedione. The clinical effects of excessive adrenal androgens may be a prominent feature of adrenal disorders in females.

## ADRENAL STEROID HORMONE BIOSYNTHESIS

The hormones secreted by the adrenal cortex are synthesized from cholesterol by a sequence of enzyme-catalyzed reactions (*Fig. 8.3*). An awareness of these pathways is important for the understanding of congenital adrenal hyperplasia, a group of conditions each caused by a lack of one of these enzymes.

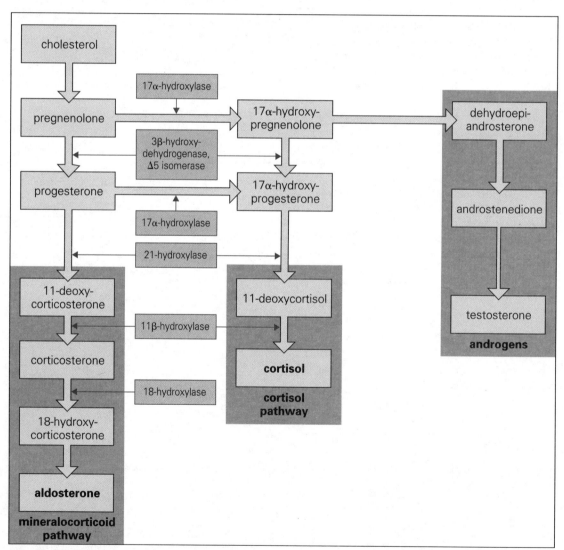

**Fig. 8.3** Biosynthesis of adrenal steroid hormones. Cortisol and the androgens are synthesized in the zona recticularis and zona fasciculata of the adrenal glands.

18-hydroxylase, required for the synthesis of aldosterone, is present only in the zona glomerulosa.

# MEASUREMENT OF ADRENAL STEROID HORMONES

The advent of sensitive and specific immunoassays for the steroid hormones has rendered obsolete the measurement of chemically related substances including hormones, for example 17-oxosteroids (adrenal androgens) and 17-oxogenic steroids (cortisol and related substances). The formerly widely used fluorometric assay for cortisol is now also obsolete. Specific immunoassays are available for the measurement of cortisol, aldosterone, 17α-hydroxyprogesterone and the principal adrenal androgens. Plasma measurements are most widely used but fluctuations in the plasma concentrations of these hormones occur for a number of reasons and the results of single estimations must be interpreted with caution.

The measurement of urinary cortisol excretion is valuable in the investigations of Cushing's syndrome. Urinary 'steroid profiling', in which steroids are separated and quantitated by gas–liquid chromatography, can be helpful in the investigation of suspected congenital adrenal hyperplasia.

## Cortisol

Ninety-five per cent of cortisol in the blood is bound to protein, principally to the cortisol-binding globulin, transcortin. Thus the amount of free cortisol that can be excreted unchanged in the urine is very small. Transcortin is almost fully saturated at normal cortisol concentrations and it follows that if cortisol production is increased, the concentration present in the plasma in the free form, and thus the amount which is excreted, increases to a disproportionately greater extent than the total. For this reason, measurement of the 24-hour urinary excretion of cortisol, provided that an accurate urine collection can be made, is a sensitive way of detecting increased, but not decreased, secretion of the hormone.

Plasma cortisol concentrations show a diurnal variation, being highest in the morning and lowest at night (*Fig. 8.4*). Blood for cortisol measurement should usually be drawn between 0800 h and 0900 h; however, samples are taken at 2300 h to detect loss of the diurnal variation, an early feature of adrenal hyperfunction (Cushing's syndrome). Random measurements are rarely of any value in the diagnosis of adrenal disease, except that a high concentration in a sick patient may reasonably be taken to exclude adrenal failure.

Cortisol is secreted in response to stress, mediated through ACTH, and thus stress must be kept to a minimum if results are to be interpreted correctly. Investigations of adrenal hypo- or hyperfunction often involve measurement of cortisol after attempting to stimulate or suppress its secretion.

When interpreting plasma cortisol results, it must be remembered that the synthetic glucocorticoid, prednisolone, can cross-react with cortisol in immunoassays for

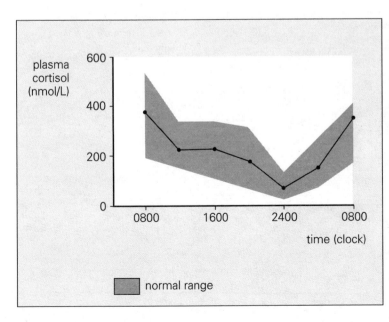

**Fig. 8.4** Diurnal variation in plasma cortisol concentration. Plasma cortisol levels are at their highest shortly after waking and then decline throughout the day to reach a nadir in the late evening. Because of this variation, it is important that blood samples are taken at times that coincide either with the peak or the trough, random samples being of little value. The graph shows mean values and the range in a sample of healthy men.

the hormone. Cross-reaction does not occur with dexamethasone. Spironolactone, an aldosterone antagonist used as a potassium-sparing diuretic, cross-reacts with cortisol in the formerly used fluorometric assay, but not in immunoassays.

## Aldosterone

Plasma aldosterone concentration varies with posture and blood should usually be drawn from patients after they have been recumbent overnight and then, for comparison, after a period of being upright. Aldosterone secretion is stimulated via the action of renin and therefore it is often appropriate to measure the plasma renin activity at the same time as the aldosterone to establish whether aldosterone secretion is autonomous or under normal control. This point is discussed further in connection with Conn's syndrome and aldosteronism (*see p. 131*).

## Androgens

Measurements of adrenal androgens are of value in the diagnosis and management of congenital adrenal hyperplasia (*see p. 133*) and in the investigation of virilization in women (*see Chapter 10*).

## DISORDERS OF THE ADRENAL CORTEX

Adrenal disorders may present with clinical features related either to hypo- or hyperfunction. In congenital adrenal hyperplasia, a combination of features may be present.

## Adrenal hypofunction (Addison's disease)

The common causes and clinical features of this disease are listed in *Fig. 8.5*. The cases originally described by Addison were caused by tuberculosis but autoimmune disease is now the major cause in the United Kingdom. In such cases, adrenal autoantibodies will usually be present and there may be associated autoimmune disease of other organs, for example, pernicious anaemia.

The commonest cause of adrenal hypofunction is suppression of the pituitary–adrenal axis by glucocorticoids used therapeutically. Although during treatment patients may develop features of Cushing's syndrome, a sudden withdrawal of steroids or failure to increase the dose during stress (e.g., surgery) may precipitate acute adrenal failure. Normal pituitary–adrenal function is regained only slowly when steroids are withdrawn and it is essential that the dosage is reduced gradually when steroid treatment is to be discontinued.

The majority of the clinical features of adrenal failure are due to the lack of glucocorticoids and mineralocorticoids. Increased pigmentation is due to the high plasma concentration of ACTH. This hormone has some melanocyte-stimulating activity and its concentration is increased as a result of the loss of negative feedback control by cortisol.

Adrenal failure usually has an insidious onset but may develop acutely. Adrenal crisis is a medical emergency. The clinical features include severe hypovolaemia, shock and hypoglycaemia. It may be precipitated by stress, e.g., due

| Adrenal hypofunction | |
|---|---|
| **Causes** | **Clinical features** |
| **Common**<br>autoimmune adrenalitis<br>tuberculosis<br>adrenalectomy | **Common**<br>tiredness, generalized weakness<br>  and lethargy<br>anorexia, nausea, vomiting<br>weight loss<br>dizziness and postural hypotension<br>pigmentation<br>loss of body hair  (women) |
| **Less common**<br>secondary tumour<br>  deposits<br>amyloidosis<br>haemochromatosis<br>histoplasmosis<br>adrenal haemorrhage | **Less common**<br>hypoglycaemia<br>depression |

**Fig. 8.5** Causes and clinical features of primary adrenal hypofunction.

to infection, trauma or surgery, in patients with incipient adrenal failure. Patients being treated with glucocorticoids, whether in physiological doses (replacement therapy) or pharmacological doses (e.g., in severe inflammatory conditions) are also susceptible to adrenal failure in these circumstances if the dosage is not increased. Haemorrhage into the adrenal glands may occur as a complication of anticoagulant treatment and in meningococcal septicaemia, and can result in acute adrenal failure.

## CASE HISTORY 8.1

A 17-year-old girl presented with a two-month history of tiredness and lethargy. She had noticed that she became dizzy when she stood up. On examination, she had pigmentation of the buccal mucosa and palmar creases and in an old appendicectomy scar. Her blood pressure was 120/80 mmHg lying down, but fell to 90/50 mmHg when she stood up.

### Investigations

| serum: | sodium | 128 mmol/L |
|---|---|---|
| | potassium | 5.4 mmol/L |
| | urea | 8.5 mmol/L |

blood glucose (fasting)      2.5 mmol/L

short Synacthen test:
  plasma cortisol:

| 0900 h | 150 nmol/L |
|---|---|
| 30 min after Synacthen | 160 nmol/L |
| 60 min after Synacthen | 160 nmol/L |

plasma ACTH (0900 h)      500 ng/L
    (normal <50 ng/L)

anti-adrenal antibodies were detectable at a titre of 1 in 20

### Comment

On the basis of these results, a diagnosis of primary adrenal failure was made. Her symptoms resolved rapidly after starting glucocorticoid and mineralocorticoid replacement and she remained well thereafter. Postural hypotension is a common finding in adrenal failure; it is due to a decrease in ECF volume caused by a lack of aldosterone leading to sodium loss. This decrease in ECF volume may also cause a degree of prerenal uraemia as demonstrated in this case. Hyponatraemia is not always present in adrenal failure, particularly in the early stages. Sodium is lost isotonically from the kidneys, but the lack of cortisol may cause water retention and with severe hypovolaemia, vasopressin (antidiuretic hormone, ADH) secretion is stimulated. Deficiency of aldosterone is also responsible for potassium retention and thus hyperkalaemia.

The fasting blood glucose is at the low end of the reference range in this patient; the unopposed action of insulin may cause symptomatic hypoglycaemia.

The 0900 h cortisol is at the lower limit of the reference range and there is virtually no response to Synacthen. Except in very severe cases, cortisol is measurable in the plasma, even though the concentration is low–normal or frankly low. However, this represents the adrenal glands' maximal output since they are already stimulated by the high level of endogenous ACTH.

Adrenal failure can occur secondarily to pituitary failure when, although the adrenal glands are normal, there is decreased stimulation by ACTH. Other features of hypopituitarism may be present (see p. 110); in contrast to patients with primary adrenal failure, abnormal pigmentation does not occur.

Hypotension may also occur in secondary adrenal failure because the sensitivity of arteriolar smooth muscle to catecholamines is reduced by a lack of cortisol. Hyponatraemia may sometimes be present since the lack of cortisol reduces the ability of the kidneys to excrete a water load, but there is no renal salt wasting since aldosterone secretion is not dependent upon ACTH.

Unless a patient is being treated with synthetic corticosteroids, a plasma cortisol concentration of <50 nmol/L in a blood sample drawn at 0900 h is effectively diagnostic of adrenal failure, while a concentration >550 nmol/L excludes the diagnosis. However, in the majority of patients with adrenal failure, whether primary or secondary, the plasma cortisol concentration lies between these extremes, and a Synacthen test must be performed to establish the diagnosis. Synacthen is a synthetic analogue of ACTH. The normal response to a single dose of soluble ACTH ('short Synacthen test') is shown in *Fig. 8.6.* If the response is in any way abnormal the patient should be assumed to have adrenal failure. In both primary and secondary adrenal failure, the response in the short Synacthen test is absent or blunted (*see Case History 8.1*). This should be regarded as a screening test for adrenal failure; unless the clinical features leave no doubt that primary adrenal disease is responsible, it should be followed by a long Synacthen test (*Fig. 8.6*). In this test, depot Synacthen, which has a longer duration of action, is given daily for three days. Plasma cortisol concentration is measured each day and again 24 hours after the last dose. In primary adrenal failure, plasma cortisol concentrations remain low; in secondary adrenal failure the concentration increases. An alternative version of the long Synacthen test involves only a single dose of depot Synacthen, with plasma cortisol estimations made at various times up to 24 hours, but this is likely to be less sensitive if secondary adrenal failure is long-standing.

Although ideally these tests should be done before starting treatment, when a severely ill patient is judged clinically to have adrenal failure, treatment should not be delayed. A blood sample can be taken immediately for later cortisol measurement. Treatment can then be commenced with a synthetic glucocorticoid which does not cross-react with

cortisol in the laboratory assay (e.g., dexamethasone) and a Synacthen test performed as soon as is convenient. The results will not be vitiated by the treatment if only a short time elapses before the test is done.

The best differentiation between primary and secondary adrenal failure is provided by measurements of plasma ACTH, if this assay is available. In primary adrenal failure, pituitary ACTH production is greatly increased because of the lack of negative feedback control by cortisol, whereas in secondary adrenal failure the plasma level of ACTH is low.

Patients with adrenal failure require life-long replacement therapy, usually with both hydrocortisone and 9α-fludrocortisone, a synthetic mineralocorticoid. Hydrocortisone replacement is usually given in two unequal doses, in the morning (the larger dose) and in the early evening. The adequacy of replacement can be assessed clinically and by measuring plasma cortisol concentration at intervals throughout the day (cortisol 'day curve'); this allows detection of a concentration that is too high shortly after a dose or too low shortly before the next dose is due. Mineralocorticoid treatment can be assessed by measuring plasma renin activity; elevated activity implies inadequate replacement and complete suppression, excessive replacement.

| Synacthen stimulation tests | |
|---|---|
| **Short test** | **Long test** |
| **Procedure**<br>take blood sample at 0900 h for measurement of cortisol<br><br>inject 250 µg Synacthen i.m.<br><br>take further blood samples after 30 and 60 min for cortisol measurement | **Procedure**<br>day 1: inject 1 mg depot Synacthen i.m.<br><br>days 2 and 3: repeat<br><br>day 4: measure plasma cortisol at 0900 h |
| **Normal results**<br>plasma cortisol:<br>  baseline        >190 nmol/L<br>  after Synacthen   increment of 200 nmol/L<br>                with peak of >550 nmol/L | **Results**<br>Primary adrenal insufficiency: plasma cortisol on day 4 <200 nmol/L (usually <100 nmol/L)<br><br>secondary adrenal insufficiency (hypothalamic or hypopituitarism): plasma cortisol on day 4 at least 200 nmol/L above baseline |

**Fig. 8.6** Synacthen stimulation tests for the diagnosis of adrenal failure. It is important to note that blood should be taken for ACTH assay (if available), before giving Synacthen. It is not necessary to withhold any treatment until after the tests are completed, provided that the drug being used does not cross-react with cortisol, since exogenous steroids do not affect the response of the adrenal gland to ACTH in the short term.

Hydrocortisone has some intrinsic mineralocorticoid activity, and occasionally patients may be free of symptoms on hydrocortisone alone, particularly if they maintain a high salt intake.

---

### CASE HISTORY 8.2

A 40-year-old woman presented with a history of tiredness, constipation and general malaise. The clinical diagnosis of hypothyroidism was confirmed by a serum TSH of 60 mU/L and she was started on replacement therapy with thyroxine. Shortly afterwards, she developed abdominal pain, vomiting and diarrhoea after a meal including cold chicken. These symptoms persisted and were unusually severe, and thus her General Practitioner referred her to the Emergency Clinic at the local hospital. On examination she was severely dehydrated and hypotensive; blood was taken for investigations and intravenous saline infusion was started.

**Investigations**

serum:  sodium        120 mmol/L
        potassium     5.6 mmol/L
        urea          12 mmol/L
        glucose       2.5 mmol/L

The medical registrar wondered if she might have adrenal failure, and on more careful examination, noticed that she had pigmentation over her knees and knuckles. He asked the laboratory to save the remaining serum for cortisol measurement and started intravenous hydrocortisone. Her condition improved rapidly; the laboratory later reported that the cortisol concentration was <50 nmol/L.

**Comment**

Adrenal failure often develops insidiously but adrenal crisis can be precipitated at any time by stress. Another factor of relevance in this case is the hypothyroidism. Organ-specific autoimmune diseases can occur in association, and treatment of hypothyroidism in a patient with coexistent incipient adrenal failure can cause this to become clinically overt.

---

## Adrenal hyperfunction

In Cushing's syndrome, there is overproduction primarily of glucocorticoids though mineralocorticoid and androgen production may also be excessive. In Conn's syndrome, mineralocorticoids alone are produced in excess.

### Cushing's syndrome

The causes and clinical features of Cushing's syndrome are listed in *Fig. 8.7*. Pituitary-dependent adrenal hyperfunction is known specifically as Cushing's disease. The clinical features are due primarily to excessive cortisol but cortisol precursors and indeed cortisol itself have some mineralocorticoid activity. Thus sodium retention, leading to hypertension, and potassium wasting, causing a hypokalaemic alkalosis, are common findings except in iatrogenic disease (synthetic glucocorticoids have no mineralocorticoid activity). Increased production of adrenal androgens may also contribute to the clinical presentation.

Pseudo-Cushing's syndrome, in which patients appear cushingoid and may have some of the biochemical abnor-

| Cushing's syndrome |
| --- |
| **Causes** |
| corticosteroid or ACTH treatment<br>pituitary hypersecretion of ACTH (Cushing's disease)<br>adrenal adenoma<br>adrenal carcinoma<br>ectopic ACTH secretion by tumours, e.g., carcinoma of bronchus and carcinoid tumours |
| **Clinical features** |
| truncal obesity ('moon face', buffalo hump and protruberant abdomen)<br>thinning of skin<br>purple striae<br>excessive bruising<br>hirsutism, especially in adrenal carcinoma<br>skin pigmentation (only if ACTH elevated)<br>hypertension<br>glucose intolerance<br>muscle weakness and wasting, especially of proximal muscles<br>menstrual irregularities, hirsutism<br>back pain (osteoporosis and vertebral collapse)<br>psychiatric disturbances:<br>    euphoria<br>    mania<br>    depression |

**Fig. 8.7** Causes and clinical features of Cushing's syndrome.

| Screening tests for Cushing's syndrome | |
|---|---|
| **Test** | **Normal result** |
| 24 h urinary cortisol excretion | <300 nmol/24 h |
| overnight/48 h low dose dexamethasone suppression test | plasma cortisol <50 nmol/L at 0900 h |
| insulin hypoglycaemia test | plasma cortisol increases by at least 200 nmol/L in response to hypoglycaemia |

**Fig. 8.8** Screening tests for Cushing's syndrome. The values for cortisol concentration used for diagnosis may vary slightly between laboratories. Cushing's syndrome is excluded by normal results in these tests.

malities of true Cushing's disease, can occur in severe depression and in alcoholics. Alcohol-related pseudo-Cushing's syndrome usually resolves rapidly on withdrawal of alcohol. Patients with severe obesity may also look cushingoid, but Cushing's syndrome is a very rare cause of obesity.

There are two diagnostic steps in the investigation of a patient with suspected Cushing's syndrome: the demonstration of high plasma cortisol levels and the elucidation of the cause. It is common to see patients who look cushingoid; however, it is much less common that Cushing's syndrome is the cause. It is therefore often useful to carry out preliminary tests on an outpatient basis, aimed at excluding those patients who do not have adrenal disease and identifying those who may, and who thus merit further investigation. Tests used for this purpose (*Fig. 8.8*) are the measurement of 24 h urinary cortisol excretion, the overnight or low-dose dexamethasone suppression test, and the insulin hypoglycaemia test. Isolated measurements of plasma cortisol concentration are of no value. They are often normal during the day in patients with Cushing's syndrome.

Normal 24 h urinary cortisol excretion is <300 nmol. Increased excretion is characteristic of Cushing's syndrome (though it can also occur in pseudo-Cushing's and severe obesity), but care is required in the interpretation of results. If the urine collection is incomplete, the true excretion will be underestimated. This problem may be obviated by expressing the results as a fraction of the urinary creatinine excretion.

Dexamethasone is a synthetic glucocorticoid which binds to cortisol receptors in the pituitary and suppresses ACTH release (and thus the secretion of cortisol by the adrenals) in normal individuals. In the overnight test, 1 mg is given at night and blood is drawn for measurement of cortisol at 0900 h the next morning. In normal individuals this should be <50 nmol/L. A failure of suppression is characteristic of Cushing's syndrome but is not specific since it may also be seen in pseudo-Cushing's syndrome and as a

result of stress. Fewer false positives occur if dexamethasone is given at a dose of 0.5 mg 6-hourly for 48 h, with cortisol being measured on the morning after the last dose. False negatives virtually never occur with either protocol. It is important that, if urinary cortisol excretion is to be measured, the period of collection does not include the time when dexamethasone is being given.

This insulin hypoglycaemia test, also used in the investigation of pituitary function (*see p. 108*) can be helpful in the diagnosis of Cushing's syndrome since the normal increase in plasma cortisol concentration which occurs in response to hypoglycaemia is abolished even in mild Cushing's syndrome, while in patients with pseudo-Cushing's, a normal response occurs.

Loss of diurnal variation of cortisol secretion is an early feature of Cushing's syndrome and the diagnosis is excluded if the plasma cortisol concentration at 2300 h or 2400 h is normal. Since the patient must be resting and not stressed, plasma cortisol measurement at night is not a practical outpatient procedure. It necessitates hospital admission, itself a stressful event, with the result that false positive results are common. However, if care is taken to minimize stress (ideally blood is taken from the sleeping patient through a previously inserted cannula after two or three days in hospital), a raised value does indicate pathological over-production of cortisol.

**CASE HISTORY 8.3**

A 35-year-old male window cleaner presented with muscle weakness. This mainly affected his thighs with the result that he sometimes had to use his hands to help himself up from a sitting position. He was also finding it difficult to climb ladders at work. He had no other complaints.

On examination, he had a cushingoid appearance with truncal obesity, proximal muscle wasting, violaceous abdominal striae and a plethoric, 'moon face'. His blood pressure was 180/110 mmHg. He admitted that he had noticed the changes in his appearance developing over the past nine months but had been too shy to seek medical advice. It was only when he became concerned that he might not be able to continue working that he consulted his doctor. He was admitted to hospital for further investigation.

## Investigations

serum: sodium             136 mmol/L
       potassium       3.2 mmol/L
       bicarbonate     33 mmol/L

blood glucose (fasting)    7.5 mmol/L

serum cortisol: (0900 h)   930 nmol/L
           (2400 h)   900 nmol/L
plasma ACTH  (0900 h)      130 ng/L
  (normal < 50 ng/L)
urine cortisol excretion  840 nmol/24 h

dexamethasone suppression test:
  0900 h serum cortisol after
    0.5 mg dexamethasone four times
    daily for two days (low dose) 880 nmol/L

  0900 h serum cortisol after
    2.0 mg dexamethasone four times
    daily for two days (high dose) 320 nmol/L

## Comment

The diagnosis is Cushing's disease. The clinical features are typical. The high 0900 h cortisol, lack of diurnal variation and high urinary cortisol excretion all suggest adrenal hyperfunction. An overnight dexamethasone suppression test was not performed, because the presentation was so typical that an outpatient screening test was considered unnecessary. However, the formal two-stage test gave a result typical of Cushing's disease, with no change at the low dose, and decreased cortisol secretion with the high dose.

In Cushing's disease, the pituitary usually remains susceptible to feedback by glucocorticoids, but is apparently less sensitive than normal (i.e., a higher concentration of cortisol is necessary to suppress ACTH; Fig. 8.9b). In Cushing's syndrome caused by adrenal tumours, whether adenomas or carcinomas, and also in ectopic ACTH secretion, there is usually no response to dexamethasone, even at the higher dose, since pituitary ACTH secretion is already suppressed by the high plasma cortisol levels (Fig. 8.9c). This patient's plasma ACTH is raised; with adrenal tumours, feedback of cortisol to the pituitary suppresses ACTH while with ectopic ACTH secretion, ACTH levels are very high (Fig. 8.9d). The results of biochemical tests in the various forms of Cushing's syndrome are summarized in Fig. 8.10.

Measurements of plasma ACTH concentration are of great value in establishing the cause of Cushing's syndrome. However, the hormone is very labile and plasma must be separated rapidly, using a refrigerated centrifuge, and kept deep-frozen until the assay is performed if meaningful results are to be obtained.

This patient has a hypokalaemic alkalosis, a result of renal potassium wasting, and hypertension, a result of sodium retention. The fasting blood glucose is a little above normal; impaired glucose tolerance is common in Cushing's syndrome but clinical features of diabetes are uncommon, except in ectopic ACTH secretion. If the patient is coincidentally diabetic there may be a marked deterioration in control.

A skull radiograph in this patient showed a normal pituitary fossa; in Cushing's disease, the pituitary tumour secreting ACTH is usually very small, but may be revealed by CT or MRI scanning.

Tests that are useful in elucidating the cause of Cushing's syndrome include the high dose dexamethasone suppression test, and measurement of plasma ACTH. The former involves giving 2 mg dexamethasone 6-hourly for 48 h; plasma cortisol concentration is measured at 0900 h on the morning following the last dose. In Cushing's disease, the cortisol concentration characteristically decreases to less than 50% of the pre-treatment value. Failure of suppression suggests ectopic ACTH secretion or an adrenal tumour. Plasma ACTH concentrations are often very high with ectopic secretion and are low with adrenal tumours. Moderately elevated values are seen in Cushing's disease.

Exceptions to these results occur frequently. Many patients with ectopic ACTH have a characteristic clinical

## Cushing's syndrome

**a. Normal**

production of cortisol by adrenal cortex
stimulated by ACTH

cortisol exerts a negative feedback effect on
release of ACTH by pituitary

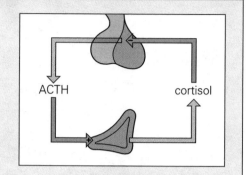

**b. Cushing's disease**

ACTH secretion increased

pituitary insensitive to feedback
by normal levels of cortisol

higher levels of cortisol required to produce
negative feedback effect on ACTH secretion

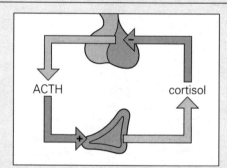

**c. Adrenal tumours**

autonomous cortisol production

high circulating cortisol inhibits ACTH secretion

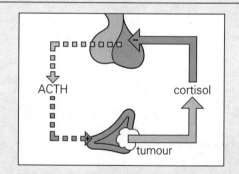

**d. Ectopic ACTH secretion**

high level of ACTH secreted by tumour
stimulates excessive cortisol production

secretion of ACTH by pituitary inhibited

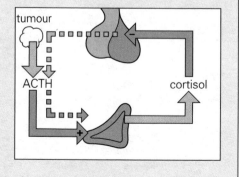

**Fig. 8.9** Pituitary–adrenal relationships in Cushing's syndrome.

| Results of adrenal function tests in Cushing's syndrome | | | | |
|---|---|---|---|---|
| Condition | Basal cortisol (nmol/L) | Dexamethasone suppression test | | Plasma ACTH (ng/L) |
| | | Low dose | High dose | |
| Cushing's disease | ↑ (<1000) | no suppression | suppression | ↑ (<200) |
| adrenal tumour | ↑ (variable) | no suppression | no suppression | ↓ |
| ectopic ACTH secretion | greatly ↑ (>1000) | no suppression | no suppression | greatly ↑ (>200) |

Fig. 8.10 Results of adrenal function tests in Cushing's syndrome. With ectopic ACTH secretion by carcinoid tumours, the results of these tests may be identical to those seen in Cushing's disease, as the tumour may have glucocorticoid receptors which will respond to dexamethasone.

presentation, with weight loss, severe muscle weakness, pigmentation, hypertension, hypokalaemic alkalosis and diabetes, but without the classical somatic manifestations of Cushing's disease. In other cases, however (particularly when due to carcinoid tumours), ectopic ACTH secretion may produce a clinical syndrome which is clinically and biochemically identical to Cushing's disease. Imaging techniques, for example, chest X-ray and pituitary and abdominal CT scanning, may reveal a tumour, while selective venous blood sampling for ACTH measurement, to locate the source of ACTH secretion, can also be helpful.

The CRH (corticotrophin releasing hormone) test can be useful to differentiate between Cushing's disease and ectopic ACTH secretion. An intravenous bolus (100 µg) of CRH causes an increase in plasma cortisol concentration in normal individuals. In the majority of patients with Cushing's disease the response is exaggerated, while in ectopic ACTH secretion and with adrenal tumours, it is usually absent.

The management of Cushing's syndrome depends upon the cause. Adrenal adenomas and, if possible, carcinomas, should be resected. The treatment of choice for Cushing's disease is transsphenoidal hypophysectomy. Bilateral adrenalectomy was formerly used and still may sometimes be required since the adrenals may become semi-autonomous. Bilateral adrenalectomy must always be followed by treatment to the pituitary (usually external irradiation) to prevent continued growth of the pituitary tumour. If this is not done, the tumour may increase in size and give rise to clinical symptoms and signs. The latter includes pigmentation, due to the secretion of excessive quantities of ACTH (Nelson's syndrome). Patients who have undergone hypophysectomy or bilateral adrenalectomy will require appropriate steroid replacement therapy for life. When surgery is not possible, and in all cases pending surgery, symptomatic relief may ensue from the use of drugs which block cortisol synthesis, such as metyrapone, which inhibits steroid-11-hydroxylase.

### Conn's syndrome

The common causes and clinical features of this condition are listed in Fig. 8.11. Conn's syndrome is characterized by excessive production of aldosterone (aldosteronism). In some 80% of cases, this is due to an adrenal adenoma, while in the remainder, there is diffuse hypertrophy of the cells of the zona glomerulosa, which produce aldosterone, in both adrenals. The majority of the clinical features are due to hypokalaemia, itself a result of renal potassium wasting.

| Conn's syndrome |
|---|
| **Causes** |
| adrenal adenoma<br>bilateral hypertrophy of zona glomerulosa cells<br>adrenal carcinoma (very rare) |
| **Clinical features** |
| hypertension<br>muscle weakness (occasionally paralysis)<br>latent tetany and paraesthesiae<br>polydipsia and polyuria |

Fig. 8.11 Causes and clinical features of Conn's syndrome.

Patients are also hypertensive, a consequence of aldosterone-induced sodium retention. Conn's syndrome is a rare cause of hypertension and accounts for only approximately 1% of all cases, but it is important since it is potentially curable.

Primary aldosteronism may be mimicked by treatment with carbenoxolone and by the ingestion of liquorice. Both these substances have metabolites with mineralocorticoid activity.

Aldosteronism is also seen in patients whose plasma renin activity is increased. This is secondary aldosteronism, since the adrenal glands are responding to their normal trophic stimulus, in contrast to the automonous secretion of aldosterone in Conn's syndrome, which is termed primary aldosteronism. In primary aldosteronism, plasma renin is low.

Secondary aldosteronism is far more common than the primary form and is associated with a variety of conditions (Fig. 8.12) in which renin secretion is stimulated. Patients may or may not be hypertensive, depending on the underlying condition.

When investigating a patient with hypokalaemia and hypertension, many possible causes of secondary aldosteronism can be eliminated either on clinical grounds or on the basis of simple tests. Plasma sodium concentration is usually high–normal or slightly elevated in primary aldosteronism; in secondary aldosteronism, the concentration is usually <138 mmol/L. The definitive test to distinguish between primary and secondary aldosteronism involves simultaneous measurement of plasma aldosterone and renin. In primary aldosteronism, plasma renin activity is reduced; in secondary, renin is the cause of the excessive aldosterone secretion and is raised. However, the measurement of renin is technically difficult and should be reserved for the further investigation of those patients in whom there is a high index of suspicion of primary aldosteronism. Such patients are selected on the basis of the results of simpler tests (Fig. 8.13).

Primary aldosteronism should be suspected in any hypertensive patient who has a low plasma potassium concentration. Diuretics are an important cause of hypokalaemia and indeed the use of diuretics in hypertension is the commonest cause of hypokalaemia and raised blood pressure. It is therefore essential that, if a hypertensive patient has been treated with a diuretic and is found to be hypokalaemic, the patient is given some other antihypertensive treatment for at least two weeks before further investigation is undertaken. Prazosin or guanethidine are suitable for this purpose. Other causes of hypokalaemia (see Fig. 2.17) should be sought and eliminated.

In Conn's syndrome, the hypokalaemia is caused by renal potassium wasting. Potassium should be absorbed maximally in the presence of hypokalaemia and in a hypokalaemic patient who is not on diuretics, renal potassium excretion of more than 30 mmol/24 h is very suggestive of primary aldosteronism. In early cases, or if patients have a low salt intake, frank hypokalaemia may be intermittent or the plasma potassium concentration only marginally abnormal. The sensitivity of diagnosis is increased if a salt intake of at least 120 mmol/24 h is maintained during the investigation of suspected aldosteronism. In equivocal cases, it may be helpful to increase the patient's sodium intake to 200 mmol/24 h and repeat the measurements of plasma potassium concentration. Sodium loading increases the amount of sodium reaching the distal renal tubules. In a normal subject, the loading inhibits aldosterone secretion but if there is autonomous secretion this sodium is reabsorbed and there is a reciprocal increase in the amount of potassium excreted.

| Conditions associated with secondary hyperaldosteronism |
|---|
| **Common**<br>congestive cardiac failure<br>cirrhosis of liver with ascites<br>nephrotic syndrome |
| **Less common**<br>renal artery stenosis<br>sodium-losing nephritis<br>Bartter's syndrome<br>renin-secreting tumours |

**Fig. 8.12** Conditions associated with secondary hyperaldosteronism.

| Screening tests for Conn's syndrome |
|---|
| potassium (off diuretics) <3.5 mmol/L<br>urine potassium >30 mmol/24 h<br>serum and urine potassium as above with<br>   sodium loading (200 mmol/24 h)<br>exclusion of other causes of hypokalaemia<br>exclusion of secondary hyperaldosteronism |

**Fig. 8.13** Screening tests for Conn's syndrome.

Plasma aldosterone concentration and renin activity are affected by posture. Standing increases renin secretion, and hence that of aldosterone, in normal subjects, due to the decrease in renal blood flow. Basal blood measurements of renin activity and aldosterone concentration must be made with the patient recumbent. After waking, he/she should remain lying down until the blood sample is drawn. A further sample is collected after 30 minutes' ambulation, for renin measurement (*see Case History 8.3*).

The response of aldosterone to posture may help to distinguish between Conn's syndrome due to a tumour or to adrenal hyperplasia. A further blood sample is taken after the patient has been ambulant for 4h. In the majority of patients with adenomas, plasma aldosterone concentration decreases by 50% in relation to the recumbent sample; with bilateral hyperplasia, there is often an increase. This differential response is due to adenomas being sensitive to ACTH (the concentration of which falls during the morning) while in adrenal hyperplasia, the adrenals are sensitive to angiotensin II (the concentration of which rises when the patient is ambulant). Plasma cortisol concentration must be measured at the same time. Only if it falls can it be certain that the predicted fall in ACTH has occurred. As in Cushing's syndrome, imaging techniques and selective blood sampling may be required to diagnose the cause of Conn's syndrome in equivocal cases.

**CASE HISTORY 8.4**

A 35-year-old woman was found to have a blood pressure of 190/110 mmHg by her general practitioner at a routine health check. He prescribed a thiazide diuretic but a week later she returned to the surgery complaining of severe muscle weakness and constipation. The doctor arranged an urgent consultation at the local hospital where her serum potassium was found to be 2.6 mmol/L. The diuretic was stopped, her blood pressure was controlled with prazosin and she was given oral potassium supplements. After three weeks her serum potassium concentration was only 3.0 mmol/L. A 24-hour urine collection contained 70 mmol potassium. Conn's syndrome was suspected and she was admitted to the hospital for further investigation.

**Investigations**

plasma aldosterone
  (0900 h, recumbent)                    1320 pmol/L
                              (normal 100–450 pmol/L)
  (1300 h, ambulant)                      510 pmol/L

plasma renin activity
(0900 h) < 0.5 pmol/min/mL
                      (normal 1.1–2.7 pmol/min/mL)
(0930 h, ambulant)            < 0.5 pmol/min/mL

**Comment**

A CT scan of the abdomen showed a small mass arising from the left adrenal gland. This was removed surgically. She made a rapid recovery after the operation and repeated checks showed her to be normokalaemic and normotensive.

Giving a diuretic may provoke symptomatic hypokalaemia in mild aldosteronism. The hypokalaemia in this condition is characteristically resistant to potassium supplementation. The diagnosis of Conn's syndrome is indicated by the high aldosterone, low renin, and the failure of plasma renin activity to rise after being upright for 30 min. In normal subjects, the decrease in renal blood flow caused by standing stimulates renin release. In aldosteronism, renin is suppressed and there is little or no increase when the patient stands up.

The fall in aldosterone concentration after 4 h is characteristic of Conn's syndrome due to an adrenal tumour.

If Conn's syndrome is shown to be due to a tumour, this should be removed surgically. In patients with bilateral adrenal hyperplasia, treatment with spironolactone, a diuretic which antagonizes the action of aldosterone, may be sufficient to control the blood pressure. Spironolactone is also used in patients with tumours while they await surgery.

## Congenital adrenal hyperplasia (CAH)

This syndrome encompasses a group of inherited metabolic disorders of adrenal steroid hormone biosynthesis. The clinical features of each depend upon the position of the defective enzyme in the synthetic pathway, which ultimately determines the pattern of hormones and precursors that is produced (*see Fig. 8.3*).

21-Hydroxylase deficiency, with an incidence of 1 in 12,000 of live births in the United Kingdom, accounts for around 95% of all cases of CAH. The majority of the remaining 5% are due to deficiency of 11β-hydroxylase. 21-hydroxylase deficiency is often incomplete and adequate cortisol synthesis can then be maintained by increased secretion of ACTH by the pituitary. It is this that causes hyperplasia of the glands. Because of the enzyme block, the substrate of the enzyme (17α-hydroxyprogesterone) accumulates and there is increased formation of adrenal androgens (*see p. 122*).

Female infants affected by CAH may be born with ambiguous genitalia but when the enzyme block is only partial the condition may not present until early adulthood with hirsutism, amenorrhoea or infertility (late onset CAH). Males may present with pseudoprecocious puberty. In about one-third of neonates with 21-hydroxylase deficiency the enzyme deficiency is complete; these present shortly after birth with a life-threatening salt-losing state in which both cortisol and aldosterone production are insufficient to maintain normal homoeostasis. The partial and complete forms of 21-hydroxylase deficiency appear to be two separate entities, the manifestations of the condition running true-to-type within affected families.

Diagnosis is made by demonstrating an elevated concentration of 17α-hydroxyprogesterone (17-OHP) in the plasma at least two days after birth (before this time maternally derived 17-OHP may still be present in the infant's blood). Treatment involves replacement of cortisol, and mineralocorticoid if necessary, which should suppress the excessive ACTH production and hence the excessive androgen synthesis. Treatment is monitored by measurement of either plasma 17-OHP or androstenedione.

Partial 11β-hydroxylase deficiency is also more common than complete deficiency of the enzyme. It is characterized by hypertension, due to the accumulation of 11-deoxycorticosterone, a substrate of the defective enzyme which has salt-retaining properties. There is excessive androgen production. The diagnosis rests upon the demonstration of an increased plasma concentration of either 11-deoxycortisol or its urinary metabolite. Treatment is with cortisol alone; aldosterone production is not defective in this type of CAH.

Other forms of CAH involving, for example, 17-hydroxylase, 18-hydroxylase (thus affecting aldosterone secretion only) and steroid 3β-hydroxydehydrogenase, Δ5 isomerase, are very rare. Some indication of their consequences, in terms of adrenal steroid metabolism, can be seen by studying *Fig. 8.3*.

# DISORDERS OF THE ADRENAL MEDULLA

The main interest in the adrenal medulla for clinical biochemistry relates to phaeochromocytomas. These are tumours which secrete catecholamines, the normal secretory product of the organ, and which are a rare (approximately 0.5% of all cases), but treatable, cause of hypertension. Approximately 10% of phaeochromocytomas are found in extramedullary tissue that shares the same embryological origin, that is, chromaffin tissue derived from neuroectoderm. Catecholamines can also be produced by tumours of embryologically related tissue, for example, the carotid bodies, and by neuroblastomas, rare tumours occurring only in infants and young children and usually presenting as a rapidly enlarging abdominal mass. These tumours form part of a group known as APUD (amine precursor uptake and decarboxylation) tumours (*see p. 269*).

Patients with phaeochromocytomas usually present with hypertension; although this may be episodic, it is usually sustained. Other features include palpitation, flushing, sweating, tremor and abdominal discomfort. Although phaeochromocytomas are rare, hypertension is common, and therefore it is important to have available a screening test that identifies those patients likely to have a phaeochromocytoma and who should be subjected to more definitive investigation, and that eliminates those in whom this probability is very low.

The metabolism of catecholamines is outlined in *Fig. 8.14*. Adrenaline (epinephrine) and noradrenaline (norepinephrine) are metabolized by catechol-O-methyltransferase (COMT) to metadrenaline and normetadrenaline, respectively. They are also converted by the consecutive action of monoamine oxidase and COMT to 4-hydroxy-3-methoxymandelic acid (HMMA), also known as vanillylmandelic acid (VMA).

Approaches to screening and diagnosis vary between laboratories, and the laboratory staff should be contacted to ensure that appropriate samples are collected. Screening tests include the measurement of urinary HMMA or metanephrines (i.e., metadrenaline and metnoradrenaline). Diagnosis is based on measurements of urinary or plasma catecholamines. All these tests have good specificity but measurement of catecholamines, although technically difficult, has the highest sensitivity. Measurement of metanephrines is more sensitive than measurement of HMMA. A number of common foodstuffs, including bananas, vanilla, tea and coffee, may react in the test for HMMA.

Following diagnosis, the site of the tumour is identified by an imaging technique, guided by the fact that extra-adrenal phaeochromocytomas tend to secrete noradrenaline in excess of adrenaline, the reverse being true of tumours of the adrenal medulla itself (*see Case History 8.5*).

---

**CASE HISTORY 8.5**

A 75-year-old woman presented with anxiety, palpitation and sweating. Her pulse was 80/min, regular, and blood pressure 160/100 mmHg. She had previously been investigated for abdominal pain, for which no cause had been found. Tests of thyroid function were normal. A 24 h urine collection was made.

**Results**

urine hydroxymethoxy-   99 μmol/24 h(ref range < 35)
    mandelic acid (HMMA)

---

urine adrenaline        1.0 mmol/24 h (ref range < 0.1)
urine noradrenaline  0.38 mmol/24 h (ref range < 0.57)

A CT scan of the abdomen showed a mass arising from the left adrenal gland, and an isotopic scan of the adrenals, using meta-[131]I-iodobenzylguanidine, showed a single left adrenal mass.

**Comment**

The clinical features suggested thyrotoxicosis but this was excluded by the results of thyroid function testing. The clinical features were also consistent with a phaeochromocytoma, but a high index of suspicion may be necessary to initiate the appropriate investigations. The screening test was positive, and the high adrenaline excretion suggested that the tumour would be of adrenal origin. The biochemical localization was confirmed by the imaging procedures, and at operation, carried out after three days' treatment with phenoxybenzamine (an adrenergic blocking drug), a 5 cm left adrenal phaeochromocytoma was removed.

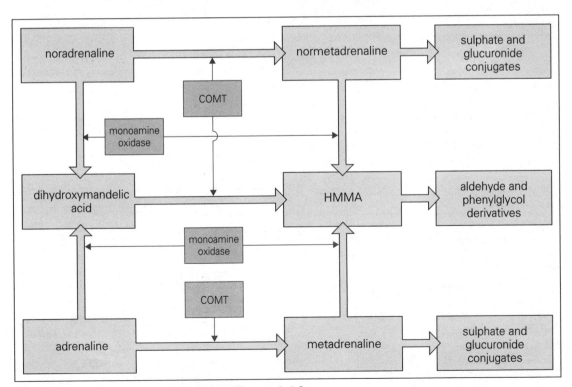

**Fig. 8.14** Metabolism of catecholamines. COMT = catechol-O-methyltransferase; HMMA = 4-hydroxy-3-methoxymandelic acid.

Provocative or suppression tests are rarely necessary for diagnosis, but when the results of catecholamine measurements are equivocal, the pentolinium test may be helpful. Pentolinium is a sympathetic ganglion-blocking drug that reduces catecholamine secretion in normal subjects but not in patients with phaeochromocytomas; in such patients, secretion is autonomous. Blood is taken for catecholamine content before and 15 minutes after giving 2.5 mg pentolinium by intravenous injection. Although still potentially dangerous, this procedure is more reliable and less hazardous than the phentolamine test which has been used in the past. This $\alpha$-adrenergic blocking drug causes dramatic hypotension in patients with phaeochromocytomas.

Although phaeochromocytomas are benign in 90% of cases, all tumours should be removed surgically. However, this is a potentially hazardous operation since large quantities of cathecolamines may be released into the circulation during the procedure. It should be noted that 10% of patients with phaeochromocytomas have multiple tumours. The tumours may be a component of the Sipple syndrome (multiple endocrine neoplasia type IIa, *see p. 275*) and thus evidence of other relevant endocrine disorders should be sought in affected patients.

## SUMMARY

The adrenal cortex secretes three classes of steroid hormones – glucocorticoids, androgens and mineralocorticoids. The secretion of glucocorticoids, of which cortisol is the most important, is controlled by adrenocorticotrophic hormone (ACTH), while ACTH secretion is subject to feedback inhibition by cortisol. Control is also exerted from the higher centres through the hypothalamus. Cortisol secretion shows a diurnal variation, with peak plasma levels in the morning and a trough in the late evening. Cortisol is essential to life; it is involved in the response to stress and with other hormones regulates many pathways of intermediary metabolism. Its metabolic action is largely catabolic. Androgen secretion is also stimulated by ACTH; these hormones have a role in determining secondary sexual characteristics in the female but do not appear to have a specific role in the male.

Aldosterone stimulates sodium reabsorption in the distal tubule of the kidneys. It is an important determinant of the extracellular fluid volume. Its secretion is controlled by the renin–angiotensin system, in response to changes in blood pressure and blood volume.

Adrenal failure is most frequently due to organ-specific autoimmune destruction of the glands although there are many other causes. It can present acutely as a medical emergency with hypoglycaemia and circulatory collapse due to renal salt wasting. In more chronic cases, lassitude, weight loss and postural hypotension are frequent clinical features. Diagnosis depends upon demonstrating a failure of the adrenal to produce cortisol in response to ACTH (Synacthen test). Pituitary disease can cause secondary adrenal failure by interfering with normal ACTH secretion.

Over-production of adrenal cortical hormones can affect predominantly cortisol (producing Cushing's syndrome), or aldosterone (Conn's syndrome). In addition, Cushing's syndrome can be secondary to excess ACTH production by a pituitary tumour or by a non-endocrine tumour (ectopic ACTH production), or be iatrogenic, due to treatment with corticosteroids or ACTH. Clinical features of Cushing's syndrome include characteristic somatic changes, muscle weakness, glucose intolerance, hypokalaemia and hypertension. Patients with Conn's syndrome develop hypertension and hypokalaemia. The diagnosis of these conditions involves first demonstrating high, non-suppressible concentrations of the hormones and then determining the cause.

The various syndromes of congenital adrenal hyperplasia are inherited metabolic disorders of adrenal steroid hormone biosynthesis. The clinical features derive from a mixture of under-production of either cortisol or aldosterone, or both, and increased production of androgens. The most common type is steroid 21-hydroxylase deficiency.

The adrenal medulla produces catecholamines but is not essential to life. There appear to be no clinical sequelae from decreased adrenal medullary activity but tumours of the glands (neuroblastomas and phaeochromocytomas) can produce excessive quantities of catecholamines. These cause hypertension and other clinical features related to increased sympathetic activity.

## FURTHER READING

Besser G M & Thorner M O (eds.) (1994) *Clinical Endocrinology: An Illustrated Text*. 2nd edition. London: Wolfe.

Aron D C & Tyrrell J B (eds) (1994) Cushing's Syndrome. *Endocrinology and Metabolism Clinics of North America*, **23**, 451–698.

Hall R & Besser M (eds) (1989) *Fundamentals of Clinical Endocrinology*. 4th edition. London: Pitman Medical.

Wilson J D & Foster D W (eds) (1992) *Williams – Textbook of Endocrinology*. 8th edition. Philadelphia: W B Saunders Company.

Bravo E L (ed.) (1994) Endocrine hypertension. *Endocrinology and Metabolism Clinics of North America*, **23**, 235–449.

# 9. The Thyroid Gland

## INTRODUCTION

The thyroid gland secretes three hormones: thyroxine (T4) and triiodothyronine (T3), both of which are iodinated derivatives of tyrosine (*Fig. 9.1*), and calcitonin, a polypeptide hormone. T4 and T3 are produced by the follicular cells but calcitonin is secreted by the C cells which are of separate embryological origin. Calcitonin is functionally unrelated to the other thyroid hormones, possibly being involved in calcium homoeostasis, and disorders of its secretion are rare (*see Chapter 12*). Thyroid disorders in which there is either over- or under-secretion of T4 and T3 are, however, common.

Thyroxine synthesis and release are stimulated by the pituitary trophic hormone, thyroid-stimulating hormone (TSH). The secretion of the trophic hormone itself is controlled by negative feedback by the thyroid hormones (predominantly T4) (*see p. 104*) which modulate the response of the pituitary to the hypothalamic hormone, thyrotrophin releasing hormone (TRH; *Fig. 9.2*). Glucocorticoids, dopamine and somatostatin inhibit TSH secretion. The physiological significance of this is not known but it may be relevant to the disturbances of thyroid hormones which can occur in non-thyroidal illness (*see p.143*).

The major product of the thyroid gland is T4. Ten times less T3 is produced (the proportion may be greater in thyroid disease), most T3 (approximately 80%) being derived from T4 by deiodination in peripheral tissues, particularly the liver and kidney. T3 is 3–4 times more potent than T4. Deiodination can also produce reverse triiodothyronine (rT3; *see Fig. 9.1*) which is physiologically inactive. It is produced instead of T3 in starvation and many non-thyroidal illnesses, and the formation of either the active or inactive metabolite of T4 appears to play an important part in the control of energy metabolism. The anterior pituitary is also active in

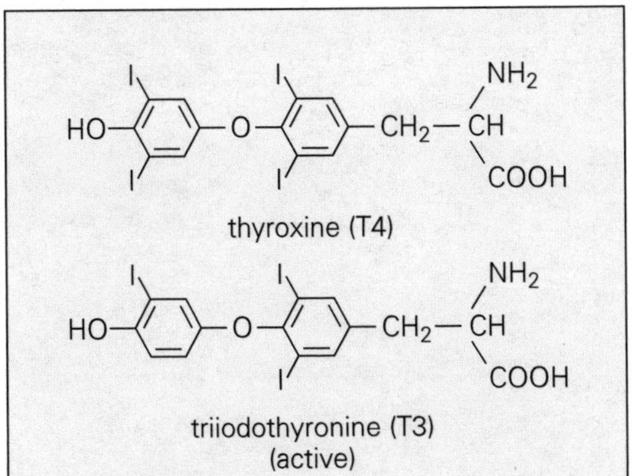

**Fig. 9.1** Chemical structure of the thyroid hormones, T4 and T3, and the inactive metabolite of T4, rT3.

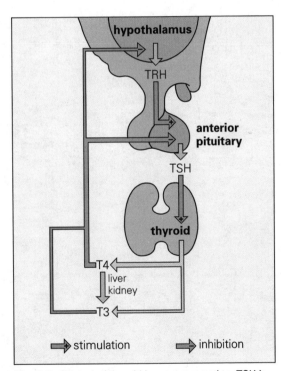

**Fig. 9.2** Control of thyroid hormone secretion. TSH is released from the pituitary in response to the hypothalamic hormone, TRH, and stimulates the synthesis and release of thyroid hormones. TSH release is inhibited by thyroid hormones which decrease the sensitivity of the pituitary to TRH. They may also inhibit TRH release by the hypothalamus.

converting T4 to T3. It is thought that the pituitary senses thyroid hormone status through a change in the concentration of T3 due to deiodination within anterior pituitary cells.

## THYROID HORMONES

### Functions

Thyroid hormones are essential for normal growth and development and have many effects on metabolic processes. They act by entering cells and binding to specific receptors in the nuclei, where they stimulate the synthesis of a variety of species of mRNA, thus stimulating the synthesis of polypeptides including hormones and enzymes. Their most obvious overall effect on metabolism is to stimulate the basal metabolic rate, but the precise molecular basis of this action is not known. Thyroid hormones also increase the sensitivity of the cardiovascular and nervous systems to catecholamines.

### Synthesis

Thyroid hormone synthesis involves a number of specific enzyme-catalyzed reactions, beginning with the uptake of iodine by the gland and culminating in the iodination of tyrosine residues in the protein, thyroglobulin (*Fig. 9.3*); these reactions are all stimulated by TSH. Rare congenital forms of hypothyroidism due to inherited deficiencies of each of the various enzymes concerned have been described.

Thyroglobulin is stored within the thyroid gland in colloid follicles. These are accumulations of thyroglobulin-containing colloid surrounded by thyroid follicular cells. Release of thyroid hormones (stimulated by TSH) involves pinocytosis of colloid by follicular cells, fusion with lysosomes to form phagocytic vacuoles and proteolysis (*Fig. 9.4*). Thyroid hormones are thence released into the blood stream. Proteolysis also results in the liberation of mono- and diiodotyrosines (MIT and DIT); these are usually degraded

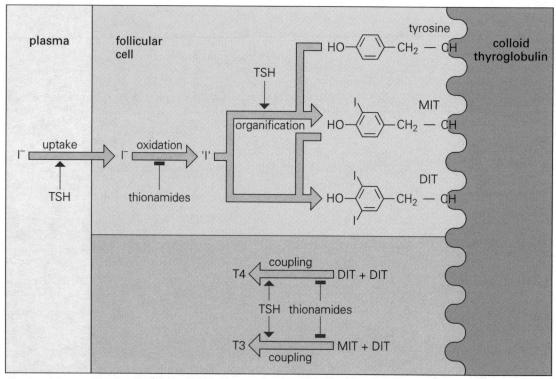

**Fig. 9.3** Biosynthesis of the thyroid hormones. The iodination and condensation reactions involve tyrosine residues that are an integral part of the thyroglobulin polypeptide. The thyroid hormones remain protein-bound until they are released from the cell. The precise nature of the active iodine moiety ('I') is not known.

Once formed, it is rapidly incorporated into tyrosine residues to form monoiodotyrosine (MIT) and diiodotyrosine (DIT). Anti-thyroid thionamide drugs, such as carbimazole, act by inhibiting the formation of the active moiety or by preventing the coupling of DIT to form T4.

within thyroid follicular cells and their iodine is retained and re-utilized. A small amount of thyroglobulin also reaches the blood stream.

## Thyroid hormones in blood

The normal plasma concentrations of T4 and T3 are 60–150 nmol/L and 1.0–2.9 nmol/L, respectively. Both hormones are extensively protein bound, some 99.98% of T4 and 99.66% of T3 being bound principally to a specific thyroxine-binding globulin (TBG) and to a lesser extent to prealbumin and albumin. TBG is approximately one-third saturated at normal concentrations of thyroid hormones (*Fig. 9.5*). It is generally accepted that only the free, non protein-bound, thyroid hormones are physiologically active. Although the total T4 concentration is normally 50 times that of T3, the different extents to which these hormones are bound to protein mean that the free T4 concentration is only 2–3 times that of free T3. In the tissues, most of the effects of T4 probably result from its conversion to T3, so that T4 itself is essentially a prohormone.

The precise physiological function of TBG is unknown; subjects who have a genetically determined deficiency of the protein show no clinical abnormality. It has, however, been suggested that the extensive binding of thyroid hormones to TBG provides a buffer which maintains the free hormone levels constant in the face of any tendency to change. The binding may also reduce the amount of thyroid hormones lost through the kidneys and it has been suggested that the binding protein may have a specific role in facilitating hormone uptake by cells. However, for the clinician and biochemist, protein binding can provide a major obstacle to the laboratory assessment of thyroid status.

Total thyroid hormone concentration is dependent upon the concentrations of binding proteins present in the blood. If these were to increase (*Fig. 9.6*), the temporary fall in free hormone concentration caused by increased protein binding would stimulate TSH release and this would restore the free hormone concentrations to normal. Conversely, if the protein concentration were to fall, the reverse would occur. In either situation, there would be a

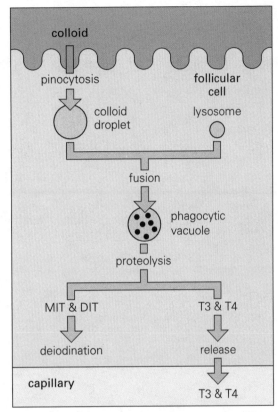

**Fig. 9.4** Secretion of the thyroid hormones. Colloid is taken up into follicular cells by pinocytosis and undergoes lysosomal proteolysis resulting in the release of thyroid hormones.

change in the concentrations of total hormones, but the free hormone concentrations would remain normal. Thus measurement of total hormone concentrations can give misleading information.

This is a matter of considerable practical importance since changes in the concentrations of the binding proteins occur in many circumstances (*Fig. 9.7*). Further, certain

| | Plasma concentration | | Extent of protein binding (%) | Half-life (days) |
|---|---|---|---|---|
| | total (nmol/L) | free (pmol/L) | | |
| T4 | 60–150 | 9.0–26.0 | 99.98 | 6–7 |
| T3 | 1.0–2.9 | 3.0–9.0 | 99.66 | 1–1.5 |

**Fig. 9.5** Thyroid hormones in blood. Each laboratory should determine its own normal range for plasma concentrations.

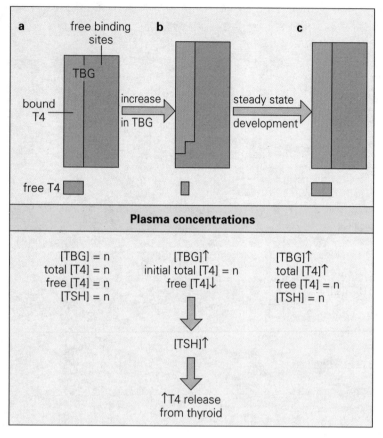

**a** free binding sites **b** **c**

TBG

bound T4 → increase in TBG → steady state development →

free T4

**Plasma concentrations**

[TBG] = n
total [T4] = n
free [T4] = n
[TSH] = n

[TBG]↑
initial total [T4] = n
free [T4]↓

↓

[TSH]↑

↓

↑T4 release
from thyroid

[TBG]↑
total [T4]↑
free [T4] = n
[TSH] = n

**Fig. 9.6** Effect of an increase in TBG concentration on plasma T4 levels. (a) In the initial steady state, TBG is one-third saturated with T4. (b) TBG levels increase causing more T4 to be bound, thus reducing the free T4 concentration. This stimulates TSH secretion which leads to an increase in the release of T4 from the thyroid. (c) The new T4 is re-distributed between the bound and the free states leading to a new steady state with the same free T4 level but an increased total T4.

drugs, for example, salicylates and phenytoin, will displace thyroid hormones from their binding proteins, thus reducing the total, but not the free, hormone concentrations once a new steady state is attained. If an attempt is made to assess thyroid status in a patient who is not in a steady state, the results may be bizarre and misleading.

Only small amounts of T4 and T3 are excreted by the kidneys due to the extensive protein binding. The major route of thyroid hormone degradation is by deiodination and metabolism in tissues, but they are also conjugated in the liver and excreted in bile.

## TESTS OF THYROID FUNCTION

Laboratory tests of thyroid function are required to assist in the diagnosis and monitoring of thyroid disease. Most laboratories offer a standard 'profile' of thyroid function tests (often TSH and free T4), and perform additional tests only if these results are equivocal or the clinical circumstances require it.

### Total thyroxine and triiodothyronine

Measurement of plasma total T4 (tT4) concentration was formerly widely used as a test of thyroid function, but has a major disadvantage in that it is dependent on binding protein concentration as well as thyroid activity. For example, a slightly elevated plasma tT4 concentration, compatible with mild hyperthyroidism, can occur with normal thyroid function if there is an increase in plasma binding protein concentration. With the introduction of more reliable assays for free T4 (fT4), there is now little if any justification for laboratories continuing to measure tT4 as a test of thyroid function.

Plasma total T3 (tT3) concentration is almost always raised in hyperthyroidism (usually to a proportionately greater extent than tT4, hence it is the more sensitive test for this condition) but may be normal in hypothyroidism. However, tT3 concentrations, like those of tT4, are dependent on the concentration of binding proteins in plasma and their measurement is being superseded by measurements of free T3 (fT3).

## Free thyroxine and triiodothyronine

The measurement of free hormone concentrations poses major technical problems since the binding of free hormones in an assay, for example, by an antibody, will disturb the equilibrium between bound and free hormone and cause release of hormone from binding proteins. Various techniques have been developed which allow the estimation of free T4 and T3 concentrations in the plasma. Such measurements, in theory, circumvent the problems associated with protein binding and have rendered obsolete the techniques for the indirect assessment of free hormone concentrations, such as the resin uptake test, calculation of the free thyroxine index or measurement of the T4/TBG ratio. However, with gross abnormalities of binding protein concentrations, the results of measurements of free hormones may be misleading due to technical problems in the test methods. Also, naturally occurring antibodies to thyroid hormones are sometimes present in the plasma and can interfere with free hormone assays. Measurement of TSH may help in both these circumstances.

In pregnancy, for reasons that are not understood, the normal range for free T4 in euthyroid women decreases as the pregnancy progresses. There is an increase in TBG, due to the increased oestrogen levels, and in total T4, but these are disproportionate, causing the level of free T4 to fall. Thyroid status, as assessed clinically, does not change.

Just as tT3 can be normal in hypothyroidism (especially in mild cases), so, too, can fT3, and its measurement is of no value in the diagnosis of this condition. Free T3 is, however, a sensitive test for hyperthyroidism. In hyperthyroid patients, both fT4 and fT3 are usually elevated (fT3 to a proportionately greater extent) but there are exceptions to this. In a small number of patients with hyperthyroidism the fT3 concentration is elevated but the fT4 is not (though it is usually high–normal) – a condition called 'T3-toxicosis'. Occasionally fT4 is elevated but not fT3. This is usually due to concomitant non-thyroidal illness resulting in decreased conversion of T4 to T3, and fT3 concentration increases when this illness resolves.

## Thyroid-stimulating hormone

Since the release of TSH from the pituitary is controlled through negative feedback by thyroid hormones, measurements of TSH can be used as an index of thyroid function. Plasma TSH concentration is increased in primary hypothyroidism, normal in euthyroid individuals and low in hyperthyroidism, and is not affected by changes in TBG concentration.

The measurement of TSH is well-established as a diagnostic test for hypothyroidism. In overt disease, plasma TSH

| Causes of abnormal plasma TBG levels |
|---|
| **Increase** |
| genetic<br>pregnancy<br>oestrogens, including<br>    oestrogen-containing oral contraceptives |
| **Decrease** |
| genetic<br>protein-losing states,<br>    e.g., nephrotic syndrome<br>malnutrition<br>malabsorption<br>acromegaly<br>Cushing's disease<br>corticosteroids (high dose)<br>severe illness<br>androgens |

**Fig. 9.7** Causes of abnormal plasma concentrations of TBG.

concentrations are unequivocally raised, often to very high values. Smaller increases are seen in borderline cases and TSH measurement is more sensitive than T4 under these circumstances. Currently available assays for TSH are sufficiently sensitive to distinguish between normal levels (0.3–5.0 mU/L) and those characteristic of overt hyperthyroidism (<0.1 mU/L), but low concentrations can also occur in individuals with sub-clinical disease and in euthyroid patients with non-thyroidal illness ('sick euthyroidism', *see below*). Indeed, in hospital patients, a low plasma TSH concentration is more often due to non-thyroidal illness than to hyperthyroidism while a slightly elevated concentration is as frequently due to recovery from such illness as to mild or incipient hypothyroidism. Thus although TSH measurements have been used on their own as a first-line test of thyroid function, they are not completely reliable and a better strategy is to measure fT4 in addition. A second reason for using this combination is to avoid misdiagnosis in patients with thyroid dysfunction secondary to a pituitary disorder, even though this is far less common than primary thyroid disease. A combination of tests may also be required to assess patients being treated for thyroid disease, particularly in the early stages.

Typical results of thyroid function tests in various conditions are shown in *Fig. 9.8*.

| Plasma fT4 | | | |
|---|---|---|---|
| | | **High** | **Normal** | **Low** |
| Plasma TSH | High | TSH-secreting tumour (rare) (fT3 = ↑) | Borderline/ compensated hypothyroidism | Hypothyroid (primary)<br><br>Recovery from sick euthyroid state |
| | Normal | Euthyroid with T4 autoantibodies (uncommon) | Euthyroid | Sick euthyroid (fT3 = ↓)<br><br>Hypopituitarism (other pituitary hormones = ↓) |
| | Low | Hyperthyroidism (fT3 = ↑) | T3 thyrotoxicosis (fT3 = ↑)<br><br>Sub-clinical hyper-thyroidism (fT3 = N/↓) | Hypopituitarism (other pituitary hormones = ↓)<br><br>Sick euthyroid (severe) (fT3 = ↓) |

**Fig. 9.8** The results of thyroid function tests in various conditions.

## Thyrotrophin releasing hormone (TRH) test

In this test, plasma TSH is measured immediately before, and 20 and 60 minutes after giving the patient 200 μg of TRH intravenously (*Fig. 9.9*). The normal response is an increase in TSH concentration of 1–20 mU/L in 20 minutes, with reversion towards the basal value at 60 minutes.

This test was formerly mainly used in the assessment of patients in whom other tests of thyroid function gave equivocal results. A normal response excludes thyroid dysfunction. The TSH response to TRH is exaggerated in hypothyroidism, even in borderline cases, while the attenuated (so-called 'flat') response characteristic of frank hyperthyroidism also occurs in incipient or borderline hyperthyroidism.

However, experience with current TSH assays has shown that the magnitude of the TSH response to TRH is a function of basal (unstimulated) TSH concentration, e.g., if the TSH is low, there will be no response to TRH. Measuring the TSH response to TRH provides no additional information over that provided by a basal TSH measurement. The TRH test is now only used in the investigation of patients with pituitary or hypothalamic disease, to assess the capacity of the pituitary to secrete TSH. TSH secretion is rarely completely lost in pituitary disease, and thus the TSH response to TRH is more usually decreased than absent

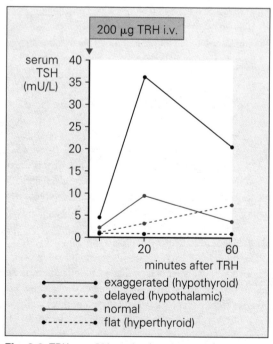

**Fig. 9.9** TRH test: 200 mg is given intravenously and serum TSH is measured at 0, 20 and 60 minutes. Typical responses are shown.

and may even be normal. In hypothalamic disease, the response is characteristically (though not invariably) delayed, plasma TSH concentration at 60 minutes exceeding that at 20 minutes.

## Other tests of thyroid function

Other biochemical disturbances, not involving the thyroid hormones, occur in thyroid disease but are of no value diagnostically; examples are hypercalcaemia and hyperphosphataemia, in some cases of thyrotoxicosis, and hypercholesterolaemia and hyponatraemia in hypothyroidism.

Techniques involving the use of radioactive isotopes for the investigation of thyroid disease are of two types. Tests involving the quantification of radioactive iodine uptake were introduced before specific tests for thyroid hormones were available but they are now little used. Thyroid scintiscanning, however, is in common use. In this technique, a dose of an isotope, usually $^{99m}Tc$, is given and its distribution within the thyroid is determined using a gamma camera. This technique allows the identification of 'hot' (active) or 'cold' (inactive and potentially malignant) nodules in patients with lumps in the thyroid. It can also distinguish between Graves' disease (uniformly increased uptake), multinodular goitre (patchy uptake) or an adenoma (single 'hot' spot) in patients with thyrotoxicosis, and can detect aberrant or ectopic thyroid tissue. A number of autoantibodies to thyroid antigens have been detected in the plasma of patients with thyroid disease. For example, thyroid-stimulating immunoglobulins are pathogenic in Graves' disease. Assays for them are not yet generally available, but it is possible that their measurement may be valuable in the diagnosis of Graves' disease as a cause of thyrotoxicosis in the absence of the characteristic eye signs, and in the prediction of relapse of Graves' disease after a course of anti-thyroid drugs. It seems probable that the antiperoxidase (formerly called anti-microsomal) antibodies present in high titre in most patients with Hashimoto's thyroiditis, and in some with Graves' disease, are also pathogenic. Anti-thyroglobulin antibodies (which also occur frequently, but are probably not pathogenic) and antibodies to thyroid hormones themselves, may bind to T4 and T3 and give rise to abnormal results in measurements of these hormones. The results are usually so bizarre that in practice they are rarely a cause of diagnostic confusion.

The measurement of thyroid autoantibodies may be helpful in patients in whom biochemical tests of thyroid function are equivocal, since their presence in high titre is consistent with thyroid disease. It is not, however, diagnostic. Most elderly individuals with thyroid autoantibodies are clinically and biochemically euthyroid.

## Problems in the interpretation of thyroid function tests

As alluded to above, no biochemical test of thyroid function can be guaranteed to be reliable in patients with non-thyroidal illness. Abnormal results may occur in patients with infections, malignancy, myocardial infarction, following surgery, etc., who do not have thyroid disease. In general, thyroid function tests should not be performed on such patients unless there is a strong suspicion that they have thyroid disease.

Typically, during the acute phase of an illness, fT3 concentration and, less often, fT4 concentration is decreased. TSH is usually normal but may be undetectable in the severely ill. During recovery, TSH may rise transiently into the hypothyroid range as free hormone concentrations return to normal. In chronic illness, for example chronic renal failure, free hormone concentrations are decreased (to an extent that may reflect the severity of the underlying disease); TSH is usually normal, but is occasionally decreased.

The occurrence of abnormalities of thyroid function tests in patients with non-thyroidal illness has been termed the 'sick euthyroid syndrome'. Causes include decreased peripheral conversion of T4 to T3; changes in the concentration of binding proteins (to an extent that may reveal technical limitations in the ability of free hormone measurements to provide a true measurement of free hormone concentrations); increased plasma concentrations of free fatty acids, which displace thyroid hormones from their binding sites, and non-thyroidal influences on the hypothalamic–pituitary–thyroid axis, for example by cortisol, which can inhibit TSH secretion.

Furthermore, many drugs can influence the results of tests of thyroid function. Some examples are given in *Fig. 9.10*.

### CASE HISTORY 9.1

Knowing that thyroid disease is common in the elderly, a house physician requested thyroid function tests on an elderly woman admitted to hospital with severe cellulitis of the leg secondary to an infected ingrowing toenail.

**Investigations**

| | |
|---|---|
| serum : TSH | 0.1 mU/L |
| fT4 | 8.0 pmol/L |
| fT3 | 2.0 pmol/L |

**Comment**

TSH, fT4 and fT3 are all low, results which at first glance might suggest thyroid failure secondary to hypopituitarism. However, a TSH this low would be unusual except in severe hypopituitarism; TSH secretion tends to be affected late in progressive pituitary disease. A random serum cortisol concentration was 950 nmol/L, indicating normal response of the hypothalamic–pituitary–adrenal axis to stress, and it was concluded that the thyroid function results were due to the 'sick euthyroid syndrome'. The infection was treated successfully and thyroid function tests were repeated prior to discharge: serum TSH concentration was 6 mU/L, fT4 was 12 pmol/L and fT3, 4.7 pmol/L.

## DISORDERS OF THE THYROID

The metabolic manifestations of thyroid disease relate either to excessive or inadequate production of thyroid hormones (hyperthyroidism and hypothyroidism, respectively). The clinical syndrome that results from hyperthyroidism is thyrotoxicosis. The term 'myxoedema' is often used to describe the entire clinical syndrome of hypothyroidism but strictly refers specifically to the dryness of the skin, coarsening of the features and subcutaneous swelling characteristic of severe hypothyroidism. Patients with thyroid disease may present with a thyroid swelling or goitre. Investigation may reveal hypo- or (more frequently) hyperthyroidism but there may be no functional abnormality. A goitre can be the presenting feature of thyroid cancer.

### Hyperthyroidism

The major causes and clinical features of hyperthyroidism are shown in *Fig. 9.11*. The commonest single cause is Graves' disease, an autoimmune disease characterized by the presence of thyroid-stimulating antibodies in the blood. These autoantibodies bind to TSH receptors in the thyroid and stimulate them in the same way as TSH, through activation of adenylate cyclase and the formation of cyclic AMP.

**CASE HISTORY 9.2**

A 24-year-old physiotherapist consulted her general practitioner because excessive moistness of her skin was causing embarrassment at work. She was also concerned that her eyes seemed to have become more prominent and that she had lost weight, although her appetite was unchanged. On examination, her doctor observed that her pulse was 92 per minute at rest and that she had a slightly enlarged thyroid gland.

| Drugs and the thyroid | |
|---|---|
| **Drug** | **Effect** |
| corticosteroids dopaminergic drugs | inhibit TSH secretion |
| lithium, iodine, carbimazole, thiouracils | inhibit T3 and T4 secretion |
| oestrogens, phenothiazines | increase TBG |
| corticosteroids, androgens | decrease TBG |
| salicylates, phenytoin | compete with T4 for binding by TBG |
| β-blockers, amiodarone | inhibit conversion of T4 to T3 |

Fig. 9.10 Drugs and the thyroid.

## Investigations

serum:  TSH        <0.1 mU/L
       fT4          34 pmol/L
       fT3          12 pmol/L

An isotopic scan of the thyroid showed an enlarged gland, with uniformly increased uptake.
Autoantibodies to thyroid peroxidase and thyroglobulin were present in the serum in high titre.

## Comment

The high fT3 and fT4 concentrations with low TSH are diagnostic of thyrotoxicosis, and the presence of autoantibodies and scan appearances are characteristic of Graves' disease. Although the clinical features are typical of thyrotoxicosis (*see Fig. 9.11*) they are often less so in milder cases and in the elderly. They may suggest an anxiety state (*see Case History 9.3*). Some clinical features are specific to Graves' disease and can have a course independent of the hyperthyroidism. Patients may present with the ocular manifestations of Graves' disease (ophthalmic Graves' disease) yet be clinically euthyroid. However, the TSH is usually suppressed even though fT3 may not be elevated, and such patients eventually become biochemically and clinically thyrotoxic. The combination of a low TSH with a normal (usually high–normal) fT3 ('sub-clinical' or 'borderline' hyperthyroidism) can occur early in the course of Graves' disease and other conditions causing thyrotoxicosis.

There are three options for the treatment of thyrotoxicosis: anti-thyroid drugs, radioactive iodine and surgery (sub-total thyroidectomy). Treatment with β-adrenergic blocking drugs may provide temporary symptomatic relief but has no effect on the underlying disease process. Very rarely, patients with thyrotoxicosis present with, or develop, thyroid storm or crisis, a medical emergency whose features include hyperpyrexia, dehydration and cardiac failure. The diagnosis of thyroid storm is made on clinical grounds and although thyroid function tests should be performed to confirm the diagnosis, treatment must not be delayed pending the results of the tests.

Unless they have a very large goitre, it is usual to treat younger patients with Graves' disease with anti-thyroid drugs. These suppress thyroid hormone synthesis, though not the release of pre-formed hormone, and thus there is usually a delay before any response is seen. Although one of the most frequently used drugs, carbimazole, is immuno-suppressive, it probably does not have a significant effect on the underlying pathogenic process in Graves' disease.

Anti-thyroid drugs are given in high doses initially, but once the patient has become euthyroid, a decrease in dosage is often possible. An alternative approach is to continue with a high dose of the chosen drug and give thyroxine at a replacement dose, e.g., 150 μg/day.

Untreated Graves' disease has a natural history of remission and relapse. Some patients (30–40%) have only a single episode of hyperthyroidism. It is usual to give

| Hyperthyroidism |
| --- |
| **Causes** |
| *Graves' disease<br>*toxic multinodular goitre<br>*solitary toxic adenoma<br>thyroiditis<br>exogenous iodine and iodine-containing drugs,<br>   e.g., amiodarone<br>excessive T4 or T3 ingestion<br>ectopic thyroid tissue,<br>   e.g., struma ovarii<br>       functioning metastatic thyroid cancer<br>pituitary tumour (very rare)<br><br>* these account for > 90% of cases |
| **Clinical features** |
| weight loss (but normal appetite)<br>sweating, heat intolerance<br>fatigue<br>palpitation; sinus tachycardia or<br>   atrial fibrillation<br>angina, heart failure (high output)<br>agitation, tremor<br>generalized muscle weakness,<br>   proximal myopathy<br>diarrhoea<br>oligomenorrhoea, infertility<br>goitre<br>eyelid retraction, lid lag |

**Fig. 9.11** Causes and clinical features of hyperthyroidism. Periorbital oedema, proptosis, diplopia, ophthalmoplegia, corneal ulceration, loss of visual acuity, pretibial myxoedema and thyroid acropachy are features of Graves' disease only.

anti-thyroid drugs for a period of one to two years. Thyroid status is monitored during this time and thereafter. If the patient relapses, a further course of drug treatment or another mode of treatment is indicated.

The laboratory diagnosis of hyperthyroidism depends on the demonstration of a high plasma concentration of fT3 (and usually fT4) with a low TSH. These tests are also used to monitor the response to treatment and for long-term follow-up. The concentrations of fT3 and fT4 fall as patients become euthyroid but some time may elapse before normal pituitary responsiveness to thyroid hormones is regained and there is an increase in TSH into the normal range. Thus while a normal TSH concentration indicates that a patient is euthyroid, a low value is not on its own indicative of persisting hyperthyroidism.

Long-term follow-up of patients treated for Graves' disease is essential. Patients treated with anti-thyroid drugs may relapse, occasionally after many years; some, on the other hand, become hypothyroid. Recurrences of the disease also occur in patients treated surgically or with radioactive iodine. Up to 35% of patients treated surgically, and the majority or patients treated with radioactive iodine, will eventually become hypothyroid, sometimes as long as ten

years or more after treatment. Hypothyroidism that develops within six months of either surgery or radioactive iodine treatment may be temporary, but abnormalities of thyroid function tests, in particular a slightly raised TSH, but normal plasma fT4 and fT3 concentrations may persist though the patient remains clinically euthyroid. This is illustrated in *Fig. 9.12*.

The pathogenic thyroid-stimulating autoantibody in Graves' disease is an IgG immunoglobulin. In a pregnant woman with Graves' disease it can cross the placenta and may cause neonatal hyperthyroidism, even if the mother is euthyroid. Neonatal hyperthyroidism is a transient phenomenon since the maternal immunoglobulins are gradually cleared from the neonatal circulation, but treatment may be required in the short term.

### CASE HISTORY 9.3

Shortly before her final examinations, a medical student experienced sleep disturbance, tachycardia with palpitation and noticed that her hands were

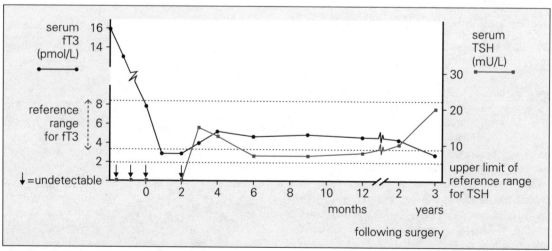

**Fig. 9.12** Changes in serum fT3 and TSH concentrations following partial thyroidectomy for Graves' disease. The patient was rendered euthyroid prior to surgery with antithyroid drugs. Initially, the TSH secretion remained suppressed but eventually rose in response to the low fT3. Normal thyroid hormone secretion by the remaining thyroid tissue was maintained by increased TSH stimulation, but eventually the patient became hypothyroid, as shown by the increased TSH. Hypothyroidism can also develop in patients treated with antithyroid drugs or radioiodine.

warm and sweaty. Her doctor was sure that her symptoms were due to anxiety, but was persuaded to take a blood sample for thyroid function tests.

### Investigations

serum: T4          165 nmol/L

      T3           2.9 nmol/L

      free T4      24 pmol/L

These results were considered to be equivocal and a TRH test was performed

serum TSH:  0 min     1.2 mU/L

           20 min     5.4 mU/L

           60 min     3.1 mU/L

### Comment

This patient was investigated before the introduction of presently available TSH assays, and exemplifies the problems posed by the effect of changes in binding protein concentration on measurements of total thyroid hormone concentration.

The total T4 is elevated and the T3 is at the upper limit of normal; the free T4 is near the upper limit of normal. Mild thyrotoxicosis could not be excluded on the basis of these results. However, the TSH response to TRH is normal, indicating that the patient is euthyroid. It transpired that she was taking an oestrogen-containing oral contraceptive pill and the resulting increase in serum TBG would explain the abnormal total hormone concentrations.

In retrospect, the normal TSH response to TRH would have been predicted from the normal basal TSH concentration, which itself suggests that the patient is euthyroid.

### CASE HISTORY 9.4

A senior civil servant was persuaded to seek medical advice because of his increasingly bizarre behaviour. He had slowed up mentally, become indecisive and had given up his daily game of squash, claiming that he no longer had the energy to play. Whereas in the past he had annoyed his colleagues by opening windows even on cold days, he now no longer objected to them remaining closed. His appearance had changed, his skin appearing sallow and his hair coarse and lacking lustre.

His general practitioner suspected hypothyroidism and elicited a history of recent constipation in addition to the other typical features. Bradycardia was present and when the peripheral reflexes were tested, slow quadriceps relaxation was noted. There was no goitre.

### Investigations

serum: TSH          >100 mU/L

### Comment

The clinical diagnosis of hypothyroidism is confirmed by the very high serum TSH concentration, reflecting the lack of negative feedback from circulating thyroid hormones. Under such circumstances, measurement of fT4 is unnecessary for diagnosis, although as discussed on p.140, most laboratories routinely measure TSH and fT4 on all samples submitted for thyroid function tests. fT4 also provides an additional index against which to assess the response to treatment.

## Hypothyroidism

There are many possible causes of primary hypothyroidism (*Fig. 9.13*) but hypothyroidism may also occur secondarily to decreased trophic stimulation both in hypopituitarism and in hypothalamic disease. It is, however, very rare for patients with pituitary failure to present with clinical features of hypothyroidism alone. The commonest cause of hypothyroidism is atrophic myxoedema, the end result of autoimmune destruction of the gland. The clinical manifestations (*Fig. 9.13*) are variable and may result in the patient being referred to almost any specialist department in a hospital.

Hypothyroidism is treated by replacement of thyroid hormones, usually T4. T3 has a short plasma half-life and is preferred when treating hypothyroid patients with ischaemic heart disease. The increase in metabolic rate and demand for oxygen prompted by hormone replacement may precipitate angina or myocardial infarction; a much more rapid response to a decrease in dosage is seen if T3 rather than T4 is used. T3 is also preferable in the initial treatment of patients in myxoedema coma (*see below*).

In the laboratory, thyroid hormone replacement can be monitored by measuring plasma TSH and, if this is abnormal, fT4 concentrations (fT3 if the patient is being treated with T3). Ideally, the replacement dosage should be sufficient to

| Hypothyroidism | |
|---|---|
| **Causes** | **Clinical features** |
| *atrophic hypothyroidism | lethargy, tiredness |
| *autoimmune hypothyroidism (Hashimoto's thyroiditis) | cold intolerance |
| | dryness and coarsening of skin and hair |
| *post-surgery, radioactive iodine, anti-thyroid drugs (e.g., carbimazole) and other agents (e.g., lithium) | hoarseness |
| | weight gain |
| congenital | slow relaxation of muscles and tendon reflexes |
| dyshormonogenic | many others including: |
| secondary (pituitary or hypothalamic disease) |   anaemia, typically macrocytic, non-megaloblastic but pernicious in 10% of cases |
| iodine deficiency |   dementia; psychosis |
| |   constipation |
| |   bradycardia, angina, pericardial effusion |
| |   muscle stiffness |
| *these account for >90% of cases |   carpal tunnel syndrome |
| |   infertility, menorrhagia, galactorrhoea |

**Fig. 9.13** Causes and clinical features of hypothyroidism. Children with hypothyroidism may present with growth failure, delayed pubertal development or a deterioration in academic performance.

maintain TSH within the reference range. Too high a level indicates inadequate replacement; a suppressed TSH suggests that replacement may be excessive. In patients treated with T4, the plasma concentrations associated with a clinically euthyroid state are generally somewhat higher than the normal euthyroid range, because there is no contribution to endogenous hormone activity by secreted T3. If the dosage is changed, the results of thyroid function tests may not reach a new steady state for some time. In particular, if the TSH has been suppressed, months may elapse before normal thyrotrophic responsiveness to T4 is regained.

Occasionally, patients with hypothyroidism present as an emergency with stupor and hypothermia. This 'myxoedema coma' has a high mortality. In addition to thyroid hormone replacement, usually with T3, possible coexistent adrenal insufficiency must be treated with hydrocortisone and appropriate measures taken to treat any infection, heart failure or electrolyte imbalance and to restore body temperature to normal.

**CASE HISTORY 9.5**

A 55-year-old businesswoman underwent the medical screening programme provided by her company. Various tests were performed, including assessment of thyroid function.

**Investigations**

| | |
|---|---|
| Serum  TSH | 8 mU/L |
| fT4 | 12 pmol/L |

**Comment**

Serum TSH concentration is slightly elevated, and fT4, though within the reference range, is near the lower end, compatible with early or borderline hypothyroidism. Thyroid failure can be an insidious condition and sufficient function of the failing thyroid may be maintained by increased secretion of TSH in the early stages. Measurement of fT4 concentration, though useful for subsequent comparison, may not be of practical help in management. The decision whether to treat the patient with thyroxine is better made on clinical grounds, although the detection of thyroid autoantibodies in serum lends weight to the diagnosis of thyroid disease. Because the clinical features of hypothyroidism can be so non-specific, patients may only appreciate, retrospectively, that they were present after replacement therapy has been started. Often, the most prudent course is to follow up the patient clinically, and repeat the tests after 3–6 months. In this case, thyroxine replacement was not given initially, but six months later serum TSH concentration had increased to 29 mU/L and fT4 was 9 pmol/L. After thyroxine replacement had been started, the patient commented that she now realized that she had been feeling 'run down' for some time beforehand.

## Thyroiditis

Inflammation of the thyroid, or thyroiditis, may be due to infection (usually viral) or autoimmune disease. In viral thyroiditis, associated with coxsackie, mumps and adenovirus, the inflammation results in a release of pre-formed colloid and there is an increase in the level of thyroid hormones in the blood stream. Patients may become transiently, and usually only mildly, thyrotoxic. This phase persists for up to six weeks and is followed by a similar period in which thyroid hormone output may be decreased, although not sufficiently to cause symptoms. Thereafter, normal function is regained.

Hashimoto's thyroiditis, an autoimmune condition, has been mentioned as a cause of hypothyroidism. Autoantibodies are present in high titre and the disease is associated with the presence of other organ-specific autoimmune diseases. Very occasionally, transient hyperthyroidism may occur early in the course of the disease due, as in viral thyroiditis, to increased release of pre-formed colloid.

## Goitre

Goitre, or enlargement of the thyroid, can occur in patients with hyperthyroidism (e.g., in Graves' disease, toxic multinodular goitre or a thyroid adenoma), hypothyroidism (e.g., in Hashimoto's disease or iodine deficiency) and in euthyroid individuals with benign or malignant tumours of the gland. Physiological enlargement of the thyroid may occur during adolescence, unaccompanied by any change in function.

Except in this latter case, thyroid function tests should be performed even in apparently euthyroid patients presenting with a goitre since the results may provide a clue to the cause. The thyroid hormone status of such patients should be investigated and may give a clue to the cause of the goitre. The laboratory has no part to play in the diagnosis of thyroid cancer, with the exception of calcitonin-secreting medullary carcinoma. When patients with thyroid cancer are treated by ablative doses of radioactive iodine and put on replacement thyroxine, the efficacy of the treatment can be assessed by measuring plasma thyroglobulin levels. Since small amounts of thyroglobulin are normally released from the gland together with thyroid hormones, persistent thyroid activity can be inferred if thyroglobulin is present in the plasma.

## SCREENING FOR THYROID DISEASE

Congenital hypothyroidism is sufficiently serious and common (1 in 4000 live births in the United Kingdom but considerably higher in some other countries) for it to be worth while to screen for the condition. Untreated, affected children become cretins, with very low intelligence and impaired growth and motor function. Treatment by replacement of T4 is simple and effective but this must be started as soon after birth as a reliable diagnosis can be made. The screening method involves measurement of TSH in a capillary blood sample collected on to a Guthrie card (see p.244) at 6–8 days of age. Screening for phenylketonuria is performed at the same time. Maternal thyroxine crosses the placenta and can affect the infant's pituitary–thyroid axis for a short period after birth.

Hypo- and hyperthyroidism are both common in the elderly (more so in the former), with a combined prevalence of approximately 5%. Since both the conditions may present insidiously, and atypically, in the elderly, attempts have been made to screen for the conditions in this population. In practice, however, the influence of non-thyroidal illness on the results of thyroid function tests renders this a far from straightforward proposition. Furthermore, while there is evidence that the presence of a slightly raised plasma TSH together with the presence of thyroid autoantibodies indicates an increased risk of future clinical hypothyroidism, patients with either one of these abnormalities alone may not be at risk.

## SUMMARY

The thyroid gland secretes two iodine-containing hormones, thyroxine (T4) and triiodothyronine (T3). T4 is secreted in the greater amount and is in part metabolized to T3 in peripheral tissues; T3 is the more active hormone. The synthesis and secretion of thyroid hormones is stimulated by the pituitary hormone, thyroid-stimulating hormone (TSH). The release of TSH is in turn controlled by thyrotrophin releasing hormone from the hypothalamus. T4 and T3 exert negative feedback inhibition on TSH release.

The thyroid hormones are essential for normal growth and development, and also control basal metabolic rate and stimulate many metabolic processes.

T4 and T3 are extensively protein-bound in the blood (T4 to an even greater extent than T3), to thyroxine-binding globulin, albumin and prealbumin, the free, physiologically active, fractions being less than 1% of the total. Factors which affect the concentration of the binding proteins can alter total hormone concentrations without affecting the free fraction, and thus erroneously suggest the presence of an abnormality of thyroid function.

Thyroid status is best assessed biochemically by measurement of plasma TSH and fT4 concentrations, with fT3 being measured in addition if hyperthyroidism is suspected. Typically, in primary hypothyroidism, thyroid hormone concentrations (fT4 more so than fT3) are low and TSH is high; in hyperthyroidism, TSH is very low and fT3 and, usually, fT4 are high. Drug treatment and non-thyroidal disease frequently cause the results of thyroid function tests to be abnormal in patients who do not have thyroid disease.

Patients with thyroid disease may present due to overactivity of the gland (hyperthyroidism, leading to thyrotoxicosis) or underactivity (hypothyroidism, leading to myxoedema).

Patients in either category may have enlargement of the gland (goitre) but patients with goitres can be euthyroid. Both hyper- and hypothyroidism are commonly the result of autoimmune disease although there are many other causes. The measurement of specific autoantibodies can provide useful diagnostic information in thyroid disease. Options for the treatment of hyperthyroidism include antithyroid drugs, radioactive iodine and surgery; patients with hypothyroidism require hormone replacement.

The thyroid also secretes calcitonin, a polypeptide hormone which may be involved in calcium homoeostasis.

## FURTHER READING

Anon (1989) Sensitive thyrotropin measurements: utility and futility, *Lancet*, **1**, 1176.

Besser G M & Thorner M O (eds.) (1994) *Clinical Endocrinology: An Illustrated Text*. 2nd edition. London: Wolfe.

Greenspan F S (ed.) (1991) Thyroid disease. *The Medical Clinics of North America*, **75**, 1–235.

Hall R & Besser M (eds) (1989) *Fundamentals of Clinical Endocrinology*. 4th edition. London: Pitman Medical.

Rae P, Farrar J, Beckett G, Toft A (1993) Assessment of thyroid status in elderly people, *British Medical Journal*, **307**, 177–180.

Wilson J D & Foster D W (eds) (1992) *Williams – Textbook of Endocrinology*. 8th edition. Philadelphia: WB Saunders Company.

# 10. The Gonads

## INTRODUCTION

### Androgens and testicular function

The testes are responsible for the synthesis of the male sex hormones (androgens) and the production of spermatozoa. The most important androgen, both in terms of potency and the amount secreted, is testosterone. Other testicular androgens include androstenedione and dehydroepiandrosterone (DHEA). These weaker androgens are also secreted by the adrenal glands but adrenal androgen secretion does not appear to be physiologically important in the male. In the female, however, it contributes to the development of certain secondary sexual characteristics, in particular the growth of pubic and axillary hair. The pathological consequences of increased adrenal androgen secretion are discussed in *Chapter 8* and on *p. 156*.

Testosterone is a powerful anabolic hormone. It is vital to the development of secondary sexual characteristics in the male and is essential for spermatogenesis. It is secreted by the Leydig cells of the testis under the influence of luteinizing hormone (LH). Spermatogenesis is also dependent on the function of the Sertoli cells of the testicular seminiferous tubules. These cells are follicle-stimulating hormone (FSH) dependent; they secrete inhibin, which inhibits FSH secretion, and androgen-binding protein, whose function is probably to ensure an adequate local testosterone concentration.

Testosterone concentrations in the plasma are very low before puberty but then rise rapidly to reach normal adult values. A slight decline in concentration may be seen in the elderly. Testosterone is also present in females, at a much lower concentration, about one-third being derived from the ovaries and the remainder from the metabolism of adrenal androgens. In the circulation, approximately 97% of testosterone is protein-bound, principally to sex hormone-binding globulin (SHBG) and to a lesser extent to albumin and other proteins. Only the free testosterone is available to tissues. Measurement of free testosterone concentration is technically difficult but calculation of the ratio of testosterone/SHBG concentrations provides an index of free testosterone status. The biological activity of testosterone is mainly due to dihydrotestosterone (DHT). This is formed from testosterone in target tissues in a reaction catalyzed by the enzyme, 5α-reductase. In a rare condition in which there is deficiency of this enzyme, DHT cannot be formed; male internal genitalia develop normally (Wolffian

duct development in the fetus is testosterone dependent) but masculinization, which requires DHT, is incomplete. In states of androgen insensitivity, defects of the receptors for either testosterone or DHT, or both, can cause a spectrum of clinical abnormalities ranging from gynaecomastia to pseudohermaphroditism.

Specific assays are available for testosterone, DHT and other androgens, and SHBG. There is no longer any indication for the measurement of urinary 17-oxosteroids in the assessment of gonadal function. These are metabolites of androstenedione, to which some testosterone is metabolized, but two-thirds of urinary 17-oxosteroids are derived from adrenal androgens.

### Oestrogens and ovarian function

The cyclical control of ovarian function during the reproductive years is discussed in *Chapter 7*. The principal ovarian hormone is 17β-oestradiol, but some oestrone is also produced by the ovaries. Oestrogens are also secreted by the corpus luteum and the placenta.

Oestrogens are responsible for the development of many female secondary sexual characteristics. They also stimulate the growth of ovarian follicles and the proliferation of uterine endometrium during the first part of the menstrual cycle. They have important effects on cervical mucus and vaginal epithelium, and on other functions associated with reproduction.

Plasma concentrations of oestrogens are low before puberty. During puberty, oestrogen synthesis increases and cyclical changes in concentration occur thereafter until the menopause, unless pregnancy occurs. After the menopause, the sole source of oestrogens is from the metabolism of adrenal androgens and plasma concentrations fall to very low levels. In the plasma, oestrogens are transported bound to protein, 60% to albumin and the remainder to SHBG. Only 2–3% remains unbound. Oestrogens stimulate the synthesis of SHBG and also that of other transport proteins, notably thyroxine-binding globulin (TBG) and transcortin, and thus increase total thyroxine and total cortisol concentrations in the plasma. Oestradiol is present in low concentrations in the plasma of normal men. Approximately one-third is secreted by the testis, the remainder being derived from the metabolism of testosterone in the liver and in adipose tissue. Slowly rising or sustained high levels of oestrogens together with progesterone inhibit pituitary gonadotrophin secretion by negative feedback, but the rapid rise in oestrogen concentration which occurs prior to ovulation stimulates LH secretion (positive feedback).

## Progesterone

Progesterone is an important intermediate in steroid hormone biosynthesis but is secreted in appreciable quantities only by the corpus luteum and the placenta. Its concentration in plasma rises during the second half of the menstrual cycle but then falls if conception does not take place. In the plasma, it is extensively bound to albumin and transcortin; only 1–2% is free. Progesterone has many important effects on the uterus, including preparation of the endometrium for implantation of the conceptus, and also on the cervix, vagina and breasts. It is pyrogenic and mediates the increase in basal body temperature that occurs with ovulation. Progesterone can be measured in plasma and this assay is used in the investigation of infertility in women (*see page 158*).

## Sex hormone-binding globulin

SHBG binds both testosterone and oestradiol in the plasma, though it has greater affinity for testosterone. The plasma concentration of SHBG in males is about half that in females. Factors which alter SHBG concentration (*Fig. 10.1*) alter the ratio of free testosterone to free oestradiol. If SHBG concentration decreases, the ratio of free testosterone to free oestradiol increases, though there is an absolute increase in the concentration of both hormones. If SHBG concentration increases, the ratio decreases. Thus in either sex, the effect of an increase in SHBG is to increase oestrogen-dependent effects while a decrease in SHBG increases androgen-dependent effects (*Fig. 10.2*).

# DISORDERS OF MALE GONADAL FUNCTION

## Hypogonadism

The term hypogonadism implies defective spermatogenesis or testosterone production or both. It can be primary (that is, due to testicular disease) or occur secondarily to pituitary or hypothalamic disease. Some of the causes are indicated in *Fig. 10.3*. Primary hypogonadism can be due to only defective seminiferous tubule function or defective Leydig cell function or both. The former leads to infertility through decreased production of spermatozoa, but masculinization is usually normal. Defective Leydig cell function, on the

| Factors affecting sex hormone-binding globulin concentration |
| --- |
| **Increase** |
| oestrogens<br>hyperthyroidism<br>liver cirrhosis |
| **Decrease** |
| androgens<br>hypothyroidism<br>glucocorticoids<br>malnutrition and malabsorption<br>protein-losing states<br>obesity, particularly in women |

**Fig. 10.1** Factors which cause an increase or a decrease in the plasma concentration of sex hormone-binding globulin (SHBG).

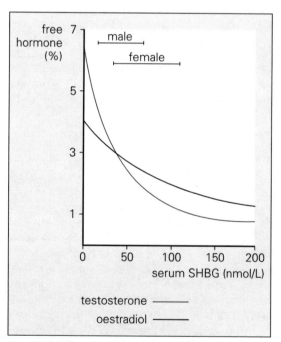

**Fig. 10.2** Effect of a change in serum SHBG concentration on free oestradiol and testosterone concentrations. A decrease in SHBG increases free testosterone concentration more than free oestradiol and thus is androgenic; an increase in the concentration of SHBG is anti-androgenic. The normal ranges of SHBG in males and females are shown.

other hand, results in a failure of testosterone-dependent functions, including spermatogenesis. The effects of decreased testosterone secretion depend upon the time of onset of the disorder. Secondary sexual characteristics are in part preserved if secretion is lost after puberty.

The basic biochemical characteristics that distinguish between primary and secondary hypogonadism are not always clear-cut. This is partly because most currently available assays for gonadotrophins are insufficiently sensitive to distinguish between low and normal concentrations. The secretion of gonadotrophins and testosterone is pulsatile. Ideally, when basal concentrations or the effects of chronic stimulation are to be measured, analyses should be performed on several blood specimens drawn over the period of an hour.

The use of provocative tests of the hypothalamo–pituitary–gonadal axis in hypogonadism is discussed in *Case History 10.1.*

---

### Causes of male hypogonadism

**Primary** (serum testosterone ↓; FSH and LH ↑)

congenital
  e.g., testicular agenesis
    Klinefelter's syndrome (47XXY)
    5α-reductase and other enzyme defects
    untreated cryptorchidism

acquired
  e.g., bilateral orchitis (mumps)
    bilateral testicular torsion
    irradiation
    cytotoxic drugs
    varicocele

**Secondary** (serum testosterone ↓; FSH and LH normal or ↓)

pituitary disorders
  e.g., tumours (especially if causing
      hyperprolactinaemia)
    panhypopituitarism

hypothalamic disorders
  e.g., Kallman's syndrome

**Fig. 10.3** Causes of male hypogonadism.

---

### CASE HISTORY 10.1

A 20-year-old man presented with impotence. On examination, he was eunuchoid; there was only sparse pubic and axillary hair, the genitalia were infantile, muscular development was poor and his span exceeded his height with a sole–pubic symphysis distance greater than symphysis to crown.

**Investigations**

| serum: | testosterone | 3 nmol/L |
| | LH | <1.5 U/L |
| | FSH | <1.5 U/L |

clomiphene test (3 mg/kg body weight clomiphene citrate daily for seven days):

| serum: | LH | <1.5 U/L |
| | FSH | <1.5 U/L |

gonadotrophin releasing hormone (GnRH) test (100 μg GnRH i.v.):

| time (min) | FSH (U/L) | LH (U/L) |
| --- | --- | --- |
| 0 | <1.5 | <1.5 |
| 20 | 2.0 | 2.0 |
| 60 | 2.5 | 3.0 |

(after 100 μg GnRH subcutaneously daily for two weeks)

| 0 | 3.5 | 4.5 |
| 20 | 8.4 | 21.5 |
| 60 | 4.5 | 8.0 |

**Comment**

The age of onset of normal puberty may sometimes be delayed until 18 years of age and hypogonadism should be diagnosed with caution in patients who are younger than this. The low testosterone and gonadotrophins in this case suggest a lesion at the level of either the pituitary or hypothalamus. This is confirmed by the failure of response to clomiphene. This drug competes with gonadal steroids for hypothalamic receptors and in normal men results in an increase in gonadotrophin secretion and thus testosterone secretion. Patients with pituitary lesions may have clinical or biochemical evidence of other pituitary abnormalities (none was present in this case).

The GnRH test is sometimes used in an attempt to distinguish between pituitary and hypothalamic causes of hypogonadism but in practice is of limited value. In pituitary disease, it might be expected that the LH and FSH responses to GnRH would be diminished or absent, but they can be normal. In hypothalamic disease, the response can be delayed (greater at 60 min than 20 min, cf. TRH test, *p.142*), normal, or decreased; in this case, it is both subnormal and delayed. The pituitary can become insensitive to exogenous GnRH in hypothalamic disease and repeated injections of the hormone may correct this. When the GnRH test was repeated after GnRH priming, this patient's response was normal, indicating a hypothalamic, rather than a pituitary defect. He was later found to be anosmic (lacking a sense of smell). The association between anosmia and hypogonadotrophic hypogonadism is called Kallman's syndrome. The eunuchoid habitus is a direct consequence of testosterone deficiency; this promotes epiphyseal fusion and when its secretion is inadequate, there is continued growth of long bones which become disproportionate to the axial skeleton.

Although biochemical tests are important in establishing that a patient has primary, rather than secondary, gonadal failure they are less useful in distinguishing between the various causes of primary hypogonadism. In general, seminiferous tubule defects are associated with a raised plasma FSH concentration; Leydig cell defects are associated with a raised plasma LH concentration. Human chorionic gonadotrophin (hCG), which has an action similar to LH, can be used to test Leydig cell function (*Fig. 10.4*). Semen analysis will provide an indication of seminiferous tubule function and testicular biopsy is valuable in patients with low sperm counts if the cause is not obvious clinically. Careful clinical examination is essential in all cases of gonadal failure.

The treatment of hypogonadism in males should be directed towards the underlying cause wherever possible. Testosterone is given in testosterone deficiency syndromes, but if fertility is required, treatment must be with gonadotrophin replacement or, in hypothalamic disorders, pulsatile GnRH administration.

## Gynaecomastia

Breast development in males is usually related to a disturbance of the balance of oestrogens to androgens. It may occur physiologically in neonates as a result of exposure to maternal oestrogens. During puberty, approximately 50% of normal boys develop gynaecomastia due to temporarily increased secretion of oestrogens relative to androgens. In both instances the gynaecomastia resolves spontaneously. Mild gynaecomastia may also occur in the elderly, as a result of a decrease in testosterone secretion.

Gynaecomastia occurring at other times should be regarded as pathological. The principal causes are shown in *Fig. 10.5*. The cause may be obvious from either the history or clinical examination. Measurement of plasma testosterone, gonadotrophins, SHBG and prolactin, and assessment of liver and possibly thyroid function will help to distinguish between them. Karyotyping is required to

| Human chorionic gonadotrophin (hCG) test | |
|---|---|
| **Procedure** | **Results** |
| day 0: 0900 h; take blood for testosterone give 2000 IU hCG i.m. | normal response: plasma testosterone level increases to above upper limit of reference range |
| day 3: 0900 h; give 2000 IU hCG i.m. | primary testicular failure: little or no response |
| day 5: 0900 h; take blood for testosterone | secondary testicular failure: response may be normal |

**Fig. 10.4** Human chorionic gonadotrophin test for primary testicular failure.

diagnose Klinefelter's syndrome in which an additional X-chromosome is present (47XXY); chest and skull radiographs, and tests of pituitary and adrenal function may be of use.

# DISORDERS OF FEMALE GONADAL FUNCTION

## The climacteric

During the climacteric, progressive ovarian failure causes a decline in ovarian oestrogen secretion and eventually menstruation ceases; the menopause is the last menstrual period. The only oestrogen produced after the menopause is the small amount derived from metabolism of adrenal androstenedione in adipose tissue. The plasma concentrations of pituitary gonadotrophins become greatly elevated, FSH tending to increase first; this change is a more reliable indication of ovarian failure than plasma oestrogen concentrations, which show considerable variability. Metabolic changes which occur after the menopause include increases in plasma low density lipoprotein concentration and plasma urate concentration. Oestrogen deficiency is a major factor contributing to the development of post-menopausal osteoporosis.

## Amenorrhoea and oligomenorrhoea

Amenorrhoea can be primary (menstruation has never occurred) or secondary. Oligomenorrhoea is sparse or infrequent menstruation; it can be due to less severe forms of some of the causes of amenorrhoea (*Fig. 10.6*).

The commonest cause of amenorrhoea in women of child-bearing age is pregnancy, and this possibility, however unlikely, must be excluded. The finding of an apparently high plasma LH concentration may suggest pregnancy before a pregnancy test is performed; chorionic gonadotrophin cross reacts in many assays for LH. Weight loss is another common cause; the frequency of the pulsatile secretion of GnRH decreases, and gonadotrophin secretion declines. Menstruation almost always ceases if weight loss falls below 75% of the ideal, but this may happen with smaller losses. Regular menstruation returns if weight is regained.

Amenorrhoea is otherwise most frequently due to a hormonal disturbance which results in a failure of ovulation. Uterine dysfunction can be responsible but can be

---

### Some causes of gynaecomastia

**Physiological**
neonatal
pubertal
old age

**Pathological**
increased oestrogens
  e.g., chronic liver disease, tumours
decreased androgens
  e.g., Klinefelter's syndrome
androgen insensitivity
  e.g., testicular feminization
refeeding after starvation
  (LH secretion increased)

**Pharmacological**
oestrogens
digoxin (binds to oestrogen receptors)
cytotoxics (testicular damage)
anti-androgens (e.g., cyproterone;
  spironolactone has some
  anti-androgenic activity)
others (phenothiazines, methyldopa,
  etc: mechanism uncertain)

**Fig. 10.5** Causes of gynaecomastia.

---

### Endocrine causes of amenorrhoea

**Primary ovarian failure**
gonadal dysgenesis, e.g., Turner's syndrome
premature menopause, e.g., autoimmune
  disease

**Pituitary disorders**
isolated gonadotrophin deficiency
tumours:
  causing decreased gonadotrophin secretion
  causing hyperprolactinaemia
panhypopituitarism, e.g., post-partum necrosis

**Hypothalamic disorders**
weight loss
intensive exercise

**Others**
thyrotoxicosis; severe hypothyroidism
congenital adrenal hyperplasia
polycystic ovary syndrome

**Fig. 10.6** Endocrine causes of amenorrhoea. Severe systemic disease of any nature can cause amenorrhoea.

excluded by the progestogen challenge test. If medroxy-progesterone acetate is given orally (10 mg daily for five days), the occurrence of vaginal bleeding 5–7 days later signifies that the uterus was adequately oestrogenized. If bleeding does not occur, the test is repeated, giving oestrogen (ethinyloestradiol, 50 μg daily for 21 days, with progestogen on the last five days). Absence of bleeding indicates uterine disease. If bleeding occurs, oestrogen deficiency is present.

The diagnosis of hormonal causes of amenorrhoea requires basal measurements of plasma FSH, LH and prolactin concentrations. Hyperprolactinaemia is responsible for about 25% of cases of amenorrhoea. A high FSH is indicative of ovarian failure (and is more sensitive in this respect than LH). If LH, but not FSH, is elevated, and the patient is not pregnant, the most likely diagnosis is polycystic ovary syndrome. If LH and FSH concentrations are normal or low, a pituitary or hypothalamic disorder should be sought, by anatomical studies and dynamic testing of the hypothalamic–pituitary axis in a manner similar to that described for male hypogonadism. As in males, however, the results of such tests do not always distinguish between pituitary and hypothalamic disorders.

The investigation of amenorrhoea accompanied by hirsutism or other features of virilization is discussed in the next section.

The management of amenorrhoea depends upon the cause, and whether fertility is required. In hyperprolactinaemia, the treatment is directed to the underlying cause wherever possible (e.g., withdrawal of drugs, treatment of hypothyroidism); when due to a pituitary tumour, bromocriptine is usually the treatment of choice.

In ovarian, pituitary or hypothalamic disease, when fertility is not required, cyclical oestrogen and (if the patient has a uterus) progestogen replacement is given. In established ovarian failure, pregnancy is only possible using donated ova.

If fertility is required in pituitary failure, treatment is with human FSH and LH; hCG may be required to mimic the mid-cycle LH peak and stimulate ovulation. Careful monitoring of plasma oestradiol concentrations is necessary to detect hyperstimulation, which carries a risk of multiple pregnancy and the production of ovarian cysts.

Patients with hypothalamic disease may respond to clomiphene. This substance blocks oestradiol receptors in the hypothalamus and may stimulate GnRH (and thus LH and FSH) secretion. Non-responders are treated with pulsatile GnRH. Clomiphene is also useful in inducing ovulation in patients with polycystic ovary syndrome. When it has not been possible to distinguish between hypothalamic and pituitary disease, a failure to respond to pulsatile GnRH suggests that amenorrhoea is due to pituitary dysfunction.

A simple protocol for the investigation of endocrine causes of amenorrhoea is given in *Fig. 10.7*.

## Hirsutism and virilism

Hirsutism is an increase in body hair in an androgen-related distribution. In most instances, menstruation is normal, but hirsutism may be accompanied by menstrual irregularity and other features of virilism, e.g., cliteromegaly, male-pattern hair loss, etc. There is considerable racial variation in the amount of body hair in women and what may be regarded as normal in some races may be thought excessive by others.

The cause is usually excessive exposure of tissues to androgens. This may be due either to increased androgen secretion or a low level of SHBG, which increases the free testosterone fraction. In some cases, there appears to be an increased sensitivity to androgens. The causes of hirsutism and virilism are indicated in *Fig. 10.8*.

The commonest cause of hirsutism is the polycystic ovary syndrome (PCOS). This condition demonstrates considerable variation in its expression, and it is likely that many patients previously described as having 'idiopathic' hirsutism have a mild form of the polycystic ovary syndrome.

The appropriate investigation of hirsutism depends on the clinical context, although if menstruation is normal, no endocrine abnormality may be found. Measurement of LH, FSH, testosterone and, if available, SHBG, is desirable in all patients. Moderately elevated testosterone concentrations (2.5–7.0 nmol/L) occur in the PCOS and in late-onset congenital adrenal hyperplasia (CAH). Concentrations in excess of 7.0 nmol/L are strongly suggestive of an androgen-secreting tumour, which may be in an adrenal or an ovary.

The presence of other clinical features (e.g., of Cushing's syndrome) in a hirsute patient may suggest a specific diagnosis and thus appropriate further investigations. In patients with severe hirsutism or if menstrual disturbance or virilism is present, adrenal androgens and 17-OH progesterone (17-OHP) should be measured. A diagnosis of late-onset CAH is supported by the finding of an elevated concentration of 17-OHP which increases to more than twice the upper limit of normal 60 minutes after an injection of Synacthen (250 μg, i.m.). High concentrations of 17-OHP, dehydroepiandrosterone sulphate and androstenedione are found in patients with adrenal tumours, but 17-OHP does not increase significantly in response to Synacthen.

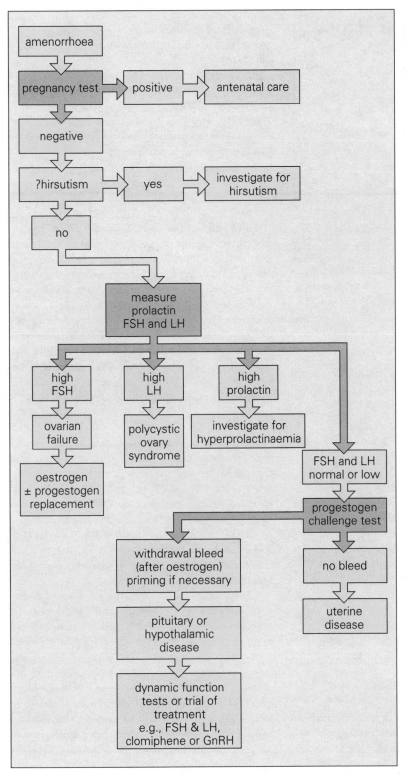

**Fig. 10.7** A protocol for the investigation of amenorrhoea; dynamic function tests (GnRH, clomiphene) may distinguish between hypothalamic and pituitary causes although in practice this may only become clear when treatment aimed at restoring fertility is instituted.

| Causes of hirsuitism and virilization |
|---|
| **Idiopathic** |
| **Ovarian**<br>polycystic ovary syndrome<br>androgen-secreting tumours<br>post-menopausal |
| **Adrenal**<br>congenital adrenal hyperplasia<br>Cushing's syndrome<br>androgen-secreting tumours |
| **Iatrogenic**<br>androgens<br>progestogens |

**Fig. 10.8** Causes of hirsutism and virilization. Idiopathic causes and the polycystic ovary syndrome account for the great majority of cases.

**CASE HISTORY 10.2**

A young woman consulted her doctor because she was embarrassed by excessive hair on her upper lip, lower abdomen and thighs. She was moderately obese. Her periods had always been irregular.

**Investigations**

serum:
testosterone      3.5 nmol/L
LH (early follicular)    14 U/L
FSH (early follicular)   3 U/L

ultrasound examination of the ovaries:
  multiple cysts present, bilaterally

**Comment**

These findings are characteristic of the polycystic ovary syndrome; testosterone concentration is slightly elevated, and LH is high in relation to FSH. The clinical features of this condition include hirsutism, acne, menstrual disturbances and obesity, but there is considerable variation in their prevalence and severity. Neither are the typical hormonal changes always present. The pathogenesis of the condition is

uncertain. The normal ovaries synthesize androgens (principally testosterone and androstenedione) but their secretion is increased in PCOS. Conversion of androgens to oestrogens in liver and adipose tissue inhibits secretion of FSH (preventing ovulation) and stimulates that of LH (further stimulating androgen secretion). Hyperinsulinaemia is frequently present and may be fundamental to the increased ovarian androgen secretion.

Conditions such as adrenal tumours and congenital adrenal hyperplasia require specific treatment. In idiopathic hirsutism and the PCOS, the management depends upon the severity of the hirsutism and whether fertility is required. In mild cases, with no menstrual disturbance, the excessive hair may be acceptably treated by cosmetic means. In more severe cases, various endocrine manipulations may be useful. These include the use of a synthetic glucocorticoid to suppress adrenal androgen excretion or, if this fails, the anti-androgen drug, cyproterone. If fertility is required, cyproterone must not be used; it may be possible to restore fertility with gonadotrophins or clomiphene.

## Infertility

Infertility – defined as failure of a couple to conceive after one year of regular, unprotected intercourse – is a common clinical problem. It can be primary (conception has never occurred) or secondary, and due to problems affecting either the male or the female. Ovulatory failure, due most frequently to hyperprolactinaemia or hypothalamic–pituitary dysfunction, is responsible in approximately 20% of cases, and defective sperm production in about one quarter. Endocrine causes of infertility are rare in males.

The investigation of infertility requires a thorough clinical and laboratory assessment of both partners. Anatomical causes, for example damage to the Fallopian tubes, are relatively common. Semen must be examined to ensure that adequate numbers of normal sperm are present. If menstruation is regular, ovulation is probably occurring. Detection of the rise in basal body temperature which follows ovulation is a useful indicator of this. More reliably, the concentration of progesterone (secreted by the corpus luteum) in plasma increases following ovulation and should exceed 30 nmol/L on day 21 of the menstrual cycle. A concentration below 10 nmol/L is very suggestive of anovulatory cycles. Intermediate values are non-diagnostic. If ovulation is confirmed, cervical mucus should be examined and a post-coital test performed to establish that motile sperm are present. If cycles are anovulatory but regular, treatment with clomiphene may restore fertility. If not, or if there is oligo- or amenorrhoea, measurements of prolactin and gonadotrophins may indicate a diagnosis (see amenorrhoea, *p. 155*). Defective sperm production should be investigated by measurements of testosterone and gonadotrophins and, if necessary, by testicular biopsy.

---

### CASE HISTORY 10.3

A couple in their late twenties were infertile in spite of regular intercourse over a two-year period. Each partner had a child by previous marriages. The woman's periods had recently become irregular. A semen sample contained a normal count of motile sperm. Physical examination revealed no abnormality. The woman was on steroid replacement treatment for adrenal failure, which had been diagnosed in her late teens.

**Investigations (woman)**

serum: prolactin     300 mU/L
      LH           12 U/L
      FSH         25 U/L

**Comment**

This is secondary infertility. The elevated FSH concentration (due to decreased negative feedback by oestrogens) indicates incipient ovarian failure. FSH is a more sensitive test for this than LH, although in established ovarian failure (after the menopause), the plasma concentrations of LH and FSH are usually both very high. The adrenal failure in the woman had been shown to be due to autoimmune disease, and there is a recognized association between autoimmune adrenal and ovarian failure (Schmidt's syndrome). Two months later she had not had a period, and a measurement of plasma LH concentration gave a value >100 U/L. It is possible for hCG to cross-react in assays for LH. A pregnancy test was positive. Ovarian failure develops gradually and occasional ovulation may still occur in the early stages.

## PREGNANCY

Many physiological and metabolic changes take place in the body during pregnancy. These include changes in the concentrations of hormones directly related to pregnancy and resulting secondary metabolic changes.

### Specific hormonal changes
#### Human chorionic gonadotrophin
Fertilization of the ovum prevents the regression of the corpus luteum. Instead, the corpus luteum enlarges, stimulated by the glycoprotein hormone hCG, produced by the trophoblast (the developing placenta). This hormone (assays usually measure the β-subunit; *see p. 277*) can be detected in maternal blood 7–9 days after conception and may be detectable in urine 1–2 days later. Its detection in the urine provides a highly sensitive and specific test for the diagnosis of pregnancy. The secretion of β-hCG begins to fall by 10–12 weeks, although it remains detectable in the urine throughout pregnancy. hCG is also produced by some tumours; its use as a tumour marker is discussed in *Chapter 19.*

#### Oestrogens
The stimulated corpus luteum secretes large amounts of oestrogens and progesterone, but after six weeks the placenta becomes the major source of these hormones. There is a massive increase in the production of oestriol during pregnancy, but production of oestrone and oestradiol increases also. Oestriol is synthesized in the placenta from androgens secreted by the fetal adrenals. Its measurement in maternal plasma or urine was formerly used to assess feto–placental function but now has been largely superseded by ultrasonography, which can be used to provide direct measurements of fetal growth and placental blood flow. The same applies to measurements of other placental products, e.g., human placental lactogen and placental alkaline phosphatase (a heat-stable isoenzyme) which have been used in the past as indicators of placental function.

### Secondary metabolic changes
Many of the metabolic changes that occur in pregnancy are discussed elsewhere in this book. Those that may suggest the presence of a pathological process are summarized in *Fig. 10.9.*

### Maternal monitoring
Patients with medical conditions may require close monitoring during pregnancy. For example, strict control of diabetes mellitus is vital and entails frequent monitoring of

| Metabolic changes during pregnancy and use of oral contraceptives | | | |
|---|---|---|---|
| Change | Cause | Pregnancy | Oral contraceptive use |
| ↓ urea | ↑ GFR; ↑ plasma volume | * | |
| ↓ albumin | ↑ plasma volume | * | |
| ↓ total protein | ↑ plasma volume | * | |
| ↑ total thyroxine | ↑ TBG | * | * |
| ↑ cortisol | ↑ transcortin | * | * |
| ↑ copper | ↑ caeruloplasmin | * | * |
| glycosuria | ↓ renal threshold | * | |
| ↓ glucose tolerance (but normal fasting levels) | | * | |
| ↑ triglyceride (VLDL) | ↑ oestrogens (antagonism of actions of insulin) | * | * |
| ↓ LDL cholesterol | | * | variable |
| ↑ HDL cholesterol | | * | variable |
| ↑ alkaline phosphatase | placental isoenzyme | * | |

Fig. 10.9 Metabolic changes which occur during pregnancy and the use of oral contraceptives. The changes refer to plasma concentrations except where indicated. Oestrogens tend to decrease low density lipoprotein (LDL) cholesterol and increase high density lipoprotein (HDL) cholesterol; progestogens have the opposite effect.

glycosylated haemoglobin and blood glucose. The close cooperation of the laboratory is also required for the monitoring of patients with thyroid disease during pregnancy.

Urine should be tested for proteinuria and glycosuria at clinic attendances; the presence of proteinuria may be an early sign of pre-eclampsia. The renal threshold for glucose is decreased during pregnancy but if more than a trace of glycosuria is detected, it is advisable to perform an oral glucose tolerance test to exclude hitherto undiagnosed diabetes.

Pre-eclampsia is a condition, peculiar to pregnancy, characterized by hypertension, proteinuria and oedema. If left untreated, it can lead to severe hypertension and renal failure. An increase in plasma urate concentration can be a sensitive indicator of deteriorating renal function in this condition. Rapid analysis of samples is necessary as pre-eclampsia can progress very quickly.

## Fetal monitoring

The antenatal diagnosis of inherited metabolic disease in early pregnancy and the use of maternal serum α-fetoprotein measurements to screen for neural tube defects are considered in *Chapter 16*.

Fetal blood can be obtained antenatally by either of two techniques: cordocentesis (aspiration of fetal blood from the umbilical cord under ultrasound control) or fetoscopy (fetal blood sampling under direct vision). Of these, cordocentesis is usually the preferred method. Analysis of fetal blood for blood gases, hydrogen ion concentration and lactate can aid in the assessment of fetal wellbeing when non-invasive studies (e.g., ultrasonic determination of umbilical artery blood flow) suggest that the fetus is at risk. Fetal blood obtained earlier in pregnancy can also be used in the antenatal diagnosis of inherited disease (*see Chapter 16*).

Premature babies are at risk of developing respiratory distress due to lack of surfactant. This is a mixture of phospholipids, including lecithin and sphingomyelin, which lowers the surface tension of the alveoli and facilitates the expansion and aeration of the fetal lungs at birth. The concentration of lecithin in amniotic fluid reflects production by fetal lungs. It increases rapidly after 32–34 weeks of gestation, corresponding to increasing fetal lung maturity and decreasing risk of development of respiratory distress. Surfactant synthesis can be stimulated by giving corticosteroids to the mother, and this is now routine practice when elective premature delivery is planned for any reason. Natural and synthetic surfactants are available for use in the baby immediately after birth. As a result, measurement of the amniotic fluid lecithin:sphingomyelin (L:S) ratio, to provide an indication of fetal lung maturity, is now rarely performed.

During labour, once the cervix is sufficiently dilated, fetal blood hydrogen ion can be measured in capillary samples obtained from the scalp. A level of more than 60 nmol/L (pH < 7.22) suggests potentially dangerous fetal hypoxaemia. A continuous, direct measurement of fetal $Po_2$ can be obtained using a transcutaneous oxygen electrode.

## Metabolic effects of oral contraceptives

Oral contraceptives contain either a combination of an oestrogen and a progestogen or a progestogen alone. In addition to suppressing ovulation, these contraceptives have a number of metabolic effects similar to some of those that occur in normal pregnancy (*Fig. 10.9*).

## SUMMARY

The principal female sex hormone, or oestrogen, is 17β-oestradiol, secreted by the ovaries. The principal male sex hormone, or androgen, is testosterone, secreted by the testes. The secretion of both these hormones is stimulated by pituitary luteinizing hormone (LH). Spermatogenesis and the maturation of ovarian follicles are dependent upon testosterone and oestradiol, respectively, and pituitary follicle-stimulating hormone (FSH). The secretion of LH and FSH is in turn controlled by gonadotrophin releasing hormone, released from the hypothalamus, and subject to feedback control by the gonadal hormones. Androgens are also produced by the adrenals and in males there is some production of oestrogens by metabolism from androgens.

Both testosterone and oestradiol are transported in the plasma bound to sex hormone-binding globulin (SHBG), with only about 3% of each hormone being in free solution. Because of the greater avidity of testosterone for SHBG, factors that increase the concentration of SHBG tend to increase oestrogen-dependent effects while those that decrease it increase androgen-dependent effects.

The secretion of all these hormones is pulsatile. The secretion of testosterone in men is maintained throughout life but in women, oestrogen secretion declines after the menopause.

Both male and female hypogonadism can be either primary or secondary to either pituitary or hypothalamic dysfunction. Measurement of the appropriate gonadal hormone and the gonadotrophins, often after attempted stimulation of their secretion, will usually indicate the correct diagnosis and permit rational treatment.

Hormone measurements are also valuable in the investigation of gynaecomastia in males and virilism in females. The commonest feature of excessive androgenization is hirsutism which is frequently idiopathic. Another common cause is the polycystic ovary syndrome, where it is associated with menstrual irregularity and infertility. Congenital adrenal hyperplasia can present for the first time in young adults, causing hirsutism, menstrual irregularity or infertility. However, the presence of severe hirsutism and virilism should suggest the possibility of an androgen-secreting tumour of the adrenals or ovaries.

The laboratory investigation of infertility also depends heavily upon hormone measurements, though many non-endocrine factors must also be considered. A prime consideration is to establish whether ovulation is taking place; this can be inferred from the finding of an increase in plasma progesterone concentration on day 21 of the menstrual cycle.

Pregnancy can be diagnosed by the detection of the β-subunit of human chorionic gonadotrophin in the urine. The formerly widely used biochemical tests of fetal well-being during pregnancy have now largely been superseded by fetal ultrasound scanning. Pregnancy causes a number of physiological changes in biochemical variables, including an increase in the plasma concentrations of hormone-binding proteins. As a result, total levels of, for example, thyroxine and cortisol, are increased during pregnancy although the free hormone concentrations are normal.

## FURTHER READING

Besser G M & Thorner M O (eds) (1994) *Clinical Endocrinology: An Illustrated Text*. 2nd edition, London: Wolfe.

Hall R & Besser M (eds) (1989) *Fundamentals of Clinical Endocrinology*. 4th edition. London: Pitman Medical.

Gow S M, Turner E I, Glasier A (1994) The clinical biochemistry of the menopause and hormone replacement therapy. *Annals of Clinical Biochemistry*, **31**, 509–528.

Wilson J D & Foster D W (eds) (1992) *Williams – Textbook of Endocrinology*. 8th edition. Philadelphia: WB Saunders Company.

# 11. Disorders of Carbohydrate Metabolism

## INTRODUCTION

Glucose is a major energy substrate. The body's sources of glucose are dietary carbohydrate and endogenous (principally hepatic) production by glycogenolysis (release of glucose stored as glycogen) and gluconeogenesis (glucose synthesis from, e.g., lactate, glycerol and most amino acids). Blood glucose concentration depends on the relative rates of influx of glucose into the circulation and of its utilization. Blood glucose concentration is normally subject to rigorous control, rarely falling below 2.5 mmol/L or rising above 8.0 mmol/L in healthy subjects whether fasted or recently fed.

Following a meal, glucose is stored as glycogen, which is mobilized during fasting. Although the blood glucose concentration falls somewhat if fasting continues, and glycogen

stores are sufficient only for about 24 hours, adaptive changes lead to the attainment of a new steady state. After approximately 72 hours, the concentration stabilizes and can then remain constant for many days. The principal source of glucose becomes gluconeogenesis, from amino acids and glycerol, while ketones, derived from fat, become the major energy substrate.

The integration of these various processes and thus the control of blood glucose concentration is achieved through the concerted action of various hormones: these are insulin and the 'counter regulatory' hormones, namely glucagon, cortisol, catecholamines and growth hormone. Their effects are summarized in *Fig. 11.1*.

Physiologically, the two most important hormones in glucose homoeostasis are insulin and glucagon. Insulin is a 53 amino acid polypeptide, secreted by the β-cells of the

| Hormones involved in glucose homoeostasis | | | |
|---|---|---|---|
| **Hormone** | **Principal actions** | | |
| Insulin | Increases | cellular glucose uptake | M, A |
| | | glycogen synthesis | L, M |
| | | *protein synthesis* | *L, M* |
| | | *fatty acid and triglyceride synthesis* | *L, A* |
| | Decreases | gluconeogenesis | L |
| | | *ketogenesis* | *L* |
| | | *lipolysis* | *A* |
| | | *proteolysis* | *M* |
| Glucagon | Increases | glycogenolysis | L |
| | | gluconeogenesis | L |
| | | *ketogenesis* | *L* |
| | | *lipolysis* | *A* |
| Adrenaline | Increases | glycogenolysis | L, M |
| | | *lipolysis* | *A* |
| Growth hormone | Increases | glycogenolysis | L |
| | | *lipolysis* | *A* |
| Cortisol | Increases | gluconeogenesis | L |
| | | glycogen synthesis | L |
| | | *proteolysis* | *M* |
| | Decreases cellular glucose uptake | | M, A |

Fig. 11.1 Hormones involved in glucose homoeostasis. Letters indicate sites of action: L = liver, M = skeletal muscle, A = adipose tissue. Normal type indicates actions directly affecting glucose; other effects are shown in italics.

pancreatic islets of Langerhans in response to a rise in blood glucose concentration. It is synthesized as a prohormone, proinsulin. This molecule undergoes cleavage prior to secretion to form insulin and C-peptide (*Fig. 11.2*). Insulin secretion is also stimulated by various gut hormones, including glucagon and gastric inhibitory peptide, GIP (glucose-dependent insulinotrophic peptide). Insulin promotes the removal of glucose from the blood and its storage in the form of glycogen. It also stimulates the synthesis of fat from glucose and its storage in adipose tissue as triglyceride. If the blood glucose level falls, insulin secretion is inhibited and stored glucose mobilized.

Glucagon is a 29 amino acid polypeptide secreted by the α-cells of the pancreatic islets; its secretion is decreased by a rise in the blood glucose concentration. In general, its actions oppose those of insulin: it stimulates glycogenolysis and gluconeogenesis and promotes lipolysis and ketogenesis (*Fig. 11.2*). The combined effects of insulin and glucagon are shown diagrammatically in *Fig. 11.3*.

The major disorders of glucose homoeostasis are diabetes mellitus, characterized by glucose intolerance and thus a tendency to hyperglycaemia, and various conditions

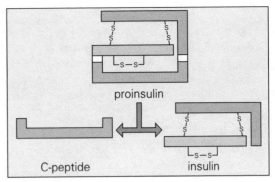

**Fig. 11.2** Biosynthesis of insulin. The cleavage of proinsulin produces insulin, consisting of two polypeptide chains linked by disulphide bridges, and C-peptide.

which can cause a pathologically low blood glucose concentration, that is, hypoglycaemia. It is to these conditions that the bulk of this chapter is devoted.

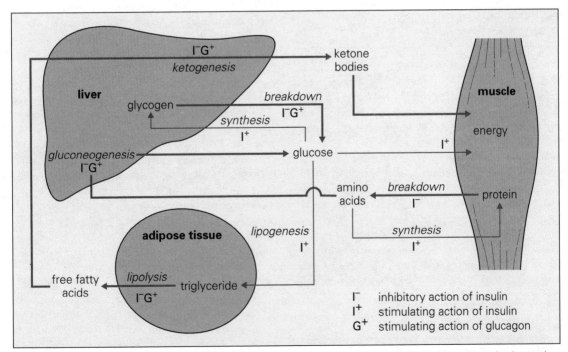

**Fig. 11.3** Combined effects of insulin and glucagon on substrate flows between liver, adipose tissue and muscle. When the ratio of the concentrations of insulin to glucagon falls (e.g., during starvation), there is increased hepatic glucose and ketone production and decreased tissue glucose utilization. When the ratio is high (e.g., after a meal), glucose is stored as glycogen and converted into fat.

| Major characteristics of IDDM and NIDDM | | |
|---|---|---|
| **Feature** | **IDDM** | **NIDDM** |
| typical age of onset | children, young adults | middle-aged, elderly |
| onset | acute | gradual |
| habitus | lean | often obese |
| weight loss | usual | uncommon |
| ketosis-prone | usually | usually not |
| plasma insulin concentration | low or absent | often normal; may be ↑ |
| family history of diabetes | uncommon | common |
| HLA association | DR3, DR4 | none |

**Fig. 11.4** Major characteristics of insulin-dependent (IDDM, Type I) and non insulin-dependent (NIDDM, Type II) diabetes mellitus.

## MEASUREMENT OF GLUCOSE CONCENTRATION

Plasma glucose concentration tends to be 10–15% higher than that of whole blood because a given volume of red cells contains less water than the same volume of plasma. The difference is of little significance at normal concentrations except in the interpretation of the results of glucose tolerance tests. However, when the glucose concentration is changing rapidly there may be a considerable discrepancy because of delayed equilibration of glucose across the red cell membranes. Red blood cells *in vitro* continue to utilize glucose, with the result that unless a blood sample can be analyzed immediately, it is essential to collect it into a tube containing sodium fluoride to inhibit glycolysis. Potassium oxalate is used as an anticoagulant in such 'fluoride–oxalate' tubes, and plasma obtained from this blood is thus unsuitable for the measurement of potassium concentration.

## DIABETES MELLITUS

### Aetiology and pathogenesis

Diabetes mellitus is a common condition, with a prevalence of approximately 1–2% in the western world. Diabetes can occur secondarily to other diseases, for example, chronic pancreatitis, following pancreatic surgery and in conditions where there is increased secretion of hormones antagonistic to insulin, e.g., Cushing's syndrome and acromegaly. Secondary diabetes is, however, uncommon. Most cases of diabetes mellitus are primary, that is, they are not associated with other conditions. There are two distinct types. In Type I (insulin-dependent diabetes mellitus – IDDM) there is destruction of pancreatic cells and effectively no insulin secretion. In Type II (non insulin-dependent diabetes mellitus – NIDDM) either insulin is secreted in amounts insufficient to prevent hyperglycaemia or there is insensitivity to its actions. Overall some 20% of patients are insulin dependent; most patients with NIDDM can be treated by diet, with or without oral hypoglycaemic drugs, for example, sulphonylureas and biguanides.

IDDM usually presents acutely in younger people, with symptoms developing over a period of days or only a few weeks; it was formerly called juvenile-onset diabetes. However, there is evidence that the appearance of symptoms is preceded by a 'prediabetic' period of several months during which growth failure, a fall in insulin response to glucose and various immunological abnormalities can be detected. NIDDM tends to present more chronically in the middle-aged and elderly with symptoms developing over months or even longer. The prevalence of NIDDM increases with increasing age and reaches over 10% in people over the age of 75 years. NIDDM was formerly called maturity-onset diabetes. The old nomenclature is inaccurate since some young diabetic patients are not insulin dependent while IDDM may occasionally present in older people. Some of the characteristics of IDDM and NIDDM are shown in *Fig. 11.4*.

The exact pathogenesis of NIDDM is uncertain. The condition shows a strong familial incidence. The concordance rate in monozygotic (identical) twins is more than 90%. However, inheritance is unpredictable. Several candidate genes have been identified, including those for glucokinase and a transmembrane glucose transporter. It seems that many genes may contribute to increased susceptibility to NIDDM. Environmental factors are also important. For example, obesity is present in approximately 40% of patients with NIDDM and the incidence in women is greater in the multiparous than the nulliparous. The pancreatic islet cells are often histologically normal in patients with NIDDM although in some (more particularly the elderly) they may contain amyloid. This is derived from amylin, a protein containing 37 amino acids, but it is uncertain if amylin has any role in the pathogenesis of NIDDM. In many patients, islet cells appear insensitive to glucose, and insulin secretion is impaired. In others, particularly the obese, plasma insulin concentrations are elevated and there is resistance to its action. In some patients, both factors may be important.

IDDM is much less frequently familial (the concordance rate in monozygotic twins is approximately 40%), but there is a strong association with certain histocompatibility antigens, for example, HLA-DR3 and DR4. An individual's HLA antigens are genetically determined and many autoimmune diseases are associated with particular HLA specificities, suggesting that IDDM is also an autoimmune disease and, further, that the susceptibility to it is in part governed by genetic factors. There is also evidence that viruses, for instance, Coxsackie B4, are aetiological agents in IDDM. Inflammation of pancreatic islets (insulitis) leads to islet cell destruction and thus a lack of insulin. Islet cell antibodies can be detected in the serum. It is suggested that activated T cells directed against viral antigens may also react with islet cell antigens in susceptible individuals and lead to cell destruction. It has been demonstrated that early treatment with cyclosporin A, an immunosuppressive agent, can induce remission in IDDM. This lends weight to an autoimmune pathogenesis and also suggests that IDDM may be preventable. Clinically overt IDDM is thought to represent the end stage of a process of gradual islet cell destruction, and if susceptible individuals could be identified at an early stage in the process, treatment might prevent its development.

## Pathophysiology and clinical features

There are two aspects to the clinical manifestations of diabetes mellitus: those related directly to the metabolic disturbance and those related to the long-term complications of the condition. The prevalence of the long-term complications (nephropathy, neuropathy, retinopathy and arteriopathy) increases with duration of the disease and there is now clear evidence that, at least in IDDM, the risk of complications is greater if glycaemic control is poor, although other factors are undoubtedly involved. There is evidence that the development of nephropathy, neuropathy and retinopathy are related to the glycation of proteins, for example, those in the glomerular basement membrane, but this is not conclusive. At high glucose concentrations, the enzyme aldose reductase catalyzes the formation of sorbitol from glucose, and the accumulation of this substance may be deleterious. Abnormalities of lipoprotein metabolism occur frequently in patients with diabetes mellitus and may predispose to atherosclerosis. Associations have also been reported between these complications and certain abnormalities of the immune system. The long-term complications of diabetes are a significant source of morbidity and mortality, but with the exception of nephropathy their diagnosis is largely clinical. In contrast, the management of the acute metabolic disturbances seen in diabetes mellitus requires close collaboration between the physician and the laboratory staff.

The hyperglycaemia of diabetes mellitus is mainly a result of increased production of glucose by the liver and, to a lesser extent, of decreased removal of glucose from the blood. In the kidneys, filtered glucose is normally completely reabsorbed in the proximal tubules, but at blood glucose concentrations much above 10 mmol/L (the renal threshold), reabsorption becomes saturated and glucose appears in the urine. There is some variation in the threshold between individuals. It is higher in the elderly and lower during pregnancy. Glycosuria results in an osmotic diuresis, increasing water excretion and raising the plasma osmolality, which in turn stimulates the thirst centre. Osmotic diuresis and thirst cause the classical symptoms of polyuria and polydipsia. Other causes of these symptoms include diabetes insipidus, hypercalcaemia, chronic hypokalaemia, chronic renal failure and excessive water intake.

Untreated, the metabolic disturbances may become profound, with the development of life-threatening ketoacidosis, non-ketotic hyperglycaemia or lactic acidosis.

## Diagnosis

The diagnosis of diabetes mellitus depends upon the demonstration of hyperglycaemia. In a patient with classical symptoms and signs, this may be inferred from the presence of glycosuria. Under these circumstances, a fasting venous plasma glucose concentration exceeding 7.8 mmol/L, or a random value exceeding 11.1 mmol/L, will confirm the diagnosis of diabetes mellitus. In patients who are asymptomatic, either of these limits must be exceeded on more than one occasion for the diagnosis to be made. In doubtful cases, it may be necessary to measure the blood glucose two hours after an oral glucose load, or perform a formal oral glucose tolerance test (OGTT). The World Health Organization (WHO) criteria for the diagnosis of diabetes mellitus are shown in *Fig. 11.5*. People whose blood glucose concentration is raised, but not sufficiently to meet these criteria, are classified as having 'impaired glucose tolerance' (IGT). Such individuals should not be stigmatized as having diabetes but they should be reviewed regularly and given dietary advice. Diabetes mellitus develops in 2–4% of people with IGT per year; a similar number revert to having normal glucose tolerance. Patients with IGT appear to have a similarly increased predisposition to myocardial infarction and stroke as patients with diabetes.

A formal OGTT needs to be carried out only when there is doubt about a diagnosis of diabetes. If the diagnosis is clear from the clinical features and confirmed by a fasting or postprandial blood glucose measurement, an OGTT is superfluous. The indications for this test, and the test protocol, are given in *Fig. 11.6*. Intravenous glucose tolerance tests are only used in research.

| Diagnostic blood glucose concentrations (mmol/L) | | | | |
|---|---|---|---|---|
| Diagnosis | Time of sample | Venous whole blood | Venous plasma | Capillary whole blood |
| diabetes mellitus | fasting<br>2 h post-glucose load | ≥6.7<br>≥10.0 | ≥7.8<br>≥11.1 | ≥6.7<br>≥11.1 |
| impaired glucose tolerance | fasting<br>2 h post-glucose load | <6.7 and<br>6.7–10.0 | <7.8 and<br>7.8–11.1 | <6.7 and<br>7.8–11.1 |

**Fig. 11.5** Diagnostic blood glucose concentrations. If a patient is asymptomatic, diabetes should only be diagnosed if two results are abnormal.

| The oral glucose test | |
|---|---|
| Indications | Procedure |
| equivocal fasting/random blood glucose concentrations<br>unexplained glycosuria, particularly in pregnancy<br>clinical features of diabetes mellitus or its complications with normal blood glucose concentrations<br>diagnosis of acromegaly *see p. 112* | patient should eat normal diet, containing at least 250 g carbohydrate per day for 3 days.<br>fast patient overnight<br>take basal blood sample for glucose determination<br>give 75 g glucose in water orally; take further blood samples at 60 and 120 min for glucose determination<br>patient should rest throughout test; smoking not permitted; drinks of water are allowed |

**Fig. 11.6** The oral glucose tolerance test. For the diagnosis of diabetes, strictly only the basal and 120 min samples are required, although it is usual to take a sample at 60 min to aid the interpretation when the 120 min result is borderline. For the diagnosis of acromegaly, and the investigation of glycosuria, samples should be taken at 30 min intervals.

## Management

There are many aspects to the management of diabetes mellitus. Education of patients is vital; they will have diabetes for the rest of their lives and must, to a considerable extent, be responsible for their own treatment, albeit with guidance from a physician. Regular follow-up is essential to monitor treatment and detect early signs of complications, particularly retinopathy which can in many cases be treated successfully, and nephropathy, since treatment may slow its progression.

The aims of treatment are twofold: to alleviate symptoms and prevent the acute metabolic complications of diabetes, and to prevent the long-term complications. The first of these objectives is usually attainable with dietary control (essentially, substitution of complex for simple carbohydrates, an increase in dietary fibre and restriction of energy intake when necessary) with or without oral hypoglycaemic agents, principally sulphonylureas, in patients with NIDDM, and with diet and insulin in patients with IDDM.

The demonstration that intensive glycaemic control reduces the risk of complications in IDDM means that the goal of treatment should be to attempt to maintain the blood glucose concentration within the physiological range. In practice, this may be difficult to achieve and intensification of treatment increases the risk of episodes of hypoglycaemia.

By inference, it is desirable to aim for physiological blood glucose concentrations in most NIDDM patients also. In the elderly, however, it may be sufficient that treatment alleviates the acute symptoms even if there is persistent hyperglycaemia (patients may be free of symptoms even with blood glucose concentrations of 15 mmol/L). Such patients are not at risk of developing ketoacidosis and attempting to improve control, perhaps by introducing a harsher dietary regime or by giving oral hypoglycaemic drugs in addition to diet, is inappropriate when the patient is unlikely to live long enough for complications to develop. Whatever the treatment, the fluctuations in blood glucose concentration that occur in most diabetic patients are still greater than those which occur in normal subjects.

## Monitoring treatment

The efficacy of treatment in diabetes is monitored clinically, by ensuring that the patient's symptoms are controlled, and in the laboratory, by semi-quantitative measurement of urine glucose concentration using reagent tablets or strips, measurement of blood glucose concentration and measurement of the concentration of glycated proteins in the blood.

Many diabetic patients test their urine for glucose at home. However, although the urine will contain glucose if the blood glucose concentration has exceeded the renal threshold at any time since the bladder was last emptied, the amount of glucose in the urine is a poor guide to the severity of any hyperglycaemia and is also dependent on the individual's renal threshold. If this is low, there may be considerable glycosuria with only slightly elevated blood glucose concentrations. In addition, testing the urine for glucose is of no value in detecting hypoglycaemia. For most diabetic patients, home blood glucose monitoring, using capillary blood and a reagent strip, preferably read using a meter designed for the purpose, is to be preferred. Urine testing for glucose should be used only in patients unable to do blood tests and in the elderly when glycaemic control need not be so strict.

The discovery that haemoglobin undergoes non-enzymatic glycation *in vivo* has facilitated assessment of diabetic control over a longer term. The rate of formation of glycated haemoglobin is proportional to the blood glucose concentration; the reaction proceeds through a reversible stage but once the major stable product ($HbA_{1c}$) is formed, it persists in that state for the lifetime of the cell. The proportion of haemoglobin in the glycated form thus effectively 'integrates' the blood glucose concentration over the previous 6–8 weeks. Normal $HbA_{1c}$ is <6%; in uncontrolled diabetes, it may exceed 10%. Caution with interpretation is required in patients with decreased red cell life spans (for example, due to haemolytic anaemia). In some of the methods used to measure glycated haemoglobin, haemoglobin variants may cross-react and give falsely high results. Other proteins also undergo glycation. Plasma fructosamine concentration is a measure of the glycation of plasma proteins, particularly albumin, and reflects glycaemic control over a shorter span than $HbA_{1c}$.

---

### CASE HISTORY 11.1

A young insulin-dependent diabetic patient attended the outpatient department for his regular follow-up and reported that he had been symptom-free since his last clinic attendance. He had not bothered to test his urine at home and did not like pricking his finger to obtain capillary blood for testing.

#### Investigations

| | |
|---|---:|
| blood glucose (two hours after breakfast) | 18 mmol/L |
| urine glucose (early morning) | 2% |
| $HbA_{1c}$ | 6.5% |

#### Comment

The $HbA_{1c}$ suggests that diabetic control is good, despite the patient's apparent lack of interest, a high

---

blood glucose concentration and glycosuria. It transpired that he had been to a party the night before and had eaten considerably more than usual. He did not want to admit this, since he was, to use his own words, 'fed up with being lectured at'.

Since the proportion of glycated haemoglobin reflects the mean blood glucose concentration over the previous few weeks, its measurement is particularly useful whenever there is a discrepancy between the patient's history and blood or urine glucose measurements. It will, for example, be high in patients who are generally poorly controlled but who make a special effort to comply with their treatment before attending a clinic, in order to please their doctor by having a normal blood glucose concentration and no glycosuria.

| Clinical and metabolic features of diabetic ketoacidosis |
| --- |
| **Clinical** |
| thirst
polyuria (but oliguria late)
dehydration
hypotension, tachycardia and
    peripheral circulatory failure
ketosis
hyperventilation
vomiting
abdominal pain
drowsiness and coma |
| **Metabolic** |
| hyperglycaemia
glycosuria
non-respiratory acidosis
ketonaemia
uraemia
hyperkalaemia
hypertriglyceridaemia
haemoconcentration |

**Fig. 11.7** Clinical and metabolic features of diabetic ketoacidosis.

# METABOLIC COMPLICATIONS OF DIABETES

## Ketoacidosis

Ketoacidosis may be the presenting feature of IDDM, or may develop in a patient known to be diabetic who omits to take his insulin or whose insulin dosage becomes inadequate because of an increased requirement, for example, as a result of infection, any acute illness such as myocardial infarction, trauma or emotional disturbance.

### CASE HISTORY 11.2

An 18-year-old girl consulted her family doctor because of tiredness and weight loss. On questioning, she admitted to feeling thirsty and had noticed that she had been passing more urine than normal. The doctor tested her urine and found glycosuria. He arranged for her to be seen at the hospital's diabetic clinic the next day. By then, however, she felt too ill to get out of bed, had started vomiting and had become drowsy. Her doctor visited her at home and arranged for immediate admission to hospital. On examination she was found to have a blood pressure of 95/60 mmHg with a pulse rate of 112/min and cold extremities. She had deep, sighing respiration (Kussmaul's respiration) and her breath smelt of acetone.

**Investigations**

| | | |
| --- | --- | --- |
| serum: | sodium | 130 mmol/L |
| | potassium | 5.8 mmol/L |
| | bicarbonate | 5 mmol/L |
| | urea | 18 mmol/L |
| | creatinine | 140 µmol/L |
| | glucose | 32 mmol/L |
| arterial blood: | hydrogen ion | 89 nmol/L (pH 7.05) |
| | $P_{CO_2}$ | 2.0 kPa (15 mmHg) |

**Comment**

The clinical and biochemical features are typical of diabetic ketoacidosis (*Fig. 11.7*). She has hypotension, tachycardia and cold extremities, suggesting marked extracellular fluid depletion (sodium depletion). The low bicarbonate and high hydrogen ion concentrations with hyperventilation and thus a decreased $P_{CO_2}$ indicate a non-respiratory acidosis with partial respiratory compensation. There is renal impairment (raised urea and creatinine) and the disproportionate increase in urea in comparison with creatinine is typical of dehydration compounded by increased urea production due to amino acid breakdown (*see below*).

Hyperkalaemia is commonly present and is a result of the combined effects of decreased renal excretion and a shift of intracellular potassium (due to insulin lack, since insulin promotes cellular potassium uptake, and to acidosis and tissue catabolism). However, in spite of the hyperkalaemia, there is always considerable potassium depletion. The plasma sodium concentration is usually decreased, because of sodium depletion and the osmotically driven shift of water from the intracellular compartment. Although this patient is markedly hyperglycaemic, clinically severe ketoacidosis can sometimes occur with only a moderate increase in the blood glucose concentration (10–15 mmol/L). The presence of ketosis can be confirmed by the detection of ketonuria using a suitable dipstick test.

The pathogenesis of the acidosis and hyperglycaemia are discussed below. Although the term 'diabetic coma' is often used synonymously with diabetic ketoacidosis, many patients have a normal level of consciousness when they present. Drowsiness is common, but only 10% of patients are actually comatose.

## Pathogenesis

The sequence of events which leads to hyperglycaemia and the consequences of this are illustrated in *Figs 11.3 and 11.8*. An increase in the ratio of the concentration of glucagon to that of insulin in the portal blood decreases the hepatic concentration of fructose 2,6-bisphosphate, a key regulatory intermediate. This results in inhibition of phosphofructokinase, and thus of glycolysis, and activation of fructose 1,6-bisphosphatase, thus stimulating gluconeogenesis. At the same time, glycogen breakdown is promoted and glycogen synthesis is inhibited. Decreased peripheral utilization of glucose, resulting from insulin lack and preferential metabolism of free fatty acids and ketones as energy substrates, contributes to the hyperglycaemia but is less important than the increased rate of glucose production.

Glycosuria causes an osmotic diuresis and hence fluid depletion which is exacerbated by the hyperventilation and vomiting. The decrease in plasma volume leads to renal hypoperfusion and prerenal uraemia. As the glomerular fil-

tration rate falls, so does the rate of urine production and the patient, initially polyuric, becomes oliguric. The loss of glucose in the urine affords some protection against the development of severe hyperglycaemia, but this is lost once oliguria develops. Established renal failure is an uncommon but recognized consequence of diabetic ketoacidosis.

Insulin lack causes increased lipolysis, with increased release of free fatty acids into the blood from adipose tissue, and decreased lipogenesis. In the liver, fatty acids normally undergo complete oxidation, are re-esterified to triglycerides or are converted to acetoacetic and β-hydroxybutyric acids (ketogenesis). Ketogenesis is promoted in uncontrolled diabetes by the high ratio of glucagon to insulin. The mechanisms involved are shown in *Fig. 11.9*. Some acetoacetate is spontaneously decarboxylated to acetone. Ketones stimulate the chemoreceptor trigger zone, causing vomiting. Acetoacetic and β-hydroxybutyric acids are the major acids responsible for the acidosis but free fatty acids and lactic acid also contribute.

## Management

Diabetic ketoacidosis is a medical emergency. Treatment entails replacement of lost fluid and minerals, and provision of insulin to reverse the metabolic disturbance. Any identifiable precipitating event, for example, infection, must also be treated.

Isotonic saline is given intravenously to replace lost fluid. The rate at which it is given will depend upon the precise circumstances, but it should usually be given rapidly, at least initially, to restore the extracellular fluid volume to normal. Careful monitoring of fluid input and output is essential, and it may be necessary to insert a central intravenous catheter to monitor central venous pressure. If there is gastric stasis, the gastric contents must be aspirated. Catheterization of the bladder may be necessary.

Potassium supplements are required; insulin causes rapid potassium uptake into cells with the result that although patients are usually hyperkalaemic at presentation, hypokalaemia will develop during treatment if potassium is not replaced. Regular monitoring of the plasma potassium concentration is essential.

Insulin is best given by constant intravenous infusion at a rate of 6–10 U/h. The blood glucose concentration must be monitored and, once it has fallen to near normal levels, the intravenous fluid is changed to 5% dextrose and the rate of insulin infusion decreased to maintain euglycaemia until it is possible to establish oral food and water intake, and a conventional regimen of subcutaneous insulin injections.

It is seldom necessary to give bicarbonate, except in the severest cases, since restoration of normal renal perfusion allows excretion of the hydrogen ion load and regeneration of bicarbonate, while restoration of normal metabolism reduces the production rate. If bicarbonate is used, it should be given in small quantities and the effect monitored by measurements of the arterial hydrogen ion concentration. Rapid correction of an acidosis may impair oxygen delivery to the tissues, through an effect on the affinity of haemoglobin for oxygen; lead to later alkalosis as the

ketoacid anions are metabolized to bicarbonate, and paradoxically increase the cerebrospinal fluid (CSF) hydrogen ion concentration because of delayed equilibration of the bicarbonate between the plasma and the CSF. The response to treatment of a typical patient with diabetic ketoacidosis is shown in *Fig. 11.10*.

The deficits present in a patient with ketoacidosis are considerable and may exceed 5 L of water and 500 mmol

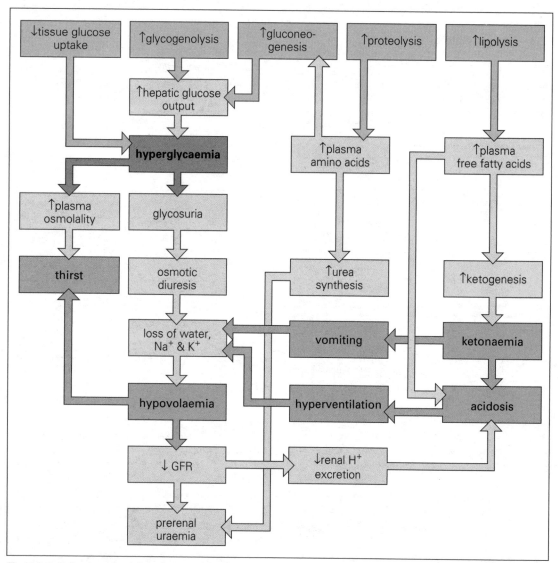

**Fig. 11.8** Pathogenesis of diabetic ketoacidosis, indicating the consequences of a decreased insulin:glucagon ratio. Hyperkalaemia is invariably present, in spite of total body potassium depletion, as a result of loss of potassium from the tissues to the ECF and, as the glomerular filtration falls, to decreased renal excretion.

each of sodium and potassium. Considerable depletion of other ions, in particular phosphate, may occur in ketoacidosis. The plasma phosphate concentration should be monitored, but specific replacement therapy is not usually required. Other biochemical abnormalities that may be seen include an increase in plasma amylase activity, hypertriglyceridaemia and, in severely shocked patients, an increase in transaminases.

## Non-ketotic hyperglycaemia

Not all patients with uncontrolled diabetes develop ketoacidosis. In NIDDM, severe hyperglycaemia can develop (blood glucose concentration >50 mmol/L) with extreme dehydration and a very high plasma osmolality, but with no ketosis and minimal acidosis. This complication is often referred to as hyperosmolar non-ketotic hyperglycaemia, but patients with ketoacidosis usually also have increased plasma osmolality, although not to the same extent.

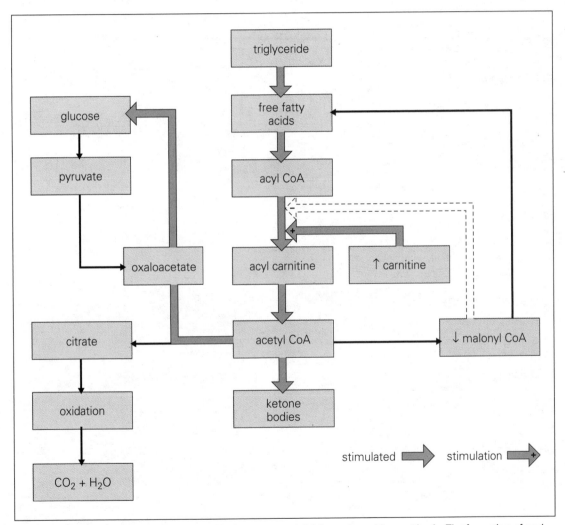

**Fig.11.9** Mechanism of increased ketogenesis in diabetic ketoacidosis. The formation of free fatty acids increases as a result of increased lipolysis. Glucagon increases carnitine formation (mechanism unknown) and inhibits the synthesis of malonyl CoA, an intermediate in fatty acid synthesis, which normally inhibits acyl-carnitine synthesis. The formation of acyl carnitine is required for transport of fatty acids into mitochondria, where ketogenesis takes place. Supplies of oxaloacetate necessary for the oxidation of acetyl CoA in the citric acid cycle are diverted instead to gluconeogenesis.

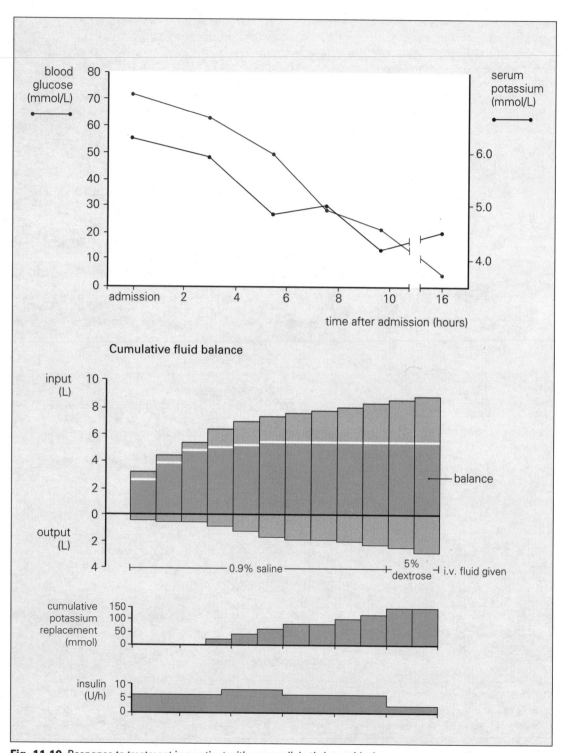

**Fig. 11.10** Response to treatment in a patient with severe diabetic ketoacidosis, indicating a fluid deficit of 6L on admission.

## CASE HISTORY 11.3

A middle-aged widow, who lived alone, was admitted to hospital after her son found her semi-conscious at home. He had not seen her for a week but she had seemed well at their last meeting. On examination, she was extremely dehydrated but not ketotic. Her respiration was normal.

### Investigations

| serum: | | |
|---|---|---|
| sodium | 149 mmol/L | |
| potassium | 4.7 mmol/L | |
| bicarbonate | 18 mmol/L | |
| urea | 35 mmol/L | |
| creatinine | 180 μmol/L | |
| glucose | 54 mmol/L | |
| total protein | 90 g/L | |
| osmolality | 370 mmol/kg | |

### Comment

The serum osmolality is very high, reflecting the severe hyperglycaemia. This has caused an osmotic diuresis, resulting in a decrease in glomerular filtration with retention of urea and creatinine and an increase in serum protein concentration due to the loss of water from the plasma. The serum bicarbonate concentration is a little below normal because of the decreased renal hydrogen ion excretion. The plasma sodium concentration is often raised in this condition, reflecting loss of water in excess of sodium as a result of the sustained osmotic diuresis.

Non-ketotic hyperglycaemia occurs only in NIDDM. There is sufficient insulin secretion to prevent the excessive lipolysis and to oppose the ketogenic action of glucagon that are essential for the generation of ketoacidosis (the concentrations of insulin required to do this are lower than those needed to prevent hyperglycaemia). Blood glucose concentrations are in general higher than in ketoacidosis. Perhaps because vomiting is not a feature, patients do not become acutely ill so quickly. A history of thirst and polyuria was subsequently obtained from this patient, who had not been previously diagnosed as having diabetes. She had also been assuaging her thirst with copious amounts of sweetened carbonated drinks.

### Management

Rehydration and the administration of insulin are the most essential aspects of treatment. Insulin is given by constant intravenous infusion but a satisfactory decrease in glucose concentration is often attained using a lower rate of infusion than that employed in ketoacidosis. In view of the hypertonicity, hypotonic ('half-normal') saline is given although it may be wise to give a litre of normal saline initially, specifically to expand the extracellular compartment and also to prevent too rapid a fall in osmolality (*see p. 15*). Potassium supplements are required, but less is needed than in ketoacidosis. Careful monitoring of the glucose concentration and fluid balance is essential. Heparin is sometimes given prophylactically in view of the hyperviscosity and attendant danger of thrombosis. In contrast to ketoacidosis, continued treatment with insulin is seldom required once the acute illness is over; patients can usually be managed either with diet alone or with diet and oral hypoglycaemic drugs.

## Lactic acidosis

Lactic acidosis is an uncommon complication of diabetes. It was formerly chiefly seen in patients treated with phenformin, a biguanide oral hypoglycaemic drug, but is now more usually associated with severe systemic illness, for example, severe shock and pancreatitis. It is discussed in more detail *on p 41*.

## Hypoglycaemia in diabetic patients

Hypoglycaemia can complicate treatment in both IDDM and NIDDM. It is discussed in more detail on *pp 175–177*.

## CASE HISTORY 11.4

A 42-year-old woman, who had been diagnosed as an insulin-dependent diabetic in childhood, complained of frequent episodes of hypoglycaemia, which had continued to occur in spite of reduction of her insulin dosage. She had also developed amenorrhoea. Her diabetes had previously been well-controlled, with only occasional episodes of hypoglycaemia and HbA$_{1c}$ in the range 6.5–7.0%. A review of her history showed that her insulin requirement had fallen from 48 to 28 U over the previous 12 months.

### Investigations

| | |
|---|---|
| HbA$_{1c}$ | 6.5% |
| serum LH | 1.2 U/L |
| serum FSH | 1.0 U/L |

**173**

**Comment**

Occasional hypoglycaemic episodes are common in patients with IDDM, and there may be obvious reasons for them, for example, a missed meal or an increase in physical activity. Recurrent hypoglycaemia can be due to over-zealous treatment, but a decrease in insulin requirements suggests a change in the activity of counter-regulatory hormones. In this instance, the development of amenorrhoea with low gonadotrophin concentrations suggested that the patient might have developed pituitary failure, with decreased production of growth hormone and ACTH causing increased sensitivity to insulin. This was confirmed by formal pituitary function testing and shown to be due to a non-functioning pituitary tumour.

## Diabetic nephropathy

The renal disease that may complicate diabetes tends to progress towards end-stage renal failure, although there is considerable variation in its time course. Proteinuria is usually present in established diabetic nephropathy, and microalbuminuria (albumin excretion 30–150 µg/min, undetectable using conventional urine dipsticks) is the earliest biochemical abnormality. There is encouraging evidence to suggest that meticulous control of the blood glucose concentration and treatment of any hypertension may abolish early microalbuminuria and prevent or delay the onset of renal impairment.

## Lipoprotein metabolism in diabetes mellitus

Both IDDM and NIDDM are associated with abnormalities of plasma lipids. In IDDM, at presentation, or if glycaemic control deteriorates, marked hypertriglyceridaemia (manifest as an increase in very low density lipoprotein, VLDL, and often by chylomicronaemia as well) may be present, due to deficiency of lipoprotein lipase and an increased flux of free fatty acids from adipose tissue which act as a substrate for hepatic triglyceride synthesis. Both these effects are directly due to insulin deficiency and are reversed by insulin treatment. Indeed, the degree of hypertriglyceridaemia correlates well with glycaemic control. Low density lipoprotein (LDL) concentration may also be increased, and that of high density lipoprotein (HDL), decreased.

In NIDDM, hypertriglyceridaemia is also common, although it is not usually as severe as in uncontrolled IDDM unless there is an additional, genetic, predisposition. It is due mainly to increased hepatic synthesis. The VLDL contains increased triglyceride and cholesteryl ester in relation to the amount of apoprotein and although LDL concentrations are not usually increased, the particles tend to be smaller and denser. These abnormalities appear to be atherogenic. As in IDDM, HDL concentration is often decreased.

Plasma lipid concentrations usually become normal in patients with well-controlled IDDM; HDL concentrations may even become increased. In contrast, the abnormalities seen in NIDDM may persist despite adequate glycaemic control. Treatment with lipid-lowering drugs may be appropriate, to reduce the risk of vascular disease.

## GLYCOSURIA

Although diabetes mellitus is the commonest cause of glycosuria, it is also seen in patients with a low renal threshold for glucose. This may occur as an isolated and harmless abnormality (renal glycosuria), can develop during pregnancy and is a feature of congenital and acquired generalized disorders of proximal renal tubular function (the Fanconi syndrome, *see p. 68*).

A positive test for reducing substances in the urine using reagent tablets (Clinitest) is given by a number of substances other than glucose, some of which are indicated in *Fig. 11.11*. Reagent sticks containing glucose oxidase are specific for glucose.

## GLUCOSE IN CEREBROSPINAL FLUID

Glucose concentration in the CSF is commonly measured in patients suspected of having bacterial meningitis, since it is usually decreased as a result of bacterial metabolism. If the CSF is frankly purulent, the measurement of CSF glucose provides no useful additional information. The CSF glucose concentration is approximately 65% of the blood glucose concentration and CSF glucose should always be interpreted in the light of the glucose concentration of a blood sample obtained at the same time.

## HYPOGLYCAEMIA

Hypoglycaemia is conventionally, though arbitarily, defined as a blood glucose concentration of less than 2.2 mmol/L.

### Causes

It is convenient, to divide the causes of hypoglycaemia into those causing a low blood glucose concentration during *fasting* and those in which it follows a stimulus (*reactive* hypoglycaemia), including the stimulus of a meal

| Substances giving a positive reducing test in urine |
|---|
| glucose |
| lactose (during lactation and the last trimester of pregnancy) |
| galactose (in galactosaemia and galactokinase deficiency) |
| fructose (in hereditary fructose intolerance and essential fructosuria) |
| pentoses (after eating certain fruits and in essential pentosuria) |
| homogentisic acid (in alkaptonuria) |
| glucuronides of drugs |
| salicylic acid (in aspirin overdose) |
| ascorbic acid (with high vitamin C intake) |
| creatinine (only in high concentration) |

**Fig. 11.11** Substances giving a positive reducing test in urine.

(post-prandial hypoglycaemia). It is usually possible to distinguish between these categories from the patient's history.

Episodes of reactive hypoglycaemia can occur in patients with fasting hypoglycaemia although fasting hypoglycaemia is virtually never a feature of conditions associated with reactive hypoglycaemia in the absence of the stimulus. The causes of hypoglycaemia are summarized in *Fig. 11.12* and the pathogenesis is indicated in each case. These conditions are discussed further in the following sections.

## Clinical features

Glucose is an essential energy substrate for the nervous system, at least in the short term; during starvation, adaptation occurs and ketone bodies can be utilized. The clinical features of hypoglycaemia are the result of dysfunction of the nervous system (neuroglycopenia) and the effects of catecholamines which are released in response to the stimulus provided by the low blood glucose.

The characteristic clinical features of acute hypoglycaemia are summarized in *Fig. 11.12*. Their development is affected by various factors, and the threshold varies between individuals. Typical signs and symptoms are more

likely to occur if the blood glucose falls rapidly and if hypoglycaemic episodes are separated by periods of normoglycaemia. If the blood glucose concentration falls rapidly, symptoms may develop at concentrations higher than 2.2 mmol/L. The clinical features of hypoglycaemia are likely to be enhanced if cerebral blood flow is impaired, while they may be attenuated in patients taking β-adrenergic blocking drugs, such as propanolol. In chronic hypoglycaemia, psychiatric manifestations may predominate, and other features may not be present, even with a glucose concentration as low as 1 mmol/L.

## Diagnosis

The two stages in the diagnosis of hypoglycaemia are confirmation of the low blood glucose concentration and elucidation of the cause. Allusion has been made to the considerable variation in the blood glucose concentration at which symptoms of hypoglycaemia begin to appear. In children and young adults, symptoms will usually be present only with a concentration of less than 2.2 mmol/L. The elderly tend to be more sensitive to a low blood glucose, perhaps because of impaired homoeostatic responses or decreased cerebral perfusion resulting from atheroma. Neonates, however, often develop symptoms only when the blood glucose is less than 1.5 mmol/L. Blood for glucose analysis must be collected in a tube containing fluoride, to inhibit glycolysis, and an anticoagulant.

That the clinical features are due to hypoglycaemia should be confirmed by giving glucose either by mouth or parenterally, as appropriate. Those which are due to acute neuroglycopenia and catecholamine release should resolve immediately, but those attributable to chronic hypoglycaemia often persist. The presence of a low blood glucose concentration and symptoms of hypoglycaemia which are abolished by giving glucose constitute 'Whipple's triad'.

The cause of the hypoglycaemia may be obvious from the patient's history, particularly in reactive hypoglycaemia. With fasting hypoglycaemia, many possible causes can be eliminated by simple tests; if this can be done, investigations should be directed towards the detection of possible excessive insulin secretion. In adults, this is invariably tumour-related, although in infants other causes need to be considered.

## HYPOGLYCAEMIC SYNDROMES

### Reactive hypoglycaemia
#### Drug-induced hypoglycaemia
Most patients with insulin-dependent diabetes experience occasional episodes of hypoglycaemia. Disturbed patients

| Hypoglycaemia | |
|---|---|
| **Causes** | **Clinical features** |
| **Reactive hypoglycaemia**<br>drug-induced:<br>  insulin<br>  sulphonylureas<br>  others<br>post-prandial:<br>  gastric surgery<br>  essential (idiopathic) reactive hypoglycaemia<br>alcohol-induced<br>inherited metabolic disorders:<br>  galactosaemia<br>  hereditary fructose intolerance<br><br>**Fasting hypoglycaemia**<br>hepatic and renal disease (rare)<br>endocrine disease:<br>  adrenal failure<br>  pituitary failure<br>  isolated ACTH or GH deficiency<br>inherited metabolic disorders:<br>  glycogen storage disease Type I<br>hyperinsulinism:<br>  insulinoma<br>  nesidioblastosis<br>non-pancreatic neoplasms<br>alcohol-induced fasting hypoglycaemia<br>various forms of neonatal hypoglycaemia<br>septicaemia | **Acute**<br>due to neuroglycopenia:<br>  tiredness<br>  confusion<br>  detachment<br>  hunger<br>  ataxia<br>  dizziness<br>  blurred vision<br>  paraesthesiae<br>  hemiparesis<br>  convulsions<br>  coma<br>due to sympathetic stimulation:<br>  palpitation and tachycardia<br>  profuse sweating<br>  facial flushing<br>  tremor<br>  anxiety<br><br>**Chronic neuroglycopenia**<br>  personality changes<br>  memory loss<br>  psychosis<br>  dementia |

**Fig. 11.12** Major causes and clinical features of hypoglycaemia. Chronic neuroglycopenia is seen mainly in patients with insulin-secreting tumours; the features of acute neuroglycopenia are classically seen in diabetic patients who have taken too much insulin, but may occur with other forms of reactive hypoglycaemia.

sometimes deliberately administer excessive insulin to draw attention to themselves. More frequently, hypoglycaemia is related to a missed meal or some other factor (*see Case History 11.4*). It should be noted that the presence of glycosuria does not exclude a diagnosis of hypoglycaemia, for the renal threshold may have been exceeded since the bladder was last emptied. The diagnosis must rest on the blood glucose concentration, but if there is any doubt, it is always safe to give glucose to a confused or unconscious diabetic patient pending the result becoming available. Glucagon can also be used to treat hypoglycaemia; it causes rapid mobilization of hepatic glycogen. Treatment with β-adrenergic blockers can mask the adrenergic symptoms of hypoglycaemia (except sweating) and delay recovery.

**CASE HISTORY 11.5**

A young male jogger collapsed during a ten-mile fun run. He was conscious but disorientated and his speech was incoherent. He was taken to hospital where a finger-prick test for blood glucose concentration showed this to be very low. Blood was sent to the laboratory for confirmation of the diagnosis. He was given 25 g glucose i.v. and recovered rapidly. He then admitted that he was an insulin-dependent diabetic; he had injected his normal dose of insulin that morning and eaten his usual breakfast. The laboratory reported a blood glucose concentration on admission of 1.6 mmol/L. He was given further carbohydrate by mouth and was discharged that evening with a normal blood glucose concentration, to be reviewed in the diabetic clinic the next day.

### Comment

Insulin requirements in insulin-dependent diabetic patients are reduced by exercise. It is an important part of the education of diabetic patients that they are aware of this and can thus reduce their insulin dose or increase their carbohydrate intake accordingly. Diabetic patients should always carry sugar and a means of identification to facilitate treatment in an emergency.

In patients with non-insulin dependent diabetes, hypoglycaemia can complicate treatment with sulphonylureas. Chlorpropamide is most frequently implicated. It has a long plasma half-life and, since it is eliminated only by the kidneys, tends to accumulate in patients with impaired renal function.

Hypoglycaemia due to drugs other than those used to treat diabetes is uncommon. β-Adrenergic blockers occasionally cause hypoglycaemia, but only when other factors such as starvation, severe exercise or liver disease are involved. Children, but not adults, poisoned with salicylates may develop severe hypoglycaemia. It has also been reported in patients who have taken overdoses of paracetamol and, in these cases, it is probably related to the severe liver damage that this drug can cause.

### Post-prandial hypoglycaemia

In patients who have undergone gastric surgery, either with a gastrointestinal anastomosis or a pyloroplasty, hypoglycaemia developing 90–150 min after a meal, particularly a meal rich in sugar, is common. There is rapid passage of glucose into the small intestine and release of hormones which stimulate insulin secretion. The insulin response is excessive and hypoglycaemia ensues as glucose absorption from the gut falls off rapidly, rather than slowly as it does when gastric emptying is normal.

Symptoms suggestive of hypoglycaemia following meals may be described by people who have not undergone surgery (essential or idiopathic post-prandial hypoglycaemia), Although transient hypoglycaemia is common from 90 to 150 min after taking 75 g glucose orally in a glucose tolerance test, it is often asymptomatic and the relevance of hypoglycaemia after this artificial stimulus is questionable. Further, low blood glucose concentrations are not always demonstrable in such subjects, nor is there objective evidence of disordered glucose homoeostasis. Nevertheless, dietary manipulations, of which the addition of guar or other vegetable fibre to the diet is the most effective, may give considerable symptomatic relief.

### Alcohol and reactive hypoglycaemia

Insulin- and drug-induced reactive hypoglycaemia are potentiated by alcohol. Alcohol also increases insulin release in response to an oral glucose load and this may enhance any tendency to post-prandial reactive hypoglycaemia. Alcohol-induced fasting hypoglycaemia is considered in *Case History 11.7.*

### Other causes of reactive hypoglycaemia

Various inherited metabolic diseases have reactive hypoglycaemia as a feature. Since these are usually first recognized in children they are considered in the discussion of neonatal and childhood hypoglycaemia (*see pp 179–180*).

Sudden cessation of hypertonic dextrose infusion, being given as part of a parenteral feeding regimen, can precipitate hypoglycaemia, especially when insulin has been given concomitantly. Hypoglycaemia may also occur after dialysis against a glucose-rich dialysate.

## Fasting hypoglycaemia

### Insulinoma

Insulinomas are tumours of the insulin-secreting β-cells of the pancreatic islets. Although uncommon, they are an important cause of fasting hypoglycaemia. The blood glucose concentration should be measured in any patient who experiences a fit, faint, transient ischaemic attack or 'funny turn' in order to exclude hypoglycaemia as a cause, although it should be realized that many patients with an insulinoma present with behavioural changes, rather than with the classical features of acute hypoglycaemia. For this reason, there is often a delay before the diagnosis is considered and appropriate investigations are performed.

Other causes of fasting hypoglycaemia are usually obvious clinically. The presence of an insulin-secreting tumour can be inferred from the presence of an inappropriately high plasma insulin concentration (>10 mU/L) at a time when the blood glucose concentration is low (<2.2 mmol/L). C-Peptide should also be measured. Although secreted in equimolar amounts with insulin, C-peptide is cleared from the circulation more slowly, so that it may be a more reliable marker of endogenous insulin secretion than insulin itself. Measurement of plasma 3-hydroxybutyrate concentration can be informative. Insulin inhibits lipolysis and hence the production of 3-hydroxybutyrate. High concentrations (>600 µmol/L) occur in hypoglycaemia with suppressed insulin secretion (e.g., cortisol deficiency, liver disease). In hyperinsulinaemia, 3-hydroxybutyrate concentrations are usually low.

Ideally, blood should be collected for these measurements while the patient is symptomatic. If this cannot be done, or symptoms of acute hypoglycaemia do not occur, blood samples should be collected after an overnight fast on three consecutive mornings; when this is done, biochemical (although often asymptomatic) hypoglycaemia is demonstrable in 90% of patients with an insulinoma. Clinical hypoglycaemia develops in almost all patients during a 72 h fast, and may be provoked by exercise during this time. Blood samples should be collected every 4–6 h and during any episode of clinical hypoglycaemia; plasma insulin and C-peptide concentrations are measured in any sample in which the blood glucose concentration is low. Although normal subjects occasionally develop hypoglycaemia during such a fast (women more frequently than men), this is asymptomatic and plasma insulin concentration is low (usually <3 mU/L).

The 72 h fast is a time-consuming procedure, and as an alternative, when required, an insulin hypoglycaemia test (p. 108) can be performed. Hypoglycaemia is induced with insulin (with the usual strict monitoring mandatory for this test) and plasma C-peptide concentration is measured. C-Peptide is not present in insulin produced for therapeutic use. In normal individuals, the induction of hypoglycaemia suppresses endogenous insulin and C-peptide secretion. In patients with an insulinoma, this does not happen; a plasma C-peptide concentration > 1.2 µg/L implies continuing, autonomous, insulin secretion. Some insulinomas secrete mainly proinsulin, but this is measured in many of the assays for insulin with the result that separate measurement of proinsulin may not be required.

## CASE HISTORY 11.6

A woman telephoned for an ambulance when she was unable to rouse her husband one morning; she noticed that his left leg and arm were jerking. In the hospital emergency room, he was seen to be pale and sweaty, with a rapid, poor-volume pulse. His blood glucose concentration was 0.8 mmol/L. He regained consciousness when given a bolus of glucose intravenously, but then became confused and required a continuous glucose infusion for several hours to prevent hypoglycaemia.

His wife revealed that she had been becoming increasingly worried about her husband. Formerly a man of equable temperament, over the past six months he had frequently arrived home in a bad mood, taken little notice of his wife and young child and sat in sullen silence until his evening meal. After eating, he would behave quite normally, apparently with no recollection of his previous behaviour. On the two mornings immediately prior to admission, she had found him sitting up in bed, apparently conscious but staring vacantly at the wall and not speaking; she had managed to get him to drink his usual cup of sweet tea and he had rapidly recovered.

A presumptive diagnosis of insulinoma was made and was confirmed by the finding of a serum insulin concentration of 80 mU/L at a time when he was hypoglycaemic. He had hepatomegaly and the serum alkaline phosphatase activity was raised. A coeliac axis angiogram demonstrated a large filling defect in the liver; at laparotomy, the liver was found to have extensive tumour deposits, shown on histological examination to be characteristic of an insulinoma. A single, small tumour was present in the pancreas. No operative treatment was possible; he initially responded well to cytotoxic drugs but relapsed and died six months later.

### Comment

This case illustrates the sometimes bizarre symptomatology of patients with insulinomas, who may be chronically hypoglycaemic. A provocative test was clearly not required to establish the diagnosis in this case. When a definitive test is required, the insulin hypoglycaemia test with measurement of C-peptide is preferable to the many other tests that have been described, using, for example, glucagon or alcohol as a secretagogue for insulin. The majority of insulinomas (approximately 90%) are, unlike the tumour in this case, benign. In some 10% of cases there are multiple pancreatic tumours and there may be associated adenomas in other endocrine organs (multiple endocrine neoplasia Type I, see p. 275).

The treatment of choice is surgical resection, when possible, and with benign tumours the prognosis is good. Diazoxide may be used to prevent hypoglycaemia pre-operatively. Its main action is to reduce insulin secretion from both normal and neoplastic β-cells. Streptozotocin, a drug which is specifically cytotoxic to β-cells, is valuable in the management of malignant insulinomas when surgical treatment is either not possible or has failed.

### Non-pancreatic neoplasms

Hypoglycaemia can also occur in association with non-pancreatic neoplasms, particularly large mesenchymal tumours such as retroperitoneal sarcomas, with hepatocellular and adrenal carcinomas and with carcinoid tumours. Patients are usually not ketotic and, except with some carcinoid tumours, plasma insulin concentrations are not increased. It has been suggested that increased glucose uptake by the tumour may be a factor but this is unlikely ever to be the sole cause. Hepatic glucose output is often reduced although there is a normal glucogenic response to glucagon. It is probable that most such tumour-related hypoglycaemia is related to the secretion of insulin-like growth factors (IGFs). Plasma IGF1 concentrations are consistently low in such patients but IGF2 is often increased, and the ratio IGF1/IGF2, decreased. Cytokines such as tumour necrosis factor (TNFα) have also been implicated.

### Hepatic and renal disease

Although the liver is central to glucose homoeostasis, its functional reserve is so great that hypoglycaemia is a rare feature of hepatic disease. It may occur, however, with the rapid, massive hepatocellular destruction that can follow poisoning with paracetamol and other toxins. The kidneys are the only organs other than the liver capable of gluconeogenesis; they are also responsible for insulin degradation. These facts may in part explain the severe hypoglycaemia that is occasionally a feature of terminal renal disease.

### Endocrine disease

Deficiency of hormones antagonistic to insulin is a recognized but uncommon cause of hypoglycaemia. Lack of cortisol can be due either to primary adrenal failure or secondary to panhypopituitarism; hypoglycaemia may be a feature of either condition. Mild hypoglycaemia can occur with isolated deficiency of ACTH or growth hormone but in the latter condition it is never symptomatic.

Rather surprisingly, in view of its role in carbohydrate metabolism, lack of adrenaline in patients who have undergone bilateral adrenalectomy and who are maintained on corticoid hormone replacement, neither causes hypoglycaemia nor interferes with the ability to recover from artificially induced hypoglycaemia.

### Alcohol-induced fasting hypoglycaemia

**CASE HISTORY 11.7**

An elderly man was found to be unrousable one morning by fellow inmates of a derelict house in which they slept. He had been drunk the previous evening and although this was not uncommon he had never before been so stuporous in the morning. An ambulance was called and he was admitted to hospital and found to be profoundly hypoglycaemic. He responded rapidly to intravenous glucose and did not then appear inebriated. He refused further treatment and discharged himself later the same day.

**Comment**

Alcohol-induced fasting hypoglycaemia is caused mainly by the inhibitory effect of alcohol on gluconeogenesis. However, acquired ACTH deficiency may be present in some alcoholics and poor nutrition and liver disease may also contribute. As in this case, hypoglycaemia characteristically develops several hours after alcohol ingestion (compare alcohol and reactive hypoglycaemia, *page 177*), when hepatic glycogen stores become exhausted. Signs of inebriation may not be present at this time and blood alcohol levels are unremarkable. Although first described, and most commonly seen, in poorly nourished chronic alcoholics, hypoglycaemia can be readily precipitated by alcohol in healthy subjects whose hepatic glycogen reserves have been depleted by lack of food.

### Inherited metabolic disease

Fasting hypoglycaemia is an important feature of glycogen storage disease Type I, discussed in more detail *on page 240*.

## HYPOGLYCAEMIA IN CHILDHOOD

## Neonatal hypoglycaemia

Although the newborn appear to have a lower threshold for the development of clinical hypoglycaemia, there is good evidence that even asymptomatic hypoglycaemia may be deleterious (particularly in relation to the central nervous system). The formerly accepted practice, whereby a lower blood glucose concentration in the newborn to that in adults was used for the definition of hypoglycaemia, should therefore be abandoned.

Hypoglycaemia may occur transiently in apparently normal babies, but is particularly common in those who have respiratory distress, severe infection, brain damage or who are small-for-dates. Premature and small-for-dates babies are particularly at risk of developing neonatal hypoglycaemia because they are born with low hepatic glycogen stores and are more likely to have feeding problems. Extensive physiological changes occur at birth and, in terms of glucose metabolism, there is a sudden interruption of the maternal glucose supply and glycogenolysis must span the period until feeding starts. Babies born to diabetic mothers may have islet cell hyperplasia which increases the risk of hypoglycaemia developing in the immediate postnatal period, though this does not persist thereafter.

## Hypoglycaemia in infancy

Any of the conditions discussed above may cause hypoglycaemia in infancy. A variety of other conditions may cause hypoglycaemia at this time (*Fig. 11.13*); these are discussed below. The inherited metabolic diseases associated with hypoglycaemia are particularly likely to present during the first few weeks of life.

The commonest form of hypoglycaemia in infancy is ketotic hypoglycaemia. This may be either primary (idiopathic) or secondary to conditions leading to relative carbohydrate deficiency, such as starvation or generalized illness in children who were small-for-dates at birth. There is reduced availability of glucogenic precursors, especially alanine, but the reason for this is unknown. The low blood glucose suppresses insulin secretion and this is the cause of the ketosis (not vice versa as used to be thought). Hypoglycaemia can be prevented by frequent feeding and the attacks become less frequent as the child grows older.

Nesidioblastosis is a rare developmental abnormality of the pancreas in which there is overgrowth of ducts and islet cells. Leucine may precipitate the hypoglycaemia in this condition, but there is doubt as to whether 'leucine-induced hypoglycaemia' is a distinct clinical syndrome. The diagnosis is made on the basis of persistent hypoglycaemia without ketosis together with an inappropriate plasma insulin concentration. No tumour is demonstrable. Treatment is by sub-total pancreatectomy, which also provides histological confirmation of the diagnosis.

The inherited metabolic diseases associated with hypoglycaemia include galactosaemia, certain glycogen storage diseases, defects of the β-oxidation of fatty acids, hereditary fructose intolerance, and some organic acidaemias and amino acidopathies.

---

**Causes of hypoglycaemia in childhood**

**Transient neonatal hypoglycaemia**

**Ketotic hypoglycaemia**
idiopathic
secondary

**Hyperinsulinaemia**
islet cell hyperplasia
nesidioblastosis
insulinoma

**Inherited metabolic disorders, including:**
glycogen storage diseases
galactosaemia
hereditary fructose intolerance
fatty acid β-oxidation defects

**Other causes**
prematurity
small-for-dates
endocrine disorders
starvation
drugs

**Fig. 11.13** Causes of hypoglycaemia in childhood.

---

**CASE HISTORY 11.8**

A healthy two-month-old female infant, who had previously been breast-fed, vomited when given supplementary feeds of sweetened cows' milk. She reacted similarly when given fruit juice and sometimes became quiet and sleepy after such a feed. Her mother experimented with various feeds and learnt to avoid those that made her child ill. The child grew up with an aversion to sweet foodstuffs and fruit. Her brother, born three years later, had a similar history.

Later, when both became medical students, they wondered if their aversion was due to hereditary fructose intolerance. Fructose tolerance tests were performed and were found to induce hypoglycaemia, vomiting and other metabolic changes characteristic of this condition.

**Comment**
If the link between a child's illness and dietary fructose (and sucrose) is not made, there may be

serious long-term consequences: failure to thrive, cirrhosis and renal tubular dysfunction, for example. If fructose is avoided and irreversible liver or kidney damage has not occurred, patients with hereditary fructose intolerance remain symptom-free. The cause of the intolerance is a lack of the B isoenzyme of fructose 1-phosphate aldolase, which catalyzes the conversion of fructose 1-phosphate and fructose 1,6-bisphosphate to trioses.

In the absence of the B isoenzyme, the other isoenzymes (A and C), which account for 15% of the catalytic activity, convert much less fructose 1-phosphate than normal but are still sufficiently active to convert fructose 1,6-bisphosphate to trioses in the glycolytic pathway. When fructose is ingested, however, it is still converted by fructokinase to fructose 1-phosphate in the normal way, but because the A and C isoenzymes have insufficient activity to metabolize it, the fructose 1-phosphate accumulates. The clinical manifestations stem from the accumulation of fructose 1-phosphate, which inhibits glucose synthesis, and the depletion of ATP and phosphate as fructose is phosphorylated but not further metabolized.

# SUMMARY

In health, the mechanisms responsible for glucose homoeostasis ensure the maintenance of blood glucose concentrations within a narrow range, whether an individual is fed or fasting.

Diabetes mellitus is a condition characterized by abnormal glucose tolerance with a tendency to hypoglycaemia and is due to a relative or absolute deficiency of insulin. It may occur secondarily to obvious pancreatic disease but the majority of cases are idiopathic. Type I, or insulin-dependent diabetes (IDDM), typically affects younger patients. It usually has an acute onset; there is strong evidence of an autoimmune pathogenesis. Type II, or non insulin-dependent diabetes (NIDDM), typically affects middle-aged and elderly people and has a more gradual onset. Genetic and environmental factors are important in its pathogenesis.

Hyperglycaemia leads to glycosuria and causes an osmotic diuresis, producing the classical clinical features of polyuria and thirst. If inadequately treated, patients with IDDM may develop diabetic ketoacidosis. In this condition, hyperglycaemia, together with increased lipolysis, proteolysis and ketogenesis, leads to severe dehydration, mineral loss, pre-renal uraemia and a profound non-respiratory acidosis. Patients with NIDDM appear to have sufficient insulin secretion to prevent the excessive lipolysis and ketogenesis which are essential to the production of ketoacidosis. Instead, inadequate treatment may lead to the development of very severe hyperglycaemia and dehydration, producing a non-ketotic, hyperosmolar state. Both ketoacidosis and non-ketotic hyperosmolar coma are medical emergencies; their management involves rehydration and insulin replacement with general supportive measures and treatment of any specific pre-existing or complicating factors.

In the longer term, patients with diabetes are at risk of developing retinopathy, neuropathy, nephropathy and vascular disease. The presence of microalbuminuria may indicate early (and potentially treatable) nephropathy. Diabetes is associated with various perturbations of lipid metabolism which predispose to atherosclerosis.

The treatment of diabetes is aimed at relieving symptoms and preventing both the short- and long-term complications. The efficacy of treatment, whether with insulin, oral hypoglycaemic drugs or dietary modification alone, can be assessed clinically and by measurements of blood and urine glucose concentrations. However, the blood glucose gives an indication of control only at a single moment and urine glucose reflects blood glucose concentration over at most only a few hours. Measurements of glycated haemoglobin ($HbA_{1c}$) provide a valuable index of glycaemic control over a period of several weeks.

The causes of hypoglycaemia fall into two groups according to whether the condition occurs in the fasting state (fasting hypoglycaemia) or is provoked by a specific stimulus, which can include food intake (reactive hypoglycaemia). Causes of fasting hypoglycaemia include insulin-secreting tumours (insulinomas) and certain other tumours producing insulin-like substances, pituitary and adrenal failure, severe liver disease and glycogen storage diseases, notably Type I (glucose 6-phosphatase deficiency). Except in patients with insulinomas, clinical features due to hypoglycaemia are rarely the only feature of any of these conditions. The diagnosis of an insulinoma depends upon the finding of inappropriately high insulin (and C-peptide) levels in the blood at a time when the patient is hypoglycaemic. This is often demonstrable after an overnight fast, precipitated if necessary by exercise. Provocative tests to stimulate insulin secretion are rarely required in patients with an insulinoma.

Reactive hypoglycaemia may be caused by drugs. Most patients with insulin-dependent diabetes experience occasional episodes of hypoglycaemia, for example, as a result of a delayed meal following an insulin injection, an error in insulin dosage or unaccustomed exercise. Oral hypoglycaemic drugs (sulphonylureas) can also cause hypoglycaemia. This is more common in patients treated with the longer acting drugs, particularly the elderly, whose capacity to metabolize or excrete the drugs may be impaired.

Following gastric surgery, rapid transit of food into the small intestine may cause inappropriate insulin secretion and lead to hypoglycaemia. Such post-prandial hypoglycaemia also occurs occasionally in normal subjects. Patients with hereditary fructose intolerance and galactosaemia develop hypoglycaemia after ingesting fructose and galactose, respectively.

Hypoglycaemia may occur following alcohol ingestion and several distinct syndromes of alcohol-related hypoglycaemia have been described. Alcohol potentiates insulin- and drug-induced hypoglycaemia and may enhance any tendency to post-prandial reactive hypoglycaemia. The hypoglycaemia that can develop 12–24 h after alcohol ingestion, particularly in chronic alcoholics, is due in part to impairment of gluconeogenesis but the presence of liver disease, poor nutrition and depletion of hepatic glycogen reserves may also be important.

Hypoglycaemia is particularly common in neonates who are small-for-dates and is a risk in those born to diabetic mothers. In addition to the conditions described, ketotic hypoglycaemia may occur in infancy. This is a condition of unknown aetiology in which there appears to be a decreased supply of glucogenic substrates.

Acutely, hypoglycaemia causes clinical features related to increased activity of the sympathetic nervous system (sweating, tachycardia) and decreased substrate supply to the central nervous system (paraesthesiae, fits, coma). These usually respond rapidly to the administration of glucose. Patients who are chronically hypoglycaemic, for example, due to an insulinoma, often present with behavioural disturbance or frank psychosis and the acute manifestations of hypoglycaemia may be absent.

## FURTHER READING

Besser G M & Thorner M O (eds.) (1994) *Clinical Endocrinology: An Illustrated Text* 2nd edition London: Wolfe.

Field J B (ed.) (1989) Hypoglycaemia. *Endocrinology and Metabolism Clinics of North America*, **18**, 1–252.

Watkins P J (1993) *ABC of Diabetes* 3rd edition London: BMJ Publishing Group.

Pickup J & Williams G (eds) (1991) *Textbook of Diabetes*. Oxford: Blackwell Scientific Publications.

# 12. Calcium, Phosphate, Magnesium and Bone

## INTRODUCTION

Calcium is the most abundant mineral in the human body. The average adult body contains approximately 25,000 mmol (1 kg), of which 99% is bound in the skeleton. The total calcium content of the extracellular fluid (ECF) is only 22.5 mmol, of which about 9 mmol is in the plasma. Bone is not metabolically inert; some of its calcium is rapidly exchangeable with the ECF, the turnover between bone and ECF being approximately 500 mmol/24 h (*Fig. 12.1*).

In the kidneys, ionized calcium is filtered by the glomeruli (240 mmol/24 h). Most of this is reabsorbed in the tubules and normal renal calcium excretion is 2.5–7.5 mmol/24 h. Obligatory renal calcium excretion is approximately 2.5 mmol/24 h. Because of the faecal loss, the minimum dietary requirement is about 12.5 mmol/L (though it is higher during growth, pregnancy and lactation). Gastrointestinal secretions contain calcium, some of which is reabsorbed together with dietary calcium. Since calcium in the ECF pool is effectively exchanged through the kidneys, gut and bone about

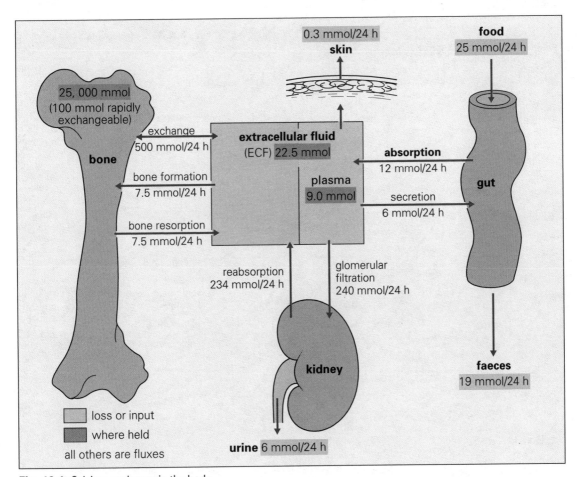

**Fig. 12.1** Calcium exchange in the body.

33 times every 24 hours, a small change in any of these fluxes will have a profound effect on ECF, and hence plasma, calcium concentration.

Calcium has many important functions in the body (*Fig. 12.2*). Its effect on neuromuscular activity is of particular importance in the symptomatology of hypocalcaemia and hypercalcaemia, as is described later in this chapter.

## BONE

Bone consists of osteoid, a collagenous organic matrix, on which is deposited complex inorganic hydrated calcium salts known as hydroxyapatites. These have the general formula:

$$Ca^{2+}_{10-x}(H_3O^+)_{2x}(PO_4^{3-})_6(OH^-)_2$$

Even when growth has ceased, bone remains biologically active. Continuous turnover occurs and bone resorption (mediated by osteoclasts) is followed by new bone formation (mediated by osteoblasts); the control of this process is poorly understood. It is probably integrated by local production of cytokines. Bone formation requires osteoid synthesis and adequate calcium and phosphate for the laying down of hydroxyapatite. Alkaline phosphatase, secreted by osteoblasts, is essential to the process, probably acting by releasing phosphate from pyrophosphate. Bone provides an important reservoir of calcium, phosphate and, to a lesser extent, magnesium and sodium.

## PLASMA CALCIUM

In the plasma, calcium is present in three forms (*Fig. 12.3*): bound to protein (mainly albumin); complexed with citrate and phosphate, and free ions. Only the latter form is physiologically active and it is the concentration of ionized calcium which is maintained by homoeostatic mechanisms.

| Functions of calcium | |
|---|---|
| **Function** | **Example** |
| structural | bone<br>teeth |
| neuromuscular | control of excitability<br>release of neurotransmitters<br>initiation of muscle contraction |
| enzymic | coenzyme for coagulation factors |
| signalling | intracellular second messenger |

**Fig. 12.2** Functions of calcium.

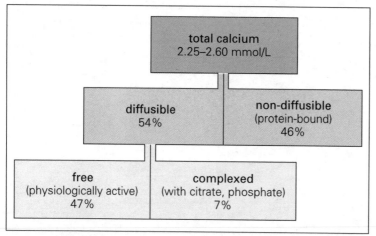

**Fig. 12.3** Distribution of calcium in human plasma. Some 80% of the amount bound to protein is bound to albumin, the remainder to γ-globulins.

In alkalosis, hydrogen ions dissociate from albumin, and calcium binding to albumin increases. There is also an increase in calcium complex formation. As a result, the concentration of ionized calcium falls, and this may be sufficient to produce clinical symptoms and signs of hypocalcaemia although total plasma calcium concentration is unchanged. In an acute acidosis, the reverse effect is observed, i.e., the ionized calcium concentration is increased.

The most commonly used methods for determining plasma calcium concentration measure the total calcium, although technology for the measurement of ionized calcium using ion-selective electrodes is becoming more widely available. No clear superiority has yet been demonstrated for measurements of ionized, as opposed to total, calcium concentration in the management of the majority of cases of disordered calcium metabolism. One undoubted advantage of ionized calcium measurements over conventional measurements of total calcium is the speed with which results are available. They may thus be useful to monitor calcium in circumstances when rapid changes in concentration can occur, for example, during exchange blood transfusion and during surgery with extra-corporeal bypass.

Changes in plasma albumin concentration will affect total calcium levels independently of the ionized calcium concentration, leading to possible misinterpretation of results in both hypoproteinaemic and hyperproteinaemic states. Various formulae have been devised to indicate the total calcium concentration to be expected if the albumin concentration were normal. One widely used formula is given in *Fig. 12.4*, but such estimates of 'corrected' calcium concentration should be interpreted with caution, especially when blood hydrogen ion concentration is abnormal. This is another instance where a direct measurement of ionized calcium may be helpful. A common cause of apparent hyperproteinaemia, and hence hypercalcaemia, is venous stasis during blood sampling; this must be avoided when determinations of plasma calcium are to be made. For example, a tourniquet should not be used. Although globulins bind calcium to a lesser extent than albumin, the increase in $\gamma$-globulin in patients with myeloma can also increase the total plasma calcium concentration. In myeloma, however, hypercalcaemia is commonly present with an increased ionized calcium concentration, due to the secretion of calcium-mobilizing substances by the tumour cells.

## CALCIUM-REGULATING HORMONES

Calcium concentration in the ECF is normally maintained within narrow limits by a control system involving two hormones, parathyroid hormone (PTH) and calcitriol (1,25-dihydroxycholecalciferol). These hormones also control the inorganic phosphate concentration of the ECF.

### Parathyroid hormone

This hormone is a polypeptide, comprising 84 amino acids; as with many hormones, it is synthesized as a larger precursor, pre-pro-PTH (115 amino acids). Prior to secretion, two amino acid sequences are lost; the removal of a 25 amino acid chain produces pro-PTH, a further six amino acids being lost to form PTH itself. The pre- and prosequences are thought to be involved in the intracellular transport of the hormone. The biological activity of PTH resides in the N-terminal 1–34 amino acid sequence of the hormone. PTH is secreted by the parathyroid glands in response to a fall in plasma (ionized) calcium concentration. Hypercalcaemia and calcitriol (see below) inhibit PTH

---

| Calculation of 'corrected' plasma calcium concentration |
| --- |
| if plasma albumin concentration is [alb] g/L and measured total calcium is [Ca] mmol/L |
| for [alb] <40, corrected calcium = [Ca] + 0.02 × {40 − [alb]} mmol/L |
| for [alb] >45, corrected calcium = [Ca] − 0.02 × {[alb] − 45} mmol/L |
| for example,    [Ca] = 1.82 mmol/L <br> [alb] = 28 g/L <br><br> 'corrected' calcium = 2.06 mmol/L |

Fig. 12.4 Correction of plasma total calcium concentration for changes in albumin concentration.

secretion and synthesis, respectively. The action of PTH tends to increase the plasma calcium concentration and reduce plasma phosphate (*Fig. 12.5*).

Although PTH increases the tubular reabsorption of calcium in the kidneys, its action on bone releases calcium into the ECF and thus increases the amount of calcium filtered by the glomeruli. However, PTH also increases the reabsorbed fraction of the filtered load and the overall effect of the hormone is to increase plasma calcium concentration.

Despite the importance of PTH in the control of phosphate excretion, changes in phosphate concentration do not directly affect secretion of the hormone. Mild hypomagnesaemia stimulates PTH secretion, but more severe hypomagnesaemia reduces it as the secretion of PTH is magnesium-dependent.

Intact PTH has a half-life in the blood of only 3–4 minutes. It is rapidly metabolized in liver and kidney, undergoing cleavage in the region of amino acids 33–37 and elsewhere. As a result, various fragments of the hormone are present in the blood as well as the intact hormone; these include an N-terminal fragment, with a similar half-life to that of the intact hormone, a C-terminal fragment (half-life 2–3 hours) and others (*Fig. 12.6*). Previously used PTH immunoassays suffered from a lack of specificity for the biologically active moieties but current immunometric assays measure only intact PTH, and provide a reliable measure of parathyroid hormone status.

## Calcitriol

This hormone is derived from vitamin D by successive hydroxylation in the liver (25-hydroxylation) and kidney (1α-hydroxylation). Hydroxylation in the liver is not subject to feedback control, but that in the kidney is closely regulated (*Fig. 12.7*). When the 1α-hydroxylation of 25-hydroxycholecalciferol is inhibited, there is an increase in 24-hydroxylation. The product of this reaction, 24,25-dihydroxycholecalciferol, has no known physiological function. Both this metabolite and calcitriol undergo further metabolism in the kidney but the products are physiologically inactive.

The principal actions of calcitriol are indicated in *Fig. 12.7*. In the gut, it stimulates absorption of dietary calcium and phosphate; this process involves the synthesis of a calcium-binding protein (calbindin D) in enterocytes. This protein is one of a widely distributed group of calcium-binding proteins which are present in many other tissues. In bone, calcitriol promotes mineralization largely indirectly, through its role in the maintenance of ECF calcium and phosphate concentrations. The binding of calcitriol to osteoblasts increases the production of alkaline phosphatase and of a calcium-binding protein, osteocalcin, the exact function of which is uncertain. At high concentrations, calcitriol stimulates osteoclastic bone resorption, which releases calcium and phosphate into the ECF. In the kidney, calcitriol inhibits its own synthesis. It may have a small stimulatory effect on calcium reabsorption, acting permissively with PTH.

Many other tissues have receptors for calcitriol, suggesting that it has roles in addition to those in calcium homoeostasis. It has been shown to influence cellular differentiation in normal and malignant tissues; it also stimulates the production of several cytokines, suggesting that it has a role in immunomodulation.

| Actions of parathyroid hormone | | | |
|---|---|---|---|
| | Target organ | Action | Effect |
| PTH | bone | rapid release of calcium | ↑ plasma [Ca$^+$] |
| | | ↑ osteoclastic resorption | |
| | kidney | ↑ calcium reabsorption | ↑ plasma [Ca$^+$] |
| | | ↓ phosphate reabsorption | ↓ plasma [Pi] |
| | | ↑ 1α-hydroxylation of 25-hydroxycholecalciferol | ↑ calcium and phosphate absorption from gut |
| | | ↓ bicarbonate reabsorption | acidosis |

**Fig. 12.5** Actions of parathyroid hormone. In bone, PTH causes rapid release of calcium to the ECF mediated by osteocytes; calcitriol has a permissive effect on this process. PTH also stimulates osteoclastic bone resorption. Although it increases renal tubular reabsorption of calcium, the amount filtered is greatly increased as a result of hypercalcaemia, and hypercalciuria is usual. The phosphaturic action of PTH causes hypophosphataemia if renal function is normal.

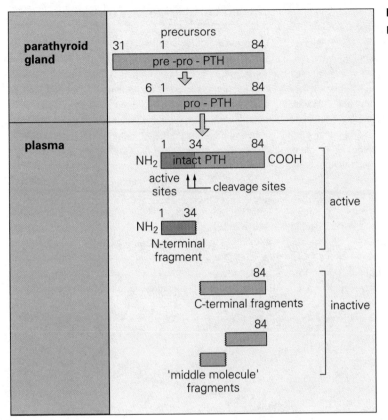

**Fig. 12.6** Parathyroid hormone: precursors and cleavage products.

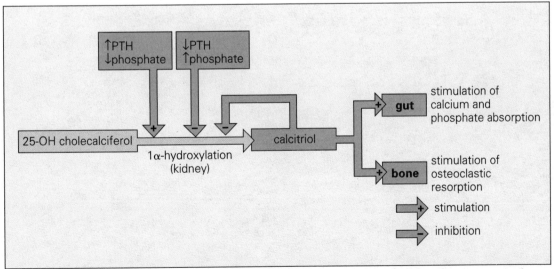

**Fig 12.7** Calcitriol (1,25-dihydroxycholecalciferol): Principal actions and control of renal synthesis. These actions increase the extracellular concentrations of calcium and phosphate. Other hormones, including growth hormone, prolactin and oestrogens, have a longer term stimulatory effect on calcitriol synthesis.

## Calcitonin

This polypeptide hormone, produced by the C cells of the thyroid, can be shown experimentally to inhibit osteoclast activity, and thus bone resorption, but it is not known if this is of any physiological significance. Subjects who have had a total thyroidectomy do not develop a clinical syndrome that can be ascribed to calcitonin deficiency. Also, calcium homoeostasis is normal in patients with medullary carcinoma of the thyroid, a tumour which secretes large quantities of calcitonin. Plasma calcitonin concentrations are elevated during pregnancy and lactation. So, too, are calcitriol concentrations, and calcitonin may block the action of calcitriol on bone and permit increased calcium uptake from the gut to take place without loss of mineral from bone.

Calcitonin has been detected in many other sites, including the gut and the central nervous system where it may act as a neurotransmitter. In some tissues, calcitonin m-RNA is translated to peptides other than calcitonin (calcitonin gene-related peptides). The function of these peptides is unknown.

## CALCIUM AND PHOSPHATE HOMOEOSTASIS

The response of the body to a fall in plasma calcium concentration, provided that this is not due to disordered homoeostasis in the first instance, is illustrated in *Fig. 12.8*. Hypocalcaemia stimulates the secretion of PTH and, through this, increases the production of calcitriol. There is an increase in the uptake of both calcium and phosphate from the gut and in their release from bone. PTH is phosphaturic, so the excess phosphate is excreted but the fractional reabsorption of calcium by the kidney is increased, some of the mobilized calcium is retained and the plasma calcium concentration tends to rise towards normal.

In hypophosphataemia (*Fig. 12.9*), calcitriol secretion is increased but PTH is not. Indeed, any tendency for calcitriol to increase the plasma calcium concentration should inhibit PTH secretion. Calcium and phosphate absorption from the gut are stimulated. Calcitriol has a much smaller effect on renal calcium reabsorption than PTH with the result that, in the absence of PTH, the excess calcium absorbed from

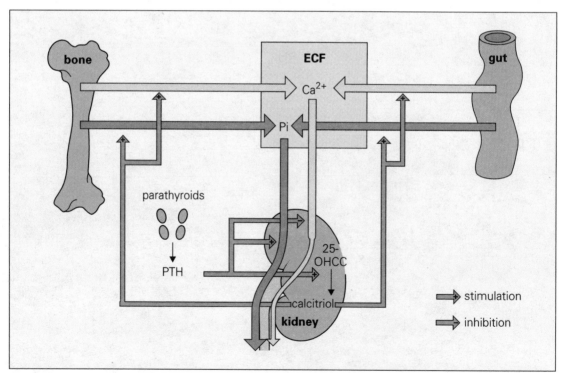

**Fig. 12.8** Homoeostatic responses to hypocalcaemia. Hypocalcaemia stimulates the release of PTH which in turn stimulates calcitriol synthesis. These hormones act together to restore plasma calcium concentration to normal, independently of phosphate concentration (25-OHCC=25-hydroxycholecalciferol.

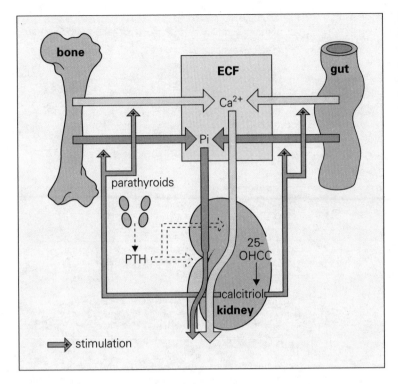

**Fig. 12.9** Homoeostatic responses in hypophosphataemia. In the absence of PTH (secretion is not affected by phosphate), an increase in calcitriol production due to stimulation of 1α-hydroxylase tends to increase the plasma phosphate independently of calcium concentration.

the gut is excreted in the urine. The net outcome is the restoration of the phosphate concentration towards normal, independently of calcium.

## DISORDERS OF CALCIUM, PHOSPHATE AND MAGNESIUM METABOLISM

### Hypercalcaemia

The causes of hypercalcaemia are listed in *Fig. 12.10*. Hypercalcaemia may be discovered during the investigation of an illness in which it is known to be a potential complication, during the investigation of clinical features suggestive of hypercalcaemia (*Fig. 12.10*) and frequently as an incidental result of calcium being measured as part of a 'biochemical profile'.

#### *Malignant disease*

This is a very common cause of hypercalcaemia particularly in patients in hospital. There may or may not be obvious metastases in bone. Patients with hypercalcaemia and malignant disease are usually symptomatic, due to the malignancy, the hypercalcaemia, or both.

Non-metastatic hypercalcaemia is discussed *on p. 271*; with most solid tumours, it is due to the secretion by the

tumour of PTH-related peptides. These are peptides having some amino acid sequence homology with PTH. They may have a role in calcium homoeostasis in the fetus but are not normally detectable in significant quantities in the adult. In patients with metastases in bone, there is often no relationship between the extent of metastasis and the severity of the hypercalcaemia, suggesting that humoral factors may be involved in the pathogenesis of hypercalcaemia in malignant disease whether or not osseous metastases are present. Other humoral factors that have been implicated include transforming growth factors, prostglandins and, particularly in haematological malignancies, osteoclast-activating cytokines (see *Case History 13.1*).

#### *Primary hyperparathyroidism*

The prevalence of this condition is of the order of one case per thousand persons. It can occur at any age and affects both men and women but is most common in postmenopausal women. It is usually due to a parathyroid adenoma, less often to diffuse hyperplasia of the glands, and only rarely to parathyroid carcinoma. Adenomas may be multiple and the condition is sometimes familial; it may occur as part of one of the syndromes of multiple endocrine neoplasia.

| Hypercalcaemia | |
|---|---|
| **Causes** | **Clinical features** |
| **Common**<br>malignant disease, with or without metastasis to bone<br><br>primary hyperparathyroidism<br><br>**Less common**<br>thyrotoxicosis<br><br>vitamin D intoxication<br><br>thiazide diuretics<br><br>sarcoidosis<br><br>idiopathic hypocalciuric hypercalcaemia<br><br>renal transplantation (tertiary hyperparathyroidism)<br><br>**Uncommon**<br>milk-alkali syndrome<br><br>lithium treatment<br><br>tuberculosis<br><br>immobilization (especially in Paget's disease)<br><br>acromegaly<br><br>adrenal failure<br><br>idiopathic hypercalcaemia of infancy<br><br>diuretic phase of acute renal failure | weakness, tiredness, lassitude, weight loss and muscle weakness<br><br>mental changes (impaired concentration, drowsiness, personality changes, coma)<br><br>anorexia, nausea, vomiting and constipation<br><br>abdominal pain (rarely peptic ulceration and pancreatitis)<br><br>polyuria, dehydration and renal failure<br><br>renal calculi and nephrocalcinosis (mainly associated with primary hyperparathyroidism)<br><br>short QT interval on ECG<br><br>cardiac arrhythmias and hypertension<br><br>corneal calcification and vascular calcification<br><br>there may also be features of the underlying disorder, such as bone pain in malignant disease and hyperparathyroidism |

**Fig. 12.10** Causes and clinical features of hypercalcaemia

immunoreactive PTH

   (intact hormone assay)           150 ng/L

      (reference range 10–65 ng/L)

bone radiographs                 normal

serum urea, albumin and alkaline

phosphatase:                    all normal

## Comment

Hyperparathyroidism may present in many ways (*see Fig. 12.10*), including renal or ureteric colic due to calculi which are themselves a result of hypercalciuria. Only about 10% of patients have clinical evidence of bone disease at presentation, although biochemical and radiological evidence is present in more than 20%. Many patients with hyperparathyroidism have no or few symptoms and are detected as a result of biochemical screening. Indeed, hyperparathyroidism is by far the most common cause of asymptomatic hypercalcaemia.

The plasma calcium concentration is nearly always raised. Exceptions to this occur if there is concomitant renal disease, vitamin D deficiency or hypothyroidism; occasionally the calcium is only raised intermittently. The phosphaturic action of PTH causes hypophosphataemia but this is not invariable; the plasma phosphate concentration may be normal or raised, particularly if there is renal damage. The plasma alkaline phosphatase is raised in only 20–30% of cases. Hypercalciuria is a reflection of the hypercalcaemia and is of no diagnostic importance.

The plasma PTH concentration (measured by a technique which detects the intact hormone only) is usually elevated but may be high–normal. Measurements of PTH should be interpreted in relation to the plasma calcium concentration. If this is elevated by any mechanism which does not involve PTH, parathyroid activity should be suppressed. Although PTH secretion does not cease completely under these circumstances, the hormone will be undetectable in plasma or present only at a low concentration.

The introduction of reliable assays for PTH has rendered obsolete several tests which were used as an aid to the diagnosis of this condition. These included measurement of renal phosphate clearance, assessment of the effects of steroids on plasma calcium concentration (a decrease usually occurs when hypercalcaemia is due to causes other than hyperparathyroidism) and multivariate analysis of several biochemical variables.

The definitive treatment for hyperparathyroidism is surgery. Although patients with mild (<3.00 mmol/L) asymptomatic hypercalcaemia may stay healthy for many years without an operation, they are at increased risk of developing osteoporosis and renal impairment and should be reassessed regularly. A high fluid intake should be maintained, to discourage renal calculus formation. Parathyroid adenomas are usually small and rarely palpable. Imaging techniques may help to localize the tumour preoperatively. A tumour may be localized by measuring PTH in blood samples obtained by selective catheterization of neck veins. This is a highly specialized technique, but is particularly useful if hypercalcaemia recurs and a second operation is required, since the normal anatomical relationships will have been distorted by the previous surgery.

### Secondary and tertiary hyperparathyroidism

Plasma PTH concentrations are also raised in many patients with chronic renal disease and with vitamin D deficiency. Both these conditions are associated with decreased synthesis of calcitriol, which causes hypocalcaemia, and the increase in PTH secretion is an appropriate physiological response. This is termed secondary hyperparathyroidism. The increase in PTH may not normalize the plasma calcium; in the absence of adequate calcitriol, there is resistance to the calcium-mobilizing effect of PTH on bone. Occasionally, patients with end-stage renal failure become hypercalcaemic, due to the development of autonomous PTH secretion, presumably as a result of the prolonged hypocalcaemic stimulus. Such hypercalcaemia may manifest for the first time in a patient given a renal transplant, who becomes able to metabolize vitamin D normally. This is termed tertiary hyperparathyroidism.

Parathyroid hormone is, in part, metabolized and excreted by the kidney. Increased plasma concentrations of PTH in renal failure reflect impairment of these processes as well as increased secretion. Much of the excess consists of C-terminal fragments, which are inactive in calcium homoeostasis. Measurement of PTH is essential to the monitoring of patients with chronic renal failure.

### Other causes of hypercalcaemia

Malignancy and hyperparathyroidism account for the majority of cases of hypercalcaemia but other conditions can be responsible. It is sometimes seen in patients with thyrotoxicosis, although thyroid hormones have no specific role in calcium homoeostasis, hypercalcaemia being due to the increased osteoclastic activity that may be present in this condition. Coincidental thyrotoxicosis may provoke symptomatic hypercalcaemia in a patient with mild, subclinical hyperparathyroidism. Thyrotoxicosis can also cause osteoporosis (*see page 197*).

Excessive intake of vitamin D itself is a rare cause of hypercalcaemia, but the 1-hydroxylated derivatives (calcitriol, alfacalcidol) are extremely potent and may cause hypercalcaemia. Plasma calcium concentration should be monitored regularly in patients treated with these agents.

In the milk-alkali syndrome, hypercalcaemia is associated with the ingestion of milk and antacids for the control of dyspeptic symptoms. The ingestion of alkali is important in the pathogenesis of the hypercalcaemia; it is thought that it decreases renal excretion of calcium but the precise mechanism is unknown. This syndrome is uncommon, and becoming more so since the introduction of drugs which inhibit gastric acid secretion for the treatment and prevention of peptic ulceration. It should also be remembered that dyspepsia itself may be a feature of hyperparathyroidism since calcium stimulates gastrin release. Occasionally, patients with parathyroid adenomas may have associated gastrin-secreting tumours (multiple endocrine neoplasia Type 1).

Thiazide diuretics are a common cause of mild hypercalcaemia, due to an effect on renal calcium excretion. Chronic lithium therapy can cause increased PTH secretion and is an occasional cause of hypercalcaemia. Approximately 10% of patients with sarcoidosis develop hypercalcaemia, as a result of 1-hydroxylation of 25-hydroxycholecalciferol by macrophages in the sarcoid granulomas. Hypercalcaemia can also complicate other granulomatous disorders (e.g., tuberculosis) for a similar reason. Hypercalcaemia (and hyperphosphataemia) is occasionally seen in acromegaly, probably due to the stimulation of renal 1-hydroxylase by growth hormone and, very rarely, in adrenal failure, particularly when it is acute.

During a period of immobilization, there is a decreased stimulus to bone formation and continued resorption (a part of normal bone turnover) results in hypercalciuria. Hypercalcaemia is usually only seen in immobilized patients if there is pre-existing increased bone turnover, as occurs during puberty and in patients with Paget's disease.

Familial hypocalciuric hypercalcaemia is a condition of unknown cause, inherited as an autosomal dominant trait. It has only recently been recognized and is probably underdiagnosed. Chronic hypercalcaemia develops from childhood and is usually asymptomatic. Hypophosphataemia is sometimes present; PTH concentrations are usually normal but may be slightly elevated. The diagnosis may be made only when hypercalcaemia persists after parathyroidectomy, but it may be inferred from finding a low rate of calcium excretion in the urine of a patient with hypercalcaemia.

The cause of idiopathic hypercalcaemia of infancy is unknown. It is associated with characteristic elfin facies and supravalvar aortic stenosis.

### Investigation

The way in which hypercalcaemia is investigated is dependent on the clinical setting. In hospital patients, malignancy is much commoner than hyperparathyroidism; the reverse is true in asymptomatic individuals with hypercalcaemia. In any patient, clinical features of the causative disorder may be present. The plasma phosphate concentration is of limited discriminative value; although low in most uncomplicated cases of primary hyperparathyroidism, it can also be decreased in hypercalcaemia due to malignancy and can be raised in either condition if there is renal impairment. Plasma alkaline phosphatase activity can be elevated in either condition, although is more frequently so in malignant disease.

Radiographic examination may reveal the characteristic subperiosteal bone reabsorption and bone cysts of hyperparathyroidism, but these are only present in a minority of cases; their absence does not exclude the diagnosis. A primary lung tumour or bony metastases will often, but not always, be revealed by radiography, but other tumours may not be so easily detected.

Measurement of PTH, using an assay for the intact hormone, is essential. Even if there is clear evidence of malignant disease or some other cause of hypercalcaemia, hyperparathyroidism is sufficiently common for there to be a real possibility of it being present coincidentally. The measurement of urinary calcium excretion is of no diagnostic value, except in the diagnosis of familial hypocalciuric hypercalcaemia.

If hyperparathyroidism and malignancy are excluded, re-assessment of the history, for both drugs and features of other conditions associated with hypercalcaemia, may prompt appropriate further investigations.

---

### CASE HISTORY 12.2

A 38-year-old man developed thirst and polyuria while on holiday in Spain. He had no other symptoms. He consulted his family doctor when he arrived home. The urine was tested but there was no glycosuria. Blood was taken for biochemical investigations.

## Investigations

serum:
| | | |
|---|---|---|
| calcium | 3.24 mmol/L | |
| phosphate | 1.20 mmol/L | |
| alkaline phosphatase | 90 IU/L | |
| urea | 10.0 mmol/L | |
| creatinine | 150 μmol/L | |

The patient, a non-smoker, was admitted to hospital for investigation. He had previously been well, apart from some joint pain and a painful rash on his legs several months before which had resolved spontaneously. The chest radiograph showed some increased hilar shadowing but was otherwise normal. No bony abnormality was seen on skeletal radiographs. He was slightly dehydrated and was given an intravenous saline infusion. Despite a good diuresis, the serum calcium was unchanged. He was then given hydrocortisone, 40 mg three times daily, and a week later the serum calcium was 2.80 mmol/L. At this time, the result of the PTH assay on blood taken on admission became available; no PTH could be detected.

## Comment

The patient presents with acute, symptomatic hypercalcaemia. The diagnosis could be hyperparathyroidism, an occult malignancy, or some other condition. In view of the slight renal impairment, the normal serum phosphate is not helpful. PTH is undetectable, implying suppression of the parathyroids by hypercalcaemia, rather than autonomous PTH secretion, and the dramatic response to hydrocortisone also militates against hyperparathyroidism. The hypercalcaemia of malignancy responds unpredictably to steroids. The clue to the diagnosis is provided by the chest radiograph and the previous history, which are suggestive of sarcoidosis. The hypercalcaemia in this condition is characteristically sensitive to steroids and is often more severe in the summer, due to increased synthesis of vitamin D by the action of ultraviolet light on the skin. The diagnosis of sarcoidosis was further supported by a positive Kveim test and the finding of a raised serum angiotensin-converting enzyme activity.

## Management

When possible, the underlying cause should be treated but the hypercalcaemia itself may require treatment in the short term. Dehydrated patients should be rehydrated with intravenous saline. Once this has been achieved, frusemide may be used; this stimulates a diuresis and inhibits the renal tubular reabsorption of calcium, thus promoting calcium excretion. Various other drugs may be used, for example, calcitonin, bisphosphonates, corticosteroids and mithramycin. Sodium phosphate, given intravenously, is potentially very dangerous, particularly in a patient with renal impairment, since it may cause extensive metastatic calcification. Life-threatening resistant hypercalcaemia may require treatment by dialysis or, exceptionally, emergency parathyroidectomy.

## Hypocalcaemia

The causes of hypocalcaemia are listed in *Fig. 12.11*. The importance of interpreting a low plasma calcium concentration in the light of the albumin concentration has already been stressed. The clinical features relate to increased neural and muscular excitability (*Fig. 12.11*).

### Vitamin D deficiency

The causes of this condition, which causes osteomalacia in adults and rickets in children, are discussed in *Chapter 21*. Deficiency may be due to inadequate endogenous synthesis or dietary supply of vitamin D, or to malabsorption. Whatever the cause, the effect is to decrease the amount of 25-hydroxycholecalciferol available for calcitriol synthesis, leading to decreased absorption of calcium and phosphate from the gut (see *Case History 6.2*). Although the 1α-hydroxylation of 25-hydroxycholecalciferol is stimulated in hypocalcaemia, with severe deficiency of the vitamin, lack of the substrate will prevent sufficient calcitriol being formed.

Vitamin D deficiency is a cause of secondary hyperparathyroidism. This further lowers the plasma phosphate concentration and patients with vitamin D deficiency usually show hypocalcaemia, hypophosphataemia and a raised plasma alkaline phosphatase activity. The plasma concentration of 25-hydroxycholecalciferol is low.

Hypocalcaemia and bone disease are occasionally seen in epileptic patients treated with phenobarbitone or phenytoin. Both drugs are inducers of hepatic microsomal hydroxylating enzymes and are thought to alter the metabolism of vitamin D in the liver. They probably also directly inhibit intestinal calcium absorption. In some forms of chronic liver disease, particularly primary biliary cirrhosis, hypocalcaemia and a metabolic bone disease with some features of osteomalacia develop. Mechanisms include malabsorption of vitamin D, decreased 25-hydroxylation and decreased synthesis of plasma binding protein.

Inherited disorders of vitamin D metabolism are discussed on *p. 196*.

| Hypocalcaemia | |
|---|---|
| **Causes** | **Clinical features** |
| artefactual (blood collected into EDTA tube)<br>vitamin D deficiency:<br>   dietary<br>   malabsorption<br>   inadequate exposure to ultraviolet light<br>disordered vitamin D metabolism:<br>   renal failure<br>   anticonvulsant treatment<br>$1\alpha$-hydroxylase deficiency<br>hypoparathyroidism<br>pseudohypoparathyroidism<br>magnesium deficiency<br>acute pancreatitis<br>treatment of metabolic bone disease<br>hyperphosphataemia (rare)<br>neonatal hypocalcaemia<br>massive transfusion with citrated blood | behavioural disturbance and stupor<br>numbness and paraesthesiae<br>muscle cramps and spasms<br>laryngeal stridor<br>convulsions<br>cataracts (chronic hypocalcaemia)<br>basal ganglia calcification (chronic<br>   hypocalcaemia)<br>Chvostek's sign positive<br>Trousseau's sign positive<br>prolonged QT interval on ECG |

**Fig. 12.11** Causes and clinical features of hypocalcaemia. Chvostek's sign (contraction of facial muscles on tapping facial nerve) and Trousseau's sign (carpal spasm when sphygmomanometer cuff applied to upper arm is inflated to midway between systolic and diastolic blood pressures for three minutes) may be positive before other signs are present (latent tetany). Additional features in patients with vitamin D deficiency include myopathy and bone pain.

### Renal disease

Hypocalcaemia is common in patients with end-stage renal disease (see *Case History 4.3*) but is rarely symptomatic. It is often associated with a complex metabolic bone disease known as renal osteodystrophy. The abnormalities of calcium and bone metabolism that occur in chronic renal failure are discussed in detail in *Chapter 4*.

### Hypoparathyroidism

This can be congenital or acquired. Acquired causes are listed in *Fig. 12.12*. The congenital form may be associated with thymic aplasia and immune deficiency, the Di George syndrome.

### CASE HISTORY 12.3

A 56-year-old woman was admitted to hospital for cataract extraction, in good health apart from her failing vision. She had undergone thyroidectomy for a multinodular goitre 20 years earlier. Routine preoperative investigations were carried out.

**Investigations**

| serum: | calcium | 1.60 mmol/L |
|---|---|---|
| | phosphate | 2.53 mmol/L |
| | albumin | 44 g/L |
| | alkaline phosphatase | 76 IU/L |

**Comment**

The combination of hypocalcaemia, hyperphosphataemia and a normal alkaline phosphatase is typical of hypoparathyroidism, probably due in this case to inadvertent removal of the glands. It is not uncommon for patients with chronic hypocalcaemia to be symptom free. In this patient, both Chvostek's and Trousseau's signs (*see Fig. 12.11*) were positive. Cataracts are a recognized complication of hypoparathyroidism, presumably because the high phosphate concentration leads to precipitation of calcium phosphate in the lens.

Patients with hypoparathyroidism are treated with vitamin D or its hydroxylated derivatives with or without calcium supplements, but care must be taken to avoid hypercalcaemia.

Pseudohypoparathyroidism superficially resembles hypoparathyroidism, but plasma concentrations of PTH are elevated. There are two types of pseudohypoparathyroidism; both are hereditary disorders. The effects of PTH are mediated through the formation of cyclic 3,5-AMP. In type 1, activation of adenyl cyclase is defective and cyclic AMP is not formed in response to the binding of PTH to its receptor. In type 2, cyclic AMP is formed, but the responses to it are blocked. The two types may be distinguished by measuring urinary cyclic AMP after administration of PTH. In normal individuals, and in patients with type 2 pseudohypoparathyroidism, there is an increase; in type 1, this does not occur. Patients with type 1 pseudohypoparathyroidism have characteristic skeletal abnormalities, including a rounded face, short stature, shortening of the fourth and fifth metacarpals and metatarsals, and a tendency for exotoses to form. Patients may be mentally retarded. In pseudo-pseudohypoparathyroidism, similar skeletal abnormalities are present but the plasma calcium concentration is normal. All these conditions are rare.

### Magnesium deficiency

Since magnesium is required for both PTH secretion and its action on target tissues, magnesium deficiency can cause hypocalcaemia or render patients insensitive to the treatment of hypocalcaemia with vitamin D or calcium, or both

### Pancreatitis

The causes of hypocalcaemia in acute pancreatitis are discussed in *Chapter 6.*.

---

| Causes of hypoparathyroidism |
|---|
| **Congenital**<br>(may be associated with immune deficiency) |
| **Acquired**<br>idiopathic<br>autoimmune (may be associated with other<br>   organ-specific endocrine disease)<br>surgery (thyroidectomy)<br>haemochromatosis<br>infiltrative conditions |

**Fig. 12.12** Causes of hypoparathyroidism.

---

### CASE HISTORY 12.4

An elderly woman who presented with weight loss and malabsorption due to amyloidosis of the small intestine was found to have osteomalacia and was hypocalcaemic. She was given parenteral nutritional support but despite what was considered to be adequate calcium and vitamin D supplementation, she remained hypocalcaemic.

**Investigations**

serum magnesium            0.35 mmol/L

**Comments**

Patients with malabsorption may develop magnesium deficiency and while this patient's parenteral feeds contained magnesium there was presumably an insufficient amount to correct her deficit. When given additional magnesium supplements her serum calcium rapidly returned to normal.

---

## Hyperphosphataemia

By far the most common cause of hyperphosphataemia is renal insufficiency; other causes are presented in *Fig. 12.13*. Hyperphosphataemia is a hazard if infants are fed undiluted cows' milk but excessive intake is an uncommon cause in adults, only occurring if excessive phosphate is given intravenously, for example, during parenteral feeding. Increased tissue catabolism, for example, in the treatment of malignant disease (particularly haematological malignancy), can cause hyperphosphataemia. Tissue catabolism is also one of its causes in diabetic ketoacidosis, but in these patients renal impairment is often also present.

Hyperphosphataemia is important clinically because it results in inhibition of the 1-hydroxylation of 25-hydroxycholecalciferol in the kidney; phosphate may also combine with calcium, resulting in metastatic calcium deposits in the tissues and hypocalcaemia.

### Management

Management should be directed at the underlying cause but, in practice, the most effective treatment is to give aluminium, calcium or magnesium salts by mouth to bind phosphate in the gut and prevent its absorption.

| Causes of hyperphosphataemia |
| --- |
| renal failure |
| hypoparathyroidism |
| pseudohypoparathyroidism |
| acromegaly |
| excessive phosphate intake/administration |
| vitamin D intoxication |
| catabolic states, e.g., tumour lysis syndrome |

**Fig. 12.13** Causes of hyperphosphataemia. This can develop *in vitro* if there is a delay in separating serum from cells prior to analysis.

## Hypophosphataemia

This is a common biochemical finding. When mild it is probably of little consequence, but severe hypophosphataemia (<0.3 mmol/L) can have important consequences on the function of all cells, particularly muscle cells (causing muscle weakness) and red and white blood cells, by limiting the formation of essential phosphate-containing compounds such as adenosine triphosphate (ATP) and 2,3-diphosphoglycerate (2,3-DPG). Chronic hypophosphataemia is a cause of rickets and osteomalacia

Causes of hypophosphataemia are given in *Fig. 12.14*. Although hyperphosphataemia is usual in diabetic ketoacidosis, hypophosphataemia is seen during the recovery phase when there is increased uptake of phosphate into depleted tissues. This is also the mechanism of hypophosphataemia seen in patients with malnutrition who are given a high calorie intake either enterally or parenterally. Hypophosphataemia is common during alcohol withdrawal and is multifactorial in origin. The causes include decreased intake, magnesium deficiency and, alkalosis.

Alkalosis (particularly respiratory) can cause hypophosphataemia by stimulating phosphofructokinase and the formation of phosphorylated glycolytic intermediates.

### Management

Hypophosphataemia should be anticipated, and prevented, in conditions where it may occur. It is treated by the administration of phosphate, either enterally or parenterally as appropriate, but intravenous phosphate should not be given to a patient who is hypercalcaemic or oliguric.

## Metabolic bone disease

Various bone diseases are characterized by disordered metabolism of the bone. They include osteomalacia and rickets, Paget's disease, renal osteodystrophy (*see p. 63*) and

osteoporosis. The biochemical changes associated with these conditions are summarized in *Fig. 12.15*.

### Rickets and osteomalacia

These conditions are characterized by defective mineralization of osteoid. Rickets occurs in infancy and childhood (while bones are growing); osteomalacia is its adult equivalent. Defective mineralization is most frequently due to an inadequate supply of calcium, usually because of deficiency or malabsorption of vitamin D. Such 'calciopenic' rickets and osteomalacia can also be due to impaired production of calcitriol or resistance to its actions. These are respectively features of two rare, inherited conditions: in vitamin D-dependent rickets type I, there is deficiency of renal 1-hydroxylase; in type II, there is resistance to the actions of calcitriol. Inheritance in both cases is autosomal recessive. Impaired production of calcitriol also occurs in chronic renal failure and contributes to the pathogenesis of renal osteodystrophy, in which features of osteomalacia are usually present.

Defective bone mineralization can also be due to an inadequate supply of phosphate. The cause is usually a renal tubular phosphate leak, such as occurs in the Fanconi syndrome, renal tubular acidosis type 1 and, as an isolated phenomenon, in familial X-linked hypophosphataemic rickets.

### Primary and secondary osteoporosis

Osteoporosis is a reduction in the quantity of normally mineralized bone. It increases the risk of fracture, which often occurs after only relatively minor trauma. It is a result of an imbalance between the processes of bone resorption and formation. With normal ageing, osteoblastic activity declines in relation to osteoclastic activity with the result that bone remodelling leads to a slow but progressive decrease in bone mass. This is rarely clinically significant in men, unless

| Causes of hypophosphataemia |
| --- |
| vitamin D deficiency |
| primary hyperparathyroidism |
| enteral/parenteral nutrition with inadequate phosphate (particularly in malnourished patients); intravenous glucose therapy |
| diabetic ketoacidosis (recovery phase) |
| alcohol withdrawal (rare) |
| renal tubular disease |
| phosphate binding agents, such as magnesium and aluminium salts (rare) |
| alkalosis |

**Fig. 12.14** Causes of hypophosphataemia.

| Plasma concentration | | | | |
|---|---|---|---|---|
| Condition | Calcium | Phosphate | Alkaline phosphatase | Other |
| osteoporosis | N | N | N | – |
| osteomalacia | ↓ or N | ↓ | ↑ (↑ ↑)† | – |
| Paget's disease | N(↑)* | N | ↑ ↑ ↑ | – |
| renal osteodystrophy | ↓ or N | ↑ | ↑ | ↑ creatinine |
| primary hyperparathyroidism | ↑ | N or ↓ | N or ↑ | – |
| secondary tumour deposits | N or ↑ | ↓ N or ↑ | ↑ | – |
| * during immobilization     † during early phase of recovery | | | | |

**Fig. 12.15** Biochemical changes in plasma in metabolic bone disease.

exacerbated by other factors, but in women is compounded by the effects of oestrogen deficiency after the menopause, which causes an accelerated rate of bone loss.

These types of osteoporosis are classified as primary. Post-menopausal osteoporosis primarily affects trabecular bone and is associated with vertebral crush fractures and radial fractures; age-related osteoporosis affects both trabecular and cortical bone and is associated with femoral neck fractures.

Osteoporosis can also occur secondarily to a variety of conditions (*see Fig. 12.16*), often in younger people. These conditions can also exacerbate primary osteoporosis.

There are as yet no generally available biochemical markers of osteoporosis. Plasma calcium and phosphate concentrations are normal, as is alkaline phosphatase activity (unless a fracture has occurred or there is concurrent osteomalacia). Urinary calcium and hydroxyproline (a component of collagen) excretion may be increased if the disease is rapidly progressive, but are often normal. The urinary excretion of peptides involved in cross-linking mature collagen ('pyridinium cross-links') is increased with increased bone resorption. Their measurement appears to provide a more sensitive test of this process than measurement of hydroxyproline. The most reliable technique for quantitating bone density for the purposes of diagnosis and management is an imaging technique, dual-energy X-ray absorptiometry (DEXA).

Because of the considerable cost of osteoporosis to individuals and society, considerable efforts are being made to detect individuals at high risk of developing the condition, and to devise effective strategies for prevention and man-

agement. The most effective technique for the prevention of post-menopausal osteoporosis is hormone replacement therapy (HRT). All patients at risk of developing osteoporosis should be counselled to avoid known risk factors, e.g., excessive alcohol intake, to maintain an adequate dietary calcium intake and, if they are able, undertake weight-bearing exercise. Coexistent vitamin D deficiency should be sought and treated if present. These measures,

---

**Causes of osteoporosis**

**Ageing**
especially post-menopausal

**Endocrine**
premature ovarian failure
thyrotoxicosis
Cushing's syndrome
diabetes mellitus
hypogonadism

**Drugs**
prolonged heparin treatment
glucocorticoids
alcoholism

**Others**
immobilization
malabsorption of calcium
weightlessness

**Fig. 12.16** Causes of osteoporosis.

and others including treatment with bisphosphonates and fluoride, are also used in the management of osteoporosis.

### Paget's disease of bone

This is a condition of unknown aetiology characterized by increased osteoclastic activity, which engenders increased osteoblastic activity and thus new bone formation. The new bone that is formed is abnormal and laid down in a disorganized fashion. As a result, bones become thickened, distorted and painful.

Paget's disease is a disease of the elderly, usually presenting with pain, although deformity, pathological fracture, the effects of new bone formation on surrounding structures (e.g., on the auditory nerve, causing deafness) or incidental radiological examination or biochemical testing may bring the condition to notice. Plasma alkaline phosphatase activity is increased and reflects disease activity; plasma calcium and phosphate concentrations are usually normal, although hypercalcaemia may develop if a patient with Paget's disease is immobilized. Treatment involves analgesics and, in more severe cases, the use of bisphosphonates or other agents to inhibit osteoclastic activity. Osteosarcoma is a rare complication of Paget's disease.

---

**CASE HISTORY 12.5**

An elderly man who complained of severe pain in his pelvis and thighs was diagnosed on radiological evidence as having Paget's disease of bone. The serum alkaline phosphatase was 750 IU/L. He was treated with oral bisphosphonates and made a good clinical recovery, though when his medication was stopped his thighs became painful again.

**Investigations**

The serum alkaline phosphatase activities are shown in *Fig. 12.17*.

**Comment**

The primary defect in Paget's disease is an increase in osteoclastic activity but this causes increased osteoblastic activity, reflected by high serum alkaline phosphatase activities. Serial measurements can be used, as in this case, to monitor the disease and its response to treatment.

Paget's disease can also be monitored by serial measurements of the urinary excretion of

---

hydroxyproline. This amino acid, a component of collagen, is not reutilized in the body and once released from bone by osteoclastic activity is excreted in the urine. Hydroxyproline is present in certain foodstuffs, for example gravies and jellies, and such substances must be avoided before and during urine collections. Other sources of collagen, notably the skin, also contribute to urinary hydroxyproline excretion.

---

## Magnesium

Magnesium is the fourth most abundant cation in the body. The adult human body contains approximately 1000 mmol, with about half in bone and the remainder distributed equally between muscle and other soft tissues. Only 15–29 mmol is found in the ECF, the plasma concentration being 0.8–1.2 mmol/L. The normal daily intake of magnesium (10–12 mmol) is greater than is necessary to maintain magnesium balance (approximately 8 mmol/day) and the excess is excreted through the kidneys.

Urinary magnesium excretion is increased by ECF volume expansion, hypercalcaemia and hypermagnesaemia, and decreased in the opposite of these states. Various hormones, including PTH and aldosterone, affect the renal handling of magnesium; the effects of aldosterone are probably secondary to changes in ECF volume but PTH, which increases the tubular reabsorption of filtered magnesium, appears to act directly.

Magnesium acts as a cofactor for some 300 enzymes, including enzymes involved in protein synthesis, glycolysis and the transmembrane transport of ions. A magnesium–ATP complex is the substrate for many ATP-requiring enzymes. Magnesium is important in the maintenance of the structure of ribosomes, nucleic acids and some proteins. It interacts with calcium in several ways and affects the permeability of excitable membranes and their electrical properties such that extracellular magnesium depletion causes hyperexcitability.

### Hypermagnesaemia

Significant hypermagnesaemia is uncommon. Cardiac conduction is affected at concentrations of 2.5–5.0 mmol/L; very high concentrations (>7.5 mmol/L) cause respiratory paralysis and cardiac arrest. Such extreme hypermagnesaemia may occasionally be seen in renal failure.

Intravenous calcium may give short-term protection against the adverse effects of hypermagnesaemia but in renal failure, dialysis may be necessary.

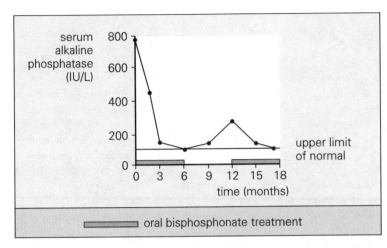

**Fig. 12.17** Serum alkaline phosphatase activities in a patient with Paget's disease of bone. Periods of treatment with oral bisphosphonates are indicated. After a good response to the first period of treatment the serum alkaline phosphatase begins to rise, indicating recrudescence of the disease; a good response was again achieved when treatment was restarted.

### Hypomagnesaemia

Hypomagnesaemia almost always indicates magnesium deficiency. Surveys have shown that it may be present in up to 10% of hospital patients; it occurs more frequently than hypermagnesaemia. The causes and clinical features are summarized in *Fig. 12.18*. Hypocalcaemia, due to decreased PTH secretion, is a clinically important consequence of hypomagnesaemia. Hypophosphataemia and hypokalaemia may also be present, but all these abnor-malities usually respond to magnesium supplementation. Plasma magnesium concentration should always be measured in patients with hypocalcaemia, or clinical features suggestive of hypocalcaemia, when these do not respond to calcium supplementation, and also in patients with refractory hypokalaemia. Other indications for its measurement include parenteral nutrition, chronic diarrhoea and other conditions listed in *Fig. 12.18*.

Mild magnesium deficiency is treated by oral supplementation; in severe deficiency, and with malabsorption, magnesium may be given by slow intravenous infusion.

| Magnesium deficiency |
|---|
| **Causes** |
| malabsorption, malnutrition and fistulae alcoholism (chronic alcoholism and alcohol withdrawal) cirrhosis diuretic therapy (especially loop diuretics) renal tubular disorders (in advanced renal disease hypermagnesaemia is usual) chronic mineralocorticoid excess |
| **Clinical features** |
| tetany (with normal or decreased calcium) agitation, delirium ataxia, tremor, choreiform movements and convulsions muscle weakness, cardiac arrhythmias |

**Fig. 12.18** Causes and clinical features of magnesium deficiency.

### CASE HISTORY 12.6

A young man presented with a short history of severe diarrhoea, abdominal pain, weight loss and rectal bleeding. He had had several previous episodes of diarrhoea and abdominal pain, but these had been much milder and he had not sought medical advice. He also complained of cramp in his arms and legs, and on testing had latent tetany.

**Investigations**

| | | |
|---|---|---|
| serum: | sodium | 142 mmol/L |
| | potassium | 3.1 mmol/L |
| | urea | 5.4 mmol/L |
| | creatinine | 96 μmol/L |
| | calcium | 2.42 mmol/L |
| | phosphate | 0.9 mmol/L |
| | albumin | 44 g/L |

**Comment**

The low potassium concentration was thought to reflect potassium loss in the stool. In view of the normal calcium, his serum magnesium was measured and found to be 0.38 mmol/L. He was given parenteral magnesium replacement (not oral, in view of his diarrhoea) and the cramps resolved. Crohn's disease was diagnosed from the appearances of a rectal biopsy.

When symptoms of hypocalcaemia occur in patients whose serum calcium is normal, hypomagnesaemia should be considered as a cause. Low concentrations of magnesium are often found in association with low concentrations of calcium, phosphate and potassium but hypomagnesaemia can occur in isolation. Other manifestations include cardiac arrhythmias and delirium.

## SUMMARY

Calcium has many functions in the body in addition to its obvious structural role in bones and teeth. It is, for example, essential for muscle contraction and its concentration affects the excitability of nerves; it is a second messenger, involved in the action of several hormones, and is required for blood coagulation. About half the calcium in the plasma is bound to protein; it is the unbound fraction that is physiologically active and whose concentration is closely regulated.

Two hormones have a central role in calcium homoeostasis. The main action of calcitriol, the hormone derived from vitamin D by successive hydroxylations in liver and kidney, is to stimulate calcium (and phosphate) uptake from the gut. Parathyroid hormone (PTH), secreted in response to a fall in plasma ionized-calcium concentration, stimulates calcitriol formation; it also stimulates calcium resorption from bone and reabsorption by the renal tubules, and has a powerful phosphaturic action. These two hormones also regulate extracellular phosphate concentration. The role of calcitonin in calcium homoeostasis has yet to be established.

The common causes of hypercalcaemia are primary hyperparathyroidism, due to parathyroid adenomas or hyperplasia, and malignant disease, with or without metastasis to bone, including myeloma. Less common causes include sarcoidosis and overdosage with vitamin D or its derivatives. Mild hypercalcaemia is often asymptomatic; when more severe, clinical features may include bone and abdominal pain, renal calculi, polyuria, thirst and behavioural disturbances.

Hypocalcaemia causes hyperexcitability of nerve and muscle, leading to muscle spasm (tetany) and, in severe cases, to convulsions. Causes include vitamin D deficiency and hypoparathyroidism. Vitamin D deficiency may be either dietary in origin, often exacerbated by poor exposure to sunlight (and hence reduced endogenous synthesis), or due to malabsorption.

Vitamin D deficiency causes osteomalacia in adults and rickets in children, both diseases being characterized by defective bone mineralization. In osteoporosis, a condition particularly common in post-menopausal women, there is a generalized loss of both bone matrix and mineral. Paget's disease of bone is common in the elderly in both sexes; there is greatly increased osteoclastic bone reabsorption which stimulates new bone formation, but this is structurally abnormal and patients present with bone pain and deformity. End-stage renal disease also leads to a metabolic bone disease. This is multifactorial in origin; features of osteomalacia and hyperparathyroidism are usually present.

Magnesium is an essential cofactor for many enzymes. Its concentration in the extracellular fluid is controlled primarily through regulation of its urinary excretion. Hypomagnesaemia can cause clinical features similar to those of hypocalcaemia and indeed can cause hypocalcaemia since the secretion of parathyroid hormone is magnesium-dependent. Deficiency of magnesium can occur with prolonged diarrhoea and malabsorption. Hypermagnesaemia is common in renal failure but it appears to be tolerated well by the body and increased concentrations rarely give rise to obvious clinical disturbances.

## FURTHER READING

Heath D & Marx S J (eds) (1982) *Calcium Disorders.* London: Butterworth.

Marcus R (ed.) (1989) Hypercalcaemia. *Endocrinology and Metabolism Clinics of North America*, **18**, 601–832.

Nordin B E C (ed.) (1984) *Metabolic Bone and Stone Disease*. 2nd edition. Edinburgh: Churchill Livingstone.

Ryan M F (1991) The role of magnesium in clinical biochemistry: an overview. *Annals of Clinical Biochemistry*, **28**, 19–26.

# 13. Plasma Proteins

## INTRODUCTION

Proteins are present in all body fluids, but it is the proteins of the blood plasma that are examined most frequently for diagnostic purposes. Over 100 individual proteins have a physiological function in the plasma (*Fig. 13.1*). Quantitatively, the single most important protein is albumin. The other proteins are known collectively as globulins. Changes in the concentrations of individual proteins occur in many conditions and their measurement can provide useful diagnostic information.

## MEASUREMENT OF PLASMA PROTEINS

### Total plasma protein

In very general terms, variations in plasma protein concentrations can be due to any of three changes: in the rate of protein synthesis; the rate of removal, and in the volume of distribution.

The concentration of proteins in plasma is affected by posture; an increase in concentration of 10–20% occurs within 30 minutes of becoming upright after a period of recumbency. Also, if a tourniquet is applied before venepuncture, a significant rise in protein concentration can occur within a few minutes. In both cases, the change in protein concentration is caused by increased diffusion of fluid from the vascular into the interstitial compartment. These effects must be borne in mind when blood is being drawn for the determination of protein concentration.

Only changes in the more abundant plasma proteins (i.e., albumin or immunoglobulins) will have a significant effect on the total protein concentration.

Except when patients have been given blood or proteins intravenously, a rapid increase in the total plasma protein is always due to a decrease in the volume of distribution (in effect, to dehydration). A rapid decrease in concentration is most usually due to an increase in plasma volume. Thus, changes in plasma protein concentration can provide a valuable aid to the assessment of a patient's state of hydration.

The total protein concentration of plasma can also fall rapidly if capillary permeability increases, since protein will diffuse out into the interstitial space. This can be seen, for example, in patients with septicaemia or generalized inflammatory conditions. Causes of increased and decreased total plasma protein concentration are summarized in *Fig. 13.2*.

| Functions of plasma proteins | |
|---|---|
| **Function** | **Example** |
| transport | thyroxine-binding globulin (thyroid hormones) apolipoproteins (cholesterol, triglyceride) transferrin (iron) |
| humoral immunity | immunoglobulins |
| maintenance of oncotic pressure | all proteins, particularly albumin |
| enzymes | renin clotting factors complement proteins |
| protease inhibitors | $\alpha_1$-antitrypsin (acts on proteases) |
| buffering | all proteins |

**Fig. 13.1** Functions of plasma proteins.

### Protein electrophoresis

This technique is widely used for the semi-quantitative assessment of serum proteins and is essential for the detection of paraproteins. Electrophoresis is usually performed on serum rather than plasma since the fibrinogen present in plasma produces a band in the $\beta_2$ region which might be mistaken for a paraprotein.

Electrophoresis, on cellulose acetate or agarose gel, separates the proteins into distinct bands: albumin, $\alpha_1$- and $\alpha_2$-globulins, $\beta$-globulins, and $\gamma$-globulins. The principal proteins comprising these groups are listed in *Fig. 13.3*. A band due to prealbumin may be visible depending on the technique used. When present in excess, C-reactive protein and $\alpha$-fetoprotein may occasionally be seen as discrete bands. Paraproteins characteristically migrate as discrete bands. The electrophoretic mobility of proteins, in particular albumin, may change when they bind drugs and other ligands, such as bilirubin, thereby producing additional bands.

Some of the more frequently seen electrophoretic patterns are shown in *Fig. 13.4*. However, whether or not

| Causes of changes in total plasma protein concentration | | | |
|---|---|---|---|
| **Increase** | | **Decrease** | |
| hypergammaglobulinaemia paraproteinaemia | ↑ protein synthesis | malnutrition and malabsorption liver disease humoral immunodeficiency | ↓ protein synthesis |
| artefactual | haemoconcentration due to stasis of blood during vene-puncture | over-hydration increased capillary permeability | ↑volume of distribution |
| dehydration | ↓ volume of distribution | protein-losing states catabolic states | ↑ excretion/ catabolism |

**Fig.13.2** Causes of changes in total plasma protein concentration.

| Principal plasma proteins | | |
|---|---|---|
| **Class** | **Protein** | **Approximate mean serum concentration (g/L)** |
| | prealbumin | 0.25 |
| | albumin | 40 |
| $\alpha_1$-globulin | $\alpha_1$-antitrypsin $\alpha_1$-acid glycoprotein | 2.9 1.0 |
| $\alpha_2$-globulin | haptoglobins $\alpha_2$-macroglobulin caeruloplasmin | 2.0 2.6 0.35 |
| $\beta$-globulin | transferrin low density lipoprotein complement components (C3) | 3.0 1.0 1.0 |
| $\gamma$-globulins | IgG IgA IgM IgD IgE | 14.0 3.5 1.5 0.03 trace |

**Fig. 13.3** Principal plasma proteins. Many other important proteins are present in only very low concentrations, for example, thyroxine-binding globulin, transcortin and vitamin-D binding globulin.

the demonstration of these patterns is of any value in the diagnosis and management of the underlying disorders is debatable, with the important exception of paraproteinaemia. For instance, pattern b in *Fig. 13.4* shows decreases in albumin and $\alpha_1$- and $\gamma$-globulins, and increases in $\alpha_2$-globulin and $\beta$-globulin (due to $\alpha_2$-macroglobulin and apolipoprotein B). While this pattern is characteristic of the nephrotic syndrome, it is only seen in very severe cases and may also be seen in other protein-losing states.

Pattern c in *Fig. 13.4* shows a decrease in the $\gamma$-globulin band which may be seen in defects of humoral immunity

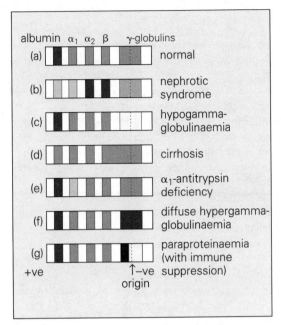

**Fig. 13.4** Some typical serum electrophoretic abnormalities.

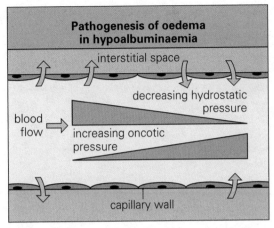

**Fig. 13.5** Pathogenesis of oedema in hypoalbuminaemia. The normal balance of hydrostatic and oncotic pressures is such that there is net movement of fluid out of the capillaries at their arteriolar ends and net movement in at their venular ends (indicated here by arrows). Oedema can thus be due to: an increase in capillary hydrostatic pressure; a decrease in plasma oncotic pressure, or an increase in capillary permeability.

involving IgG, the major component of the γ-globulins. However, because IgA and IgM are quantitatively minor components of the total γ-globulin, their concentrations can be low without the γ-globulin band appearing diminished.

In liver cirrhosis, a characteristic electrophoretic pattern may be seen (pattern d in *Fig. 13.4*), with lowered albumin, a diffuse increase in γ-globulins, and β–γ-fusion (a merging of the β and γ bands due to the increase in IgA that occurs in some forms of the condition). This pattern is often only present in advanced cases and is of little diagnostic value.

A deficiency of α$_1$-antitrypsin may be detectable by electrophoresis (pattern e in *Fig. 13.4*). This protein is the major component of the α$_1$-globulin band and in patients with α$_1$-antitrypsin deficiency who are homozygous for the Z gene this band may be very faint. It can appear normal in heterozygotes, and a technique such as isoelectric focusing, which specifically identifies the variant proteins, must be used for the determination of phenotypes when screening the relatives of patients, in genetic counselling and in antenatal diagnosis.

Pattern f in *Fig. 13.4* shows the electrophoretic appearance in diffuse hypergammaglobulinaemia. This condition is discussed later in the chapter, as is paraproteinaemia (pattern g in *Fig. 13.4*), for the detection of which serum protein electrophoresis is an essential technique.

The plasma proteins of clinical interest can all be measured using specific assays and, in general, such measurements will provide more precise diagnostic information. Preliminary electrophoresis is not helpful and may even be misleading. For example, IgA deficiency, the most frequently occurring congenital immunodeficiency disorder, is often not apparent on electrophoresis.

## SPECIFIC PLASMA PROTEINS

### Albumin

Albumin, the most abundant plasma protein, makes the major contribution (about 80%) to the oncotic pressure of plasma. Oncotic pressure is the osmotic pressure due to the presence of proteins and is an important determinant of the distribution of extracellular fluid (ECF) between the intravascular and extravascular compartments.

In hypoalbuminaemic states, the decreased plasma oncotic pressure disturbs the equilibrium between plasma and interstitial fluid with the result that there is a decrease in the movement of the interstitial fluid back into the blood at the venular end of the capillaries (*Fig. 13.5*). The accumulation of interstitial fluid is seen clinically as oedema. The relative decrease in plasma volume results in a fall in renal blood flow. This stimulates the secretion of renin, and hence of aldosterone through the formation of angiotensin (secondary aldosteronism, *see p. 132*). This results in sodium retention and thus an increase in ECF volume which potentiates the oedema.

There are many possible causes of hypoalbuminaemia (*Fig. 13.6*), a combination of which may be important in individual cases. For example, in a patient with malabsorption due to Crohn's disease, a low albumin may reflect both decreased synthesis (decreased supply of amino acids due to malabsorption) and increased loss (directly into the gut from ulcerated mucosa).

Hyperalbuminaemia may be either an artefact, for instance, as a result of venous stasis during blood collection, or due to over-infusion of albumin or to dehydration. Albumin synthesis is increased in some pathological states but never causes hyperalbuminaemia.

Plasma albumin measurements are often used to assess a patient's response to nutritional support. Albumin is useless for this purpose in the short term, though it may help with the assessment of fluid balance, since it has a half-life in the plasma of approximately 20 days. However, it is of use in the assessment of patients receiving long-term (several weeks or more) nutritional support.

The plasma albumin concentration is also used as a test of liver function. Because of its relatively long half-life in the plasma, albumin concentration is usually normal in acute hepatitis. Low concentrations are characteristic of chronic liver disease, being due to both decreased synthesis and an increase in the volume of distribution as a result of fluid retention and the formation of ascites.

Albumin is a high capacity, low affinity transport protein for many substances, such as thyroid hormones, calcium and fatty acids. The influence of a low plasma albumin on measurement of thyroid hormones and calcium is considered *on pp 139 and 184*, respectively. Albumin binds unconjugated bilirubin and hypoalbuminaemia increases the risk of kernicterus in infants with unconjugated hyperbilirubinaemia. Salicylates, which displace bilirubin from albumin, can have a similar effect.

Many drugs are bound to albumin in the blood stream and a decrease in albumin concentration can have important pharmacokinetic consequences, for example, increasing the concentration of free drug and thus the risk of toxicity.

A number of molecular variants of albumin exist. In bisalbuminaemia, the variant protein has a slightly different electrophoretic mobility from normal albumin and a pair of albumin bands are seen on electrophoresis; there are no clinical consequences. Analbuminaemia is a rare, inherited condition where the plasma albumin concentration is 250 mg/L or less. People with this condition tend to suffer episodic mild oedema but are otherwise well.

## $\alpha_1$-Antitrypsin

This $\alpha_1$-globulin is a naturally occurring inhibitor of proteases. Its significance is related to the clinical consequences of inherited disorders of $\alpha_1$-antitrypsin synthesis. These can cause emphysema, occurring at a younger age (third and fourth decades) than is usual for this condition, and neonatal hepatitis which can progress to cirrhosis.

Homozygotes for the normal protein are termed Pi (protease inhibitor) MM, and over thirty alleles of the gene have been described. $\alpha_1$-Antitrypsin deficiency is most frequently due to homozygosity for the Z allele (PiZZ), this genotype having a frequency of about 1 in 3000 in the United Kingdom. In affected individuals, the plasma $\alpha_1$-antitrypsin level is reduced to between 10 and 15% of normal. The defect is due to a single amino acid substitution which causes the protein to form aggregates which cannot be secreted from the liver and cause liver damage. The abnormal protein shows decreased glycation, but this is probably a consequence, not the cause, of its retention in hepatocytes.

---

### Causes of hypoalbuminaemia

**Decreased synthesis**
malnutrition
malabsorption
liver disease

**Increased volume of distribution**
over-hydration
increased capillary permeability:
   septicaemia
   hypoxaemia

**Increased excretion/degradation**
nephrotic syndrome
protein-losing enteropathies
burns
haemorrhage
catabolic states:
   severe sepsis
   fever
   trauma
   malignant disease

**Fig. 13.6** Causes of hypoalbuminaemia.

The development of emphysema is believed to be due to a lack of natural inhibition of the enzyme, elastase, which results in destructive changes in the lung. Not all PiZZ homozygotes will develop liver or lung disease. The risk of developing emphysema is greatly increased by smoking; cigarette smoke oxidizes a thiol group at the active site of $\alpha_1$-antitrypsin, decreasing the activity of what small amounts of the enzyme are present.

PiMZ heterozygotes have plasma $\alpha_1$-antitrypsin levels which are about 60% of normal; there is probably only a very slightly increased tendency for these individuals to develop lung disease, when compared with the normal PiMM homozygotes. Neither homozygotes for the other relatively common alleles, F and S (that is, PiFF and PiSS) nor heterozygotes (PiMF, PiMS), appear to be at increased risk of developing liver or lung disease, although PiSZ heterozygotes seem to show some susceptibility.

Accurate phenotyping is required for the screening of an affected individual's family members and for antenatal diagnosis. This involves the use of special techniques such as isoelectric focusing, to allow identification of individual proteins. Genotypic antenatal screening is now possible, using the polymerase chain reaction (PCR) to amplify fetal DNA obtained by chorionic villus sampling.

$\alpha_1$-Antitrypsin is an acute phase protein. Its concentration increases in acute inflammatory states and this may be sufficient to bring a genetically determined low level of the protein, for example, in a PiMZ heterozygote, into the normal range. However, even with an acute phase response, the $\alpha_1$-antitrypsin level in PiZZ homozygotes never rises above 50% of the lower limit of the normal range.

## Haptoglobin

Haptoglobin is an $\alpha_2$-globulin. Its function is to bind free haemoglobin released into the plasma during intravascular haemolysis. The haemoglobin–haptoglobin complexes formed are removed by the reticuloendothelial system and the concentration of haptoglobin falls correspondingly. Thus, a low plasma haptoglobin concentration can be indicative of intravascular haemolysis. However, low concentrations due to decreased synthesis are seen in chronic liver disease, metastatic disease and severe sepsis.

Haptoglobin is an acute phase protein and its concentration also increases in hypoalbuminaemic states such as the nephrotic syndrome. It demonstrates considerable genetic polymorphism; the molecule consists of pairs of two types of subunit, $\alpha$ and $\beta$, and whilst the $\beta$-chain is constant, there are three alleles for the $\alpha$-chain. However, as far as is known, these different proteins are functionally similar and their existence is not known to be of clinical significance.

## $\alpha_2$-Macroglobin

$\alpha_2$-Macroglobin is a high molecular weight protein (820,000 daltons) that constitutes approximately one-third of the $\alpha_2$-globulins. Its increased synthesis in hypoalbuminaemic states contributes to the increased $\alpha_2$-globulin band seen on electrophoresis (see pattern b in *Fig. 13.4*). Like $\alpha_1$-antitrypsin, $\alpha_2$-macroglobulin is an inhibitor of proteases, though it has a broader spectrum of activity.

## Caeruloplasmin

A deficiency of this copper-carrying $\alpha_2$-globulin is characteristic of Wilson's disease. Its concentration is increased in pregnancy and by oestrogen-containing oral contraceptives. It is also an acute phase protein.

## Transferrin

This $\beta$-globulin is the major iron-transporting protein in the plasma; normally about 30% saturated with iron, it is characteristically 100% saturated with iron in haemochromatosis. Its measurement may be useful in the assessment of a patient's response to nutritional support (*see Chapter 21*).

Transferrin and ferritin are discussed in more detail in *Chapter 17*. Ferritin is also an iron-carrying protein and measurement of its plasma concentration is the best single test now available for determining body iron stores.

## Other acute phase proteins

Characteristic changes in the concentrations of plasma proteins occur in clinical conditions where there is an acute inflammatory response, for example, trauma, burns, myocardial infarction and exacerbations of inflammatory bowel and joint disease. The proteins involved include inflammatory mediators and inhibitors, and scavengers of potentially dangerous substances. The changes typically cause an increase in $\alpha_1$- and $\alpha_2$-globulins as a result of increases of $\alpha_1$-antitrypsin, $\alpha_1$-acid glycoprotein and haptoglobin. At the same time, there is often a rapid fall in plasma albumin concentration, due primarily to redistribution as a result of increased vascular permeability. Falls in the concentrations of prealbumin and transferrin are also characteristic.

Similar changes may be seen in malignancy and in chronic inflammatory conditions, but more usually the $\alpha_1$-globulin remains normal, the $\alpha_2$-globulin is somewhat elevated and there is a diffuse increase in $\gamma$-globulins.

Although these changes, if gross, are readily apparent on electrophoresis of serum, this method is an insensitive means of monitoring the acute phase response. During this response, the concentration of C-reactive protein (a protein with $\alpha_2$ mobility, quantitatively a minor component of the plasma proteins) may increase by as much as thirty-fold.

Sufficiently sensitive methods of measuring C-reactive protein are available for it to be the test of choice in monitoring the acute phase response, of particular value in monitoring patients with inflammatory joint disease such as rheumatoid arthritis. Measurements of C-reactive protein are a more sensitive and specific means of detecting and monitoring the acute phase response than measurement of erythrocyte sedimentation rate (ESR) or plasma viscosity.

## Other plasma proteins

Measurements of other plasma proteins may provide useful information in particular circumstances. Measurement of coagulation factors (fibrinogen, factor VIII and others) is usually carried out in haematology laboratories and is essential in the investigation of some bleeding disorders. Measurement of the proteins of the complement system is of considerable value in the investigation of some diseases with an immunological basis. The apolipoproteins and tumour markers such as α-fetoprotein are considered in detail in *Chapters 14* and *19*, respectively. The importance of hormone-binding proteins, such as cortisol-binding globulin and sex hormone-binding globulin, is considered in *Chapters 8* and *10*, respectively. Plasma proteins used in the assessment of nutritional status are discussed in *Chapter 21*.

## IMMUNOGLOBULINS

The immunoglobulins are a group of plasma proteins that function as antibodies, recognizing and binding foreign antigens. This facilitates the destruction of these antigens by elements of the cellular immune system.

Since every immunoglobulin molecule is specific for one antigenic determinant, or epitope, there are vast numbers of different immunoglobulins. All share a similar basic structure (*Fig. 13.7*), consisting of two identical 'heavy' polypeptide chains and two identical 'light' chains, linked by disulphide bridges. There are five types of heavy chain (γ, α, μ, δ, ε) and two types of light chain (κ, λ), the immunoglobulin class being determined by the type of heavy chain that the molecule contains (*Fig. 13.8*).

The N-terminal amino acid sequence of both the heavy and light chains shows considerable variation between individual immunoglobulin molecules; these form the part of the immunoglobulin molecule responsible for recognition of the antigen (the antigen binding site). The amino acid sequence of the rest of the chain varies little within one immunoglobulin class; this constant part of the molecule is concerned with complement activation and interaction with the cellular elements of the immune system. The characteristics and functions of the immunoglobulins are summarized in *Fig. 13.8*.

On electrophoresis, the immunoglobulins behave mainly as γ-globulins but IgA and IgM may migrate with the β- or α₂-globulins. Because the normal plasma concentration of IgG is much higher than that of the other immunoglobulins, the γ-globulin band seen on electrophoresis of normal serum is largely due to IgG.

Increases and decreases of plasma immunoglobulin concentrations can be either physiological or pathological in origin.

## Hypogammaglobulinaemia

### Physiological causes

At birth IgA and IgM concentrations are low and rise steadily thereafter (*Fig. 13.9*), although IgA may not reach the normal adult concentration until the end of the first decade.

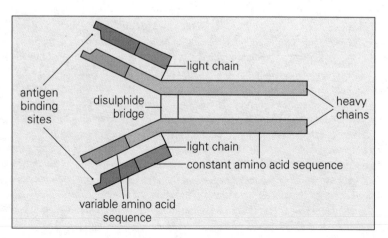

**Fig. 13.7** Structure of immunoglobulins. It is basically similar in all immunoglobulins. IgM consists of a pentamer of the basic structure and IgA is secreted as a dimer.

antigen binding sites

disulphide bridge

light chain

heavy chains

light chain

constant amino acid sequence

variable amino acid sequence

| Characteristics of the immunoglobulins | | | | |
|---|---|---|---|---|
| Class | Heavy chain | Mean plasma concentration (g/L) | Molecular weight (daltons) | Function |
| IgG | γ | 14.0 | 146,000 | the major antibody of secondary immune responses |
| IgA | α | 3.5 | 160,000 | secreted as a dimer (molecular weight 385,000 daltons) the major antibody in seromucous secretions, e.g., saliva, bronchial mucus |
| IgM | μ | 1.5 | 970,000 | a pentamer, confined to the vascular spaces the major antibody of the primary immune response |
| IgD | δ | 0.03 | 184,000 | present on the surface of B lymphocytes, involved in antigen recognition |
| IgE | ε | trace | 188,000 | present on surface of mast cells and basophils probable role in immunity to helminths and associated with immediate hypersensitivity reactions |

**Fig. 13.8** Characteristics of the immunoglobulins. Immunoglobulins of each class contain either κ- or λ-light chains. In IgA and IgG, slight variations in the structure of the constant regions of the heavy chains give rise to different subclasses.

IgG is transported across the placenta during the last trimester of pregnancy and levels are high at birth (except in premature infants). The IgG concentration then declines, as maternal IgG is cleared from the body, before rising again as it is slowly replaced by the infant's own IgG.

Physiological hypogammaglobulinaemia is one of the reasons for the susceptibility of infants (especially the premature) to infection.

***Pathological causes***

Various inherited disorders of immunoglobulin synthesis are known, ranging in severity from X-linked agammaglobulinaemia (Bruton's disease), in which there is a complete absence of immunoglobulins and affected children develop recurrent bacterial infections, to milder dysgammaglobulinaemias, in which there is a defect or partial defect of only one or two immunoglobulins. The commonest of these, IgA deficiency, has an incidence of about 1 in 400.

Hypogammaglobulinaemia may also be acquired. It commonly occurs in haematological malignancies, such as

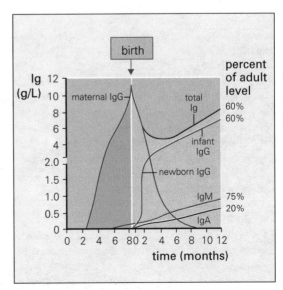

**Fig. 13.9** Changes in plasma immunoglobulin concentrations with age.

chronic lymphatic leukaemia, multiple myeloma and Hodgkin's disease. It can be a complication of the use of cytotoxic drugs and is a feature of severe protein-losing states, for example, the nephrotic syndrome. Increased catabolism also contributes to hypogammaglobulinaemia in protein-losing states.

Measurement of the specific class of immunoglobulin is essential for the diagnosis of hypogammaglobulinaemia. As previously discussed, electrophoresis is not sufficient for this purpose since the normal concentrations of the immunoglobulins, with the exception of IgG, are low and the effect of any decrease on the γ-globulin peak is too small to be detectable. IgG deficiency can be inferred if the γ-globulin band is faint, but possible coexistent deficiencies of other immunoglobulins will be missed.

## Hypergammaglobulinaemia

### Physiological causes

Increased levels of immunoglobulins are seen in both acute and chronic infections. Measurement of a particular immunoglobulin class, such as IgM, is of no value diagnostically. However, the detection and measurement of an immunoglobulin directed against a specific antigen provides an important aid to the diagnosis of many infectious diseases. Such investigations are usually performed in departments of medical microbiology.

### Pathological causes

Increases in plasma immunoglobulin concentrations are common in autoimmune diseases, for example, rheumatoid disease and systemic lupus erythematosus (SLE), and in chronic liver diseases, some of which have an autoimmune basis.

The quantification of immunoglobulin classes is rarely of diagnostic use in such conditions, although the measurement of specific auto-antibodies, such as the rheumatoid factor, an IgM directed against the body's own IgG, is of immense diagnostic value in many autoimmune diseases. Many different immunoglobulins are produced in these conditions and they give rise to a diffuse (polyclonal) increase in the γ-globulin band on electrophoresis (see Fig. 13.4, pattern f).

## Paraproteins

A paraprotein is an immunoglobulin produced by a single clone of cells of the B lymphocyte series, most frequently plasma cells. Since all the molecules are identical, the paraprotein is seen on electrophoresis of serum as a discrete band, usually in the γ-region (see Fig. 13.4, pattern g). The band may migrate elsewhere, particularly if the protein is

an IgA or IgM, or if complex formation with another plasma protein has occurred. More than one paraprotein band may occasionally be seen; this may be due to dimerization, as frequently occurs with IgA paraproteins, or to the presence of complexes or fragments of paraproteins in addition to the intact molecule.

If plasma is electrophoresed, the presence of a fibrinogen band may mimic or mask a paraprotein. Even with serum, a paraprotein may be missed on electrophoresis if, as occasionally happens, it coincides exactly with a normal band, for example, $\alpha_2$-globulin.

Paraproteins (usually IgG or IgA) occur most frequently in multiple myeloma (disseminated malignant proliferation of plasma cells) and solitary plasmacytoma, and in Waldenström's macroglobulinaemia (IgM). Paraprotein secretion (usually IgM) occurs less frequently, and to a lesser extent, in chronic lymphatic leukaemia and B cell lymphomas.

While serum protein electrophoresis is essential for the detection of paraproteins, the urine must also be examined. In approximately 20% of cases of myeloma, the tumour produces light chains only. Since these are of low molecular weight they are cleared rapidly from the blood stream and may be undetectable in serum. They are, however, detectable in urine; immunoglobulin light chains found in the urine are known as Bence Jones protein and this is present in some 50% of all cases of myeloma.

Paraproteins can also be benign, that is, not associated with malignant disease. The incidence of benign paraproteinaemias increases with age and has been reported to be as high as 3% in people over the age of 70.

Although benign paraproteins occur frequently, especially in the elderly, this diagnosis should not be made without vigorous investigation to exclude malignancy (Fig. 13.10). The most definitive diagnostic criterion is a failure of the paraprotein concentration to increase with time and this necessitates regular follow-up of the patient. There are no absolute criteria; the diagnosis of a benign paraprotein is essentially one of exclusion.

### CASE HISTORY 13.1

A 70-year-old man presented with back pain and loss of weight. Although a non-smoker, he had had several recent chest infections and was increasingly short of breath on exercise. On examination, he was anaemic but there were no other obvious abnormalities.

**Investigations**

serum: sodium          130 mmol/L
       urea             15.3 mmol/L
       creatinine       212 μmol/L
       calcium         2.75 mmol/L
       total protein      85 g/L
       albumin         30 g/L
       urate            0.51 mmol/L
       ESR (in first hour)    >100 mm
       haemoglobin      8.5 g/dL

A blood film showed normochromic, normocytic anaemia; rouleaux were present on the blood film and there was increased background staining.

Serum protein electrophoresis revealed a paraprotein in the γ-globulin region (*Fig. 13.4*, pattern g); this was typed by immunofixation and shown to be IgG-κ. There was a decrease in the normal γ-globulin band. Bence Jones protein was present in the urine and identified as κ in type.

Radiological examination showed the typical punched-out lytic lesions of myeloma in the lumbar vertebrae, ribs and pelvis.

**Comment**

This is a typical presentation of multiple myeloma. The paraprotein is an IgG in 55% of cases (*Fig. 13.11*). Replacement of normal bone marrow by malignant plasma cells frequently results in anaemia and in decreased synthesis of normal immunoglobulins.

The diagnosis rests on the demonstration of any two of the following: the presence of a paraprotein; typical radiological appearances; and the presence of increased numbers of abnormal plasma cells in the bone marrow. However, it is normal practice to confirm the diagnosis by examination of a bone marrow smear, even if the diagnosis is already obvious. Occasionally, if the marrow involvement is not widespread, an aspirate may not contain any abnormal cells.

---

**Diagnostic criteria for benign paraproteinaemia**

- no clinical features of myeloma or associated disorder
- no suppression of normal immunoglobulins
- no lytic lesions in bone on radiography
- normal bone marrow
- paraprotein concentration <10 g/L
- no Bence Jones proteinuria
- no increase in paraprotein concentration with age
- no positive evidence of malignancy on follow-up (at least three years)

**Fig. 13.10** Diagnostic criteria for benign paraproteinaemia

| Paraproteins in myeloma | |
|---|---|
| **Protein** | **Incidence (%)** |
| IgG | 55 |
| IgA | 22 |
| IgD | 1.5 |
| Bence Jones | 75 |
| Bence Jones only | 20 |

**Fig. 13.11** Paraproteins in myeloma. IgE and IgM myelomas occur, but are very rare. In about 1% of all cases, no paraprotein can be detected.

---

The presence of paraprotein causes red cells to adhere to each other (rouleaux formation) and may be sufficient to cause an increase in the background staining of the blood film. Hyponatraemia often occurs in sick people and in hyperproteinaemic states it may be 'spurious' in origin (*see p. 20*).

Renal failure is the cause of death in approximately one-third of patients with myeloma. It is often multifactorial in origin; contributory factors include obstruction of nephrons by protein, hypercalcaemia, pyelonephritis and amyloid. Hypercalcaemia is common in myeloma; its cause is discussed elsewhere (*see pp 189 and 271*).

| Laboratory findings in multiple myeloma |
|---|
| **Biochemical** |
| serum:  paraprotein |
| ↓ normal immunoglobulins |
| ↑ urea |
| ↑ creatinine |
| ↑ $\beta_2$-microglobulin |
| ↑ calcium |
| ↑ urate |
| normal alkaline phosphatase |
| urine:  Bence Jones protein |
| |
| **Haematological** |
| ↑ erythrocyte sedimentation rate (ESR) |
| anaemia (usually normochromic, normocytic) |
| rouleaux formation |

**Fig. 13.12** Laboratory findings in multiple myeloma.

Despite the extensive lytic lesions of bone, there is no increase in osteoblastic activity and the plasma alkaline phosphatase is usually normal. The laboratory findings in myeloma are summarized in *Fig. 13.12*. It should be appreciated that metabolic abnormalities may not be present when the condition is first diagnosed; they may develop subsequently and so patients should be periodically monitored for these complications. Serum $\beta_2$-microglobulin concentration is a good prognostic indicator in myeloma, presumably because it reflects both the activity of the tumour and renal function; a high level (>6 µg/mL) implies a poor prognosis; other features correlated with a poor prognosis include anaemia, renal impairment, hypercalcaemia, hypoalbuminaemia and tumour bulk as indicated by the amount of paraprotein (e.g., IgG >70 g/L, IgA > 50 g/L, Bence Jones protein >12 g/24 h). Quantitation of the paraprotein is also used as a tumour marker (*see p. 277*).

Myeloma is treated using cytotoxic drugs but the prognosis is generally poor. Local radiotherapy may be useful for isolated lesions (plasmacytomas) and for localized bone pain.

Waldenström's macroglobulinaemia is also a B cell tumour. The paraprotein is an IgM, and a hyperviscosity syndrome, causing sludging of red cells in capillaries and predisposing to thrombus formation, is a prominent feature. It is much less common than myeloma.

Rarer still is Franklin's (heavy chain) disease, in which the paraprotein produced is immunoglobulin heavy chain only. This is usually an α-chain, but may also be a γ- or µ-chain. Patients with α-chain disease present with malabsorption due to infiltration of the gut by malignant cells.

Some paraproteins precipitate out of solution when cooled to 4°C And redissolve on warming. These proteins are known as cryoglobulins and are associated with Raynaud's phenomenon, although the majority of patients with this condition do not have cryoglobulinaemia. The latter may also occur in other conditions where there are abnormalities of immunoglobulin production, for instance, systemic lupus erythematosus.

## Cytokines

Cytokines are low molecular weight (<80 kDa) peptides secreted by cells involved in inflammation and immunity, which control the activity and growth of these cells. Most of their functions are local, either on nearby cells (paracrine) or on the cell that secretes the peptide (autocrine), but some have remote (endocrine) effects. They show some functional overlap with peptide growth factors which influence the growth of non-immune cells. The two groups of factors are collectively known as peptide regulatory factors.

Four classes of cytokines are recognized.
- Interleukins (IL), which are regulators of inflammation;
- Interferons (IF), naturally occurring anti-viral agents which in general have an inhibitory effect on cell growth.
- Colony-stimulating factors (CF), which stimulate the growth of macrophages and white blood cells.
- Tumour necrosis factors (TNF), which stimulate the proliferation of many cells, including cytolytic T-cells.

Many cytokines have multiple properties and some cytokine-mediated responses can be brought about by more than one cytokine. Cytokines interact with each other with the result that the effect of an individual cytokine depends upon which other cytokines are present. They are also capable of inducing and inhibiting each other's secretion.

Cytokines are without doubt of extreme importance in the coordination of the immune response and the control of myelopoiesis. Some cytokines are secreted by tumours and can contribute to the effects of those tumours. They can be measured in serum by sensitive and specific assays, although as yet there are no clear clinical indications for doing so. Possible applications for cytokine measurements include the early diagnosis of sepsis and graft reaction, for which TNF and IL-6 show promise.

Growth factors (GF) include epidermal GF, platelet-derived GF, transforming GF and the insulin-like GFs. Secretion of the latter by mesenchymal tumours is a cause of tumour-associated hypoglycaemia.

## PROTEINS IN OTHER BODY FLUIDS

### Cerebrospinal fluid

Cerebrospinal fluid (CSF) is usually obtained for diagnostic purposes by lumbar puncture. The protein concentration is normally 0.1–0.4 g/L and the protein is predominantly albumin; higher concentrations are found in neonates (up to 0.9 g/L) and the elderly. It is important that the CSF is not contaminated with blood since the presence of plasma proteins will completely invalidate the results of CSF protein measurement.

Examination of the CSF is most often performed in cases of suspected meningitis. The diagnosis of this condition is primarily the concern of the medical microbiologist, but it is usual also to request biochemical analysis for glucose and protein. The significance of the CSF glucose concentration is considered in *Chapter 11* . In meningitis, there is secretion of IgG into the CSF but this has little effect on the total amount of protein. However, meningeal inflammation may lead to an increase in capillary permeability and, therefore, a marked increase in CSF protein content. It is important to note that, in suspected meningitis, a normal CSF protein does not exclude the diagnosis.

CSF protein concentration is increased in patients with tumours of the central nervous system and may exceed 5 g/L in patients with tumours which obstruct the normal circulation of the CSF (spinal block or Froin's syndrome).

Examination of the CSF can be of great value in the diagnosis of multiple sclerosis. Although the total protein concentration is usually only slightly raised, there is increased local synthesis of IgG and the ratio of IgG to albumin is increased from less than 10% to as much as 50%. Greater sensitivity is provided if the IgG/albumin ratio of the CSF is compared with that of plasma. The ratio is abnormal in approximately 80% of cases of multiple sclerosis but may also be abnormal in neurosyphilis, with tumours of the central nervous system and after cerebrovascular accidents.

An even more sensitive test is provided by electrophoresis of CSF on polyacrylamide gel. In multiple sclerosis, only a small number of clones of B cells produce IgG, which is seen as discrete 'oligoclonal' bands when CSF is electrophoresed. The methodology is technically demanding and considerable experience is necessary for interpretation of the results. Oligoclonal bands can be detected in over 95% of cases of multiple sclerosis, although they may also be seen in other, less common, demyelinating diseases, such as subacute sclerosing panencephalitis, and in neurosyphilis.

### Transudates and exudates

The protein concentration of pleural fluid or abdominal ascites is occasionally measured to determine whether the sample is a transudate (fluid with a low protein content derived by filtration across capillary endothelium) or an exudate (fluid with a high protein content actively secreted in response to inflammation). A value of 30 g/L is often taken as the dividing line between the two types of fluid, but this is not a reliable criterion as the protein content of both is very variable.

The important diagnostic differentiation is whether the ascites or pleural fluid is infected or if it is related to the presence of a tumour. This can only be determined by microbiological and cytological examination, so protein measurement is of little value.

### Urine

The investigation and significance of proteinuria is discussed in *Chapter 4*.

## SUMMARY

The most abundant protein in plasma is albumin, which is synthesized in the liver. Through its contribution to the colloid osmotic pressure, albumin has an important role in determining the distribution of the extracellular fluid between the vascular and extravascular spaces. It is also an important transport protein for several hormones, drugs, free fatty acids, unconjugated bilirubin and various ions. Its concentration is, however, affected by so many pathological processes (decreases occur in chronic liver disease, protein-losing states, malabsorption, following trauma and when capillary permeability is increased) that measurements must be interpreted with caution.

Most of the other plasma proteins are classified as globulins. The immunoglobulins are synthesized by plasma cells and constitute the humoral arm of the immune system. Five main classes are known of which the most abundant are IgG, IgM and IgA. IgM is the main antibody of the primary immune response and is largely confined to the vascular compartment; IgG is involved in the secondary response and is distributed throughout the extracellular fluid; IgA is secreted onto mucosal surfaces. An increase in total immunoglobulins is characteristic of chronic inflammatory conditions, for example, chronic infection and autoimmune disease. The measurement of specific immunoglobulins is of value in the investigation of immunodeficiency syndromes and certain autoimmune diseases.

Myelomas are malignant tumours of plasma cells which produce large amounts of identical, monoclonal, immunoglobulin molecules or fragments thereof, known as paraproteins. Serum and urine protein electrophoresis is essential for the detection of paraproteins but other abnormalities of plasma proteins are better investigated by specific measurement of the protein, or proteins, in question. Metabolic features of myeloma include renal impairment, hypercalcaemia and hyperuricaemia. Patients are frequently anaemic and may have an immune paresis. Causes of death include infection and renal disease.

Other plasma proteins include the coagulation factors, complement components and various transport proteins, for example, thyroxine-binding globulin, transcortin, sex hormone-binding globulin, transferrin and caeruloplasmin. Increases in the concentration of certain proteins occur in association with acute inflammatory reactions. These 'acute phase proteins' include $\alpha_1$-antitrypsin, C-reactive protein and haptoglobins. Measurement of C-reactive protein is valuable in following the course of conditions characterized by episodes of acute inflammation, such as rheumatoid arthritis and Crohn's disease. $\alpha_1$-Antitrypsin is a protease inhibitor; inherited deficiency of the protein can cause neonatal hepatitis, which may progress to cirrhosis, and emphysema in adults, particularly those who smoke. The condition can now be diagnosed antenatally, by examination of fetal blood or tissue.

The cytokines are a large group of autocrine and paracrine regulatory peptides, which modulate the activity of the immune system and are involved in the coordination of acute inflammation and the immune response. They can be measured in serum but there are as yet no clear-cut indications for doing so in diagnosis and management.

The investigation of proteins in cerebrospinal fluid is a valuable technique in the diagnosis of multiple sclerosis; the presence of oligoclonal immunoglobulin bands is characteristic of, although not specific to, this condition. Total cerebrospinal fluid protein is frequently measured in patients with suspected meningitis but is of limited diagnostic value.

## FURTHER READING

Galvani D W (1988) Cytokines: biological function and clinical use. *Journal of the Royal College of Physicians of London*, **22**, 226–231.

Thompson D, Milford-Ward A, Whicher J T (1992) The value of acute phase protein measurements in clinical practice. *Annals of Clinical Biochemistry*, **29**, 123–131.

Whicher J T (1983) Abnormalities of plasma proteins. In *Biochemistry in Clinical Practice*. D L Williams and V Marks (eds), pp 221–251. London: Heinemann.

# 14. Lipids and Lipoproteins

## INTRODUCTION

The major lipids present in the plasma are fatty acids, triglycerides, cholesterol and phospholipids. Other lipid-soluble substances, present in much smaller amounts but of considerable physiological importance, include steroid hormones and fat-soluble vitamins; these are discussed in *Chapters 9* and *21* respectively.

## TRIGLYCERIDES, CHOLESTEROL AND PHOSPHOLIPIDS

Triglycerides (strictly, triacylglycerols) consist of glycerol esterified with three long-chain fatty acids, such as stearic (18 carbon atoms) or palmitic (16 carbon atoms) acids. Triglyceride is present in dietary fat, and can be synthesized in the liver and adipose tissue to provide a source of stored energy, which can be mobilized when required, for example, during starvation. Although the majority of fatty acids in the body are saturated, certain unsaturated fatty acids are important as precursors of prostaglandins and in the esterification of cholesterol. Triglycerides containing both saturated and unsaturated fatty acids are important components of cell membranes.

Cholesterol is also important in membrane structure and is the precursor of steroid hormones and bile acids. Cholesterol is present in dietary fat, and can be synthesized in many tissues, including the liver, by a mechanism that is under close metabolic regulation. Cholesterol can be excreted in the bile either *per se*, or after metabolism to bile acids.

Phospholipids are compounds similar to the triglycerides but with one fatty acid residue replaced by phosphate and a nitrogenous base.

Because they are not water-soluble, lipids are transported in the plasma in association with proteins. Albumin is the principal carrier of free fatty acids (FFA) while the other lipids circulate in complexes known as lipoproteins. These consist of a non-polar core of triglyceride and cholesteryl esters surrounded by a surface layer of phospholipids, cholesterol and proteins known as apolipoproteins (*Fig. 14.1*). The latter are important both structurally and in the metabolism of lipoproteins (*Fig. 14.2*).

## CLASSIFICATION OF LIPOPROTEINS

Lipoproteins are classified on the basis of their densities as demonstrated by their ultracentrifugal separation. Density increases from chylomicrons (CM, of lowest density) through lipoproteins of very low density (VLDL), intermediate density (IDL), low density (LDL), to high density lipoproteins (HDL). HDL can be separated, on the basis of

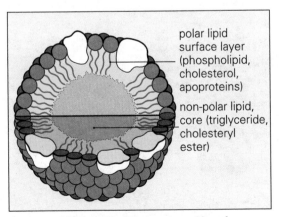

**Fig. 14.1** Diagram showing the composition of a lipoprotein particle. A segment has been removed to reveal the non-polar core of cholesteryl ester and triglyceride surrounded by phospholipids and apoprotein.

polar lipid surface layer (phospholipid, cholesterol, apoproteins)

non-polar lipid, core (triglyceride, cholesteryl ester)

| Apolipoprotein | Function |
|---|---|
| A-I | cofactor for LCAT structural (in HDL) |
| A-II | activator of hepatic lipase structural (in HDL) |
| B-100 | structural (in LDL and VLDL) receptor binding |
| B-48 | structural (in chylomicrons) |
| C-I | cofactor for LCAT? |
| C-II | activator of LPL |
| C-III | inhibitor of LPL? |
| E | receptor binding |

**Fig. 14.2** Functions of the major apolipoproteins.

density, into two metabolically distinct subtypes, HDL2 (density 1.064–1.125) and HDL3 (density 1.126–1.210). Distinct sub-types of LDL are also recognized. IDL are normally present in the blood stream in only small amounts but can accumulate in pathological disturbances of lipoprotein metabolism. This classification is illustrated in *Fig. 14.3* and the approximate lipid and apolipoprotein content in *Fig. 14.4*. However, it is important to appreciate that the composition of the circulating lipoproteins is not static. They are in a dynamic state with continuous exchange of components between the various types. The principal functions

of these lipoproteins are summarized in *Fig. 14.3* and discussed in greater detail in the next section.

Lipoprotein(a), or Lp(a), is an atypical lipoprotein of unknown function. It is larger and more dense than LDL but has a similar composition, except that it contains in addition one molecule of apo(a) for every molecule of apo B-100. Apo(a) shows considerable homology with plasminogen. The concentration of Lp(a) in the plasma varies considerably between individuals, in the range 0–100 mg/dL, and is genetically determined. An elevated concentration of Lp(a) appears to be an independent risk factor for coronary

| Classification and characteristics of lipoproteins | | | | | |
|---|---|---|---|---|---|
| lipoprotein | density (g/mL) | mean diameter (nm) | electrophoretic mobility | source | principal function |
| CM | <0.95 | 500 | remains at origin | intestine | transport of exogenous triglyceride |
| VLDL | 0.96–1.006 | 43 | pre-β | liver | transport of endogenous triglyceride |
| IDL | 1.007–1.019 | 27 | 'broad β' | catabolism of VLDL | precursor of LDL |
| LDL | 1.02–1.063 | 22 | β | catabolism of VLDL, via IDL | cholesterol transport |
| HDL | 1.064–1.21 | 8 | α | liver, intestine; catabolism of CM & VLDL | reverse cholesterol transport |

**Fig. 14.3** Classification and characteristics of lipoproteins.

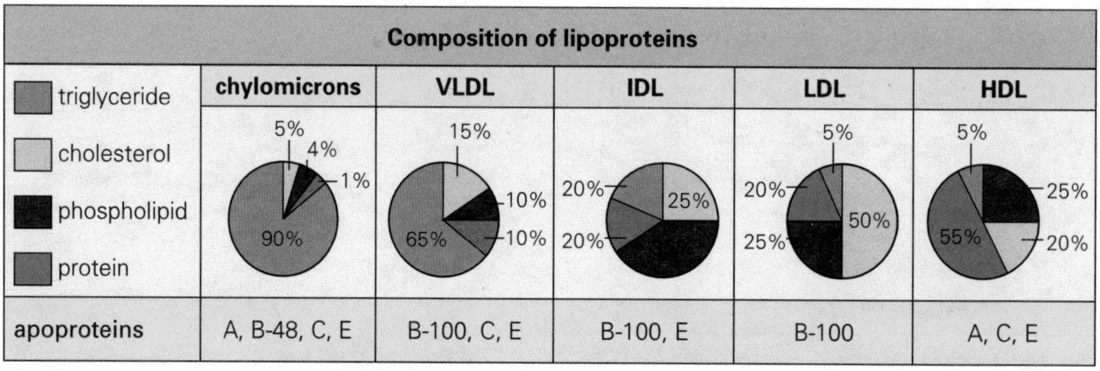

**Fig. 14.4** Composition of lipoproteins; although the composition in each class is similar, the particles are heterogeneous so the percentages given are approximate. Figures shown for HDL are for HDL3; HDL2 contains less protein and more lipid. Only the principal apoproteins are shown.

heart disease. Conventional drug treatments that lower LDL have little effect on Lp(a) concentration.

## LIPOPROTEIN METABOLISM

### Chylomicrons (CM)

Chylomicrons (*Fig. 14.5*) are formed from dietary fat (principally triglyceride, but also cholesterol) in enterocytes; they enter the lymphatics and reach the systemic circulation via the thoracic duct. Chylomicrons are the major transport form of exogenous (dietary) fat. Triglyceride constitutes about 90% of the lipid. Triglyceride is removed from chylomicrons by the action of the enzyme lipoprotein lipase (LPL), located on the luminal surface of the capillary endothelium of adipose tissue, skeletal and cardiac muscle

and lactating breast, with the result that free fatty acids are delivered to these tissues either to be used as energy substrates or, after re-esterification to triglyceride, for energy storage. LPL is activated by apo C-II.

Apo A and apo B-48 are synthesized in the gut and are present in newly formed chylomicrons; apo C-II and apo E are transferred to chylomicrons from HDL. As triglyceride is removed from chylomicrons, they become smaller; cholesterol, phospholipids, apo A and apo C-II are released from the surface of the particles and taken up by HDL. Esterified cholesterol is transferred to the chylomicron remnants from HDL, in exchange for triglyceride, by cholesteryl ester transfer protein. The core chylomicron remnants, depleted of triglyceride and enriched in cholesteryl ester, are cleared from the circulation by hepatic parenchymal

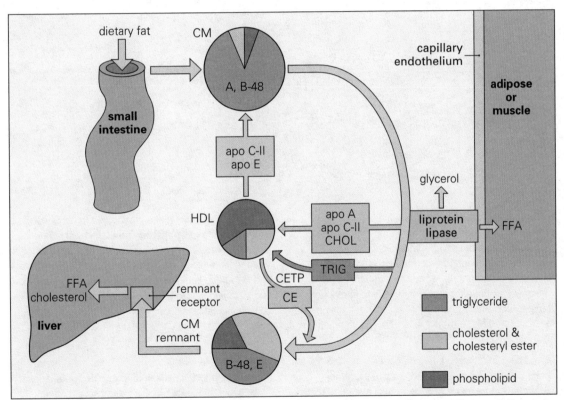

**Fig. 14.5** Chylomicrons transport dietary triglyceride to tissue where it is removed by the action of lipoprotein lipase. The resulting remnant particles are removed by the liver. They bind to remnant receptors (which recognize apo E) on hepatic cells, are internalized and catabolized. Apolipoproteins A and B-48 are synthesized in intestinal cells; apo C and apo E are acquired, together with cholesteryl esters (CE), from HDL. Apolipoprotein C-II activates lipoprotein lipase. As triglyceride is removed from chylomicrons, apo A, apo C, cholesterol and phospholipids are released from their surfaces and transferred to HDL where the cholesterol is esterified. Cholesteryl ester is transferred back to the remnant particles in exchange for triglyceride by cholesteryl ester transport protein (CETP).

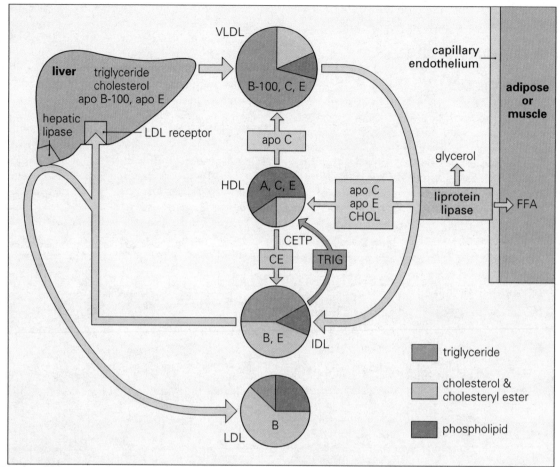

**Fig. 14.6** VLDL are synthesized in the liver and transport endogenous triglyceride from the liver to other tissues where it is removed by the action of lipoprotein lipase. At the same time, cholesterol, phospholipids and apo C and apo E are released and transferred to HDL. By this process VLDL are converted to IDL. Cholesterol is esterified in HDL and cholesteryl ester is transferred to IDL by cholesteryl ester transfer protein. Some IDL is removed by the liver but most has more triglyceride removed by hepatic triglyceride lipase and is thereby converted into LDL. Thus the triglyceride-rich VLDL are precursors of LDL, which comprise mainly cholesteryl ester and apo B-100.

cells. This hepatic uptake depends on the recognition of apo E in the remnants by hepatic remnant receptors.

Although their major function is the transport of dietary triglyceride, chylomicrons also transport dietary cholesterol and fat-soluble vitamins to the liver. Under normal circumstances, chylomicrons cannot be detected in plasma in the fasting state (>12 h after a meal).

## Very low density lipoproteins (VLDL)

Very low density lipoproteins (*Fig. 14.6*) are formed from triglyceride synthesized in the liver either *de novo* or by re-esterification of free fatty acids. VLDL also contain some cholesterol, apo B, apo C and apo E; the apo E and some of the apo C is transferred from circulating HDL.

VLDL are the principal transport form of endogenous triglyceride and initially share a similar fate to chylomicrons, triglyceride being stripped off by the action of LPL. As the VLDL particles become smaller, phospholipids, free cholesterol and apolipoproteins are released from their surfaces and taken up by HDL, thus converting the VLDL to denser particles, IDL. Cholesterol that has been transferred to HDL is esterified and the cholesteryl ester is transferred back to

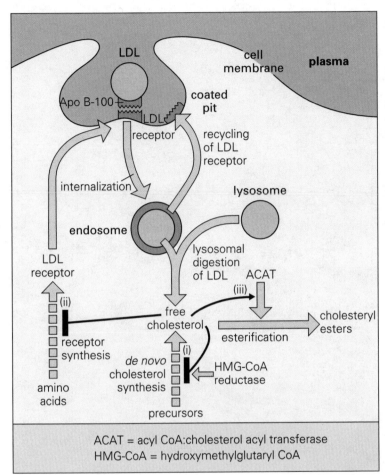

**Fig. 14.7** LDL metabolism. LDL are derived from VLDL, via IDL. They are removed by the liver and other tissues by a receptor-dependent process involving the recognition of apo B-100 by the LDL receptor. The LDL particles are hydrolyzed by lysosomal enzymes, releasing free cholesterol which (i) inhibits HMG-CoA reductase, the rate-limiting step in cholesterol synthesis, (ii) inhibits LDL receptor synthesis and (iii) stimulates cholesterol esterification by augmenting the activity of the enzyme, acyl-CoA: cholesterol acyl transferase (ACAT).

IDL by cholesteryl ester transfer protein in exchange for triglyceride. Further triglyceride is removed by hepatic triglyceride lipase located on hepatic endothelial cells, and IDL are thereby converted to LDL, composed mainly of cholesteryl esters, apo B-100 and phospholipid. Some IDL are taken up by the liver via LDL receptors. These receptors, also known as apo B, apo E recepors, are capable of binding apo B and apo E. Under normal circumstances, there are very few IDL in the circulation, because of their rapid removal or conversion to LDL.

## Low density lipoproteins (LDL)

LDL are the principal carriers of cholesterol, mainly in the form of cholesteryl ester. They are formed from VLDL via IDL (*Fig. 14.7*). LDL can pass through the junctions between capillary endothelial cells and attach to LDL receptors on cell membranes that recognize apo B-100. This is followed by internalization and lysosomal degradation with release

of free cholesterol. Cholesterol can also be synthesized in these tissues but the rate-limiting enzyme, HMG-CoA reductase (hydroxymethylglutaryl-CoA reductase), is inhibited by cholesterol with the result that, in the average adult, cholesterol synthesis in peripheral cells probably does not occur. Free cholesterol also stimulates its own esterification to cholesteryl ester by stimulating the enzyme acyl-CoA:cholesterol acyl transferase (ACAT).

LDL receptors are saturable and subject to down regulation by an increase in intracellular cholesterol. Macrophages derived from circulating monocytes can take up LDL via scavenger receptors. This process occurs at normal LDL concentrations but is enhanced when LDL concentrations are increased and by modification, e.g., oxidation, of LDL. Uptake of LDL by macrophages in the arterial wall is an important event in the pathogenesis of atherosclerosis. When macrophages become overloaded with cholesteryl esters, they are converted to 'foam cells',

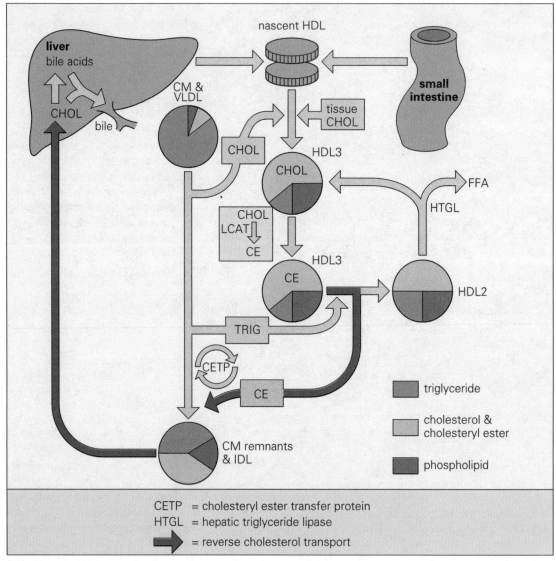

**Fig. 14.8** HDL metabolism and reverse cholesterol transport. Nascent HDL acquires free cholesterol from extra-hepatic cells, chylomicrons and VLDL and is thereby converted to HDL3. The cholesterol is esterified by the enzyme LCAT and cholesteryl ester is transferred to remnant lipoproteins by CETP in exchange for triglyceride. Remnant particles are removed from the circulation by the liver whence the cholesterol is excreted in bile both *per se* and as bile acids. Much HDL is recycled although some is probably taken up by the liver and catabolized. Apoprotein transfers have been omitted for clarity.

the classic components of atheromatous plaques. In human neonates, plasma LDL concentrations are much lower than in adults and cellular cholesterol uptake is probably all receptor-mediated and controlled.

LDL concentrations increase during childhood and reach adult levels after puberty.

## High density lipoproteins (HDL)

High density lipoprotein (*Fig. 14.8*) is synthesized primarily in the liver and, to a lesser extent, in small intestinal cells as a precursor ('nascent HDL') comprising phospholipid, cholesterol, apo E and apo A. Nascent HDL is disc-shaped; in the circulation, it acquires apo C and apo A from other lipoproteins and from extra-hepatic tissues, and in doing so assumes a spherical conformation. The free cholesterol is esterified by the enzyme lecithin-cholesterol acyltransferase (LCAT), which is present in nascent HDL and activated by its cofactor, apo A-I. This increases the density of the HDL particles which are thus converted from HDL3 to HDL2.

Cholesteryl ester is transferred from HDL2 to remnant particles in exchange for triglyceride, this process being mediated by cholesteryl ester transfer protein. Cholesteryl ester is taken up by the liver in chylomicron remnants and IDL and excreted in bile, partly after metabolism to bile acids.

The triglyceride-enriched HDL2 is converted back to HDL3 by the removal of triglyceride by the enzyme hepatic triglyceride lipase, located on the hepatic capillary endothelium. Some HDL2 is probably removed from the circulation by the liver, through receptors which recognize apo A-I.

Thus HDL has two important functions: it is a source of apoproteins for chylomicrons and VLDL, and it mediates reverse cholesterol transport, taking up cholesterol from senescent cells and other lipoproteins and transferring it to remnant particles which are taken up by the liver. Cholesterol is excreted by the liver in bile, both as cholesterol and after metabolism to bile acids.

The essential features of lipoprotein metabolism are as follows:

- Dietary triglyceride is transported in chylomicrons to tissues where it may be used as an energy source or stored.
- Endogenous triglyceride, synthesized in the liver, is transported in VLDL and is also available to tissues as an energy source or for storage.
- Cholesterol synthesized in the liver is transported to tissues in LDL, derived from VLDL; dietary cholesterol reaches the liver in chylomicron remnants.
- HDL acquire cholesterol from peripheral cells and other lipoproteins and this is esterified by LCAT. Cholesteryl ester is transferred to remnant particles which are taken up by the liver, whence the cholesterol is excreted.

## REFERENCE RANGES AND LABORATORY INVESTIGATIONS

At birth, the plasma cholesterol concentration is very low (total cholesterol less than 2.6 mmol/L, LDL cholesterol less than 1.0 mmol/L). There is a rapid increase in concentration in the first year of life, but in childhood that total does not usually exceed 4.1 mmol/L. In affluent societies particularly, concentrations rise further in early adulthood. The

reference range, as conventionally defined, for plasma cholesterol varies for different populations, but in the United Kingdom the upper limit, based on measurements on apparently healthy adults, is 6.5 mmol/L. However, it is inappropriate to quote a reference range for plasma cholesterol concentration. Epidemiological studies indicate that the risk of coronary heart disease (CHD) increases significantly with cholesterol levels of more than 5.2 mmol/L, with the result that 'normal' levels are in fact associated with a significant risk. It is thus preferable to consider a measured cholesterol concentration in relation to what is desirable, or ideal, in an individual, rather than to relate it to any reference range.

While there is an undoubted association between high plasma cholesterol concentrations (and in particular, LDL cholesterol) and an increased risk of CHD, there is an inverse correlation between HDL cholesterol and CHD risk. Many physiological factors influence LDL and HDL cholesterol levels, of which some are indicated in *Fig. 14.9.*

It cannot be overemphasized, however, that hypercholesterolaemia is only one of several risk factors for CHD. Others include hypertension, smoking, male sex, a family history of CHD, and diabetes mellitus. In assessing the risk of CHD due to hypercholesterolaemia as a guide to management, all other risk factors must be taken into account.

Hypertriglyceridaemia is also a risk factor for CHD (probably more so in women than in men), albeit a less important one. Hypertriglyceridaemia due to small, dense, triglyceride-rich LDL-particles, which are particularly associated with non insulin-dependent diabetes (NIDDM), is of particular significance, since these particles appear to be more atherogenic than other LDL sub-types. Plasma triglyceride concentrations >10 mmol/L carry a risk of pancreatitis.

Total triglyceride and cholesterol concentrations can easily be measured in the laboratory; HDL cholesterol can be determined after first using a simple precipitation technique to separate HDL from LDL. LDL cholesterol can be calculated using the formula:

$$\text{LDL CHOL} = \text{TOTAL CHOL} - \left( \text{HDL CHOL} + \frac{\text{TRIG}}{2.2} \right)$$

where all quantities are expressed in mmol/L. This formula should not be used if the triglyceride concentration exceeds 4.5 mmol/L.

*Fig. 14.10* indicates the generally accepted ideal plasma concentrations of cholesterol that may be used as a basis for assessing both the need for, and efficacy of, treatment. In practice, what is ideal should be determined on

| Influences on plasma lipoproteins | | | |
|---|---|---|---|
| Variable | HDL cholesterol | LDL cholesterol | Triglyceride |
| sex | F > M | M = F | F < M |
| age | slight ↑ in F | ↑ | ↑ |
| high P:S ratio | – or ↓ | ↓ | – or ↓ |
| exercise | ↑ | ↓ | ↓ |
| obesity | ↓ | – | ↑ |
| alcohol | ↑ | – | ↑ |
| exogenous oestrogens | ↑ | ↓ | ↑ |

**Fig. 14.9** Some physiological and external influences on plasma lipoproteins. P:S is the ratio of polyunsaturated to saturated fats in the diet.

| Interpretation of lipid results | | | |
|---|---|---|---|
| Plasma concentration (mmol/L) | Ideal | Borderline | Abnormal |
| Total cholesterol | <5.2 | 5.2–6.5 | >6.5 |
| LDL cholesterol | <4.0 | 4.0–5.0 | >5.0 |
| HDL cholesterol | >1.0 | 0.9–1.0 | <0.9 |
| HDL/total cholesterol ratio | >0.25 | 0.20–0.25 | <0.20 |
| Triglycerides (fasting) | <2.0 | 2.0–2.5 | >2.5 |

**Fig. 14.10** Interpretation of lipid results. HDL/total cholesterol ratio = HDL CHOL/(total CHOL – HDL CHOL). (See text for explanation.)

an individual basis; in patients with established CHD, even lower values for total and LDL cholesterol may be desirable. In the absence of CHD, or other CHD risk factors, higher levels are acceptable.

## Ultracentrifugation and electrophoresis

Ultracentrifugation is not a convenient technique for routine use but separation of lipoproteins by electrophoresis is a simple procedure. An example of normal fasting lipid electrophoresis is included in *Fig. 14.11*. The β-band on electrophoresis corresponds to LDL, pre-β to VLDL and the α-band to HDL. Chylomicrons, if present, remain at the ori-

gin. Electrophoresis provides only qualitative information and direct measurement of HDL cholesterol and calculation of LDL cholesterol is more informative, except for the diagnosis of remnant hyperlipidaemia (*see p. 225*).

Simple visual inspection of plasma, which has been standing overnight at 4°C, is useful (*Fig. 14.12*); chylomicrons, being less dense than plasma, float to the top giving a creamy supernatant layer; VLDL remain in suspension and impart an opalescence or turbidity to the plasma, while both LDL and HDL are too small to scatter light, with the result that even when they are present in excess the plasma remains clear.

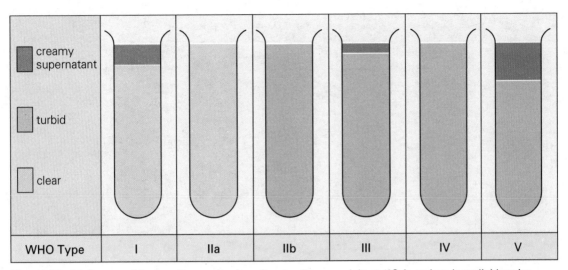

**Fig. 14.12** Appearance of fasting plasma samples, after standing overnight at 4°C, in various hyperlipidaemias.

## Blood for lipid studies

Blood for lipid studies should be drawn after an overnight fast (14 h), when chylomicrons, being derived from dietary fat, should normally have been cleared; a pathological dis-

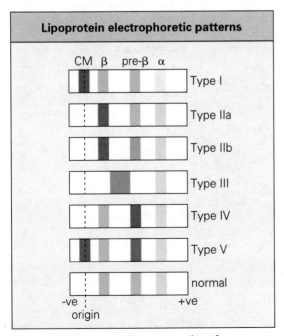

**Fig. 14.11** Diagrammatic representation of electrophoretic patterns characteristic of various lipoprotein disorders, based on the WHO classification.

turbance may thus be inferred if they are present. The patient should have kept to his own normal diet for two weeks before the blood is taken. Alcohol should not have been taken on the evening before blood sampling. This is a common cause of hypertriglyceridaemia even in patients who have otherwise fasted. When lipid studies are done on a patient who has had a myocardial infarct, blood should either be taken within 24 h or after an interval of three months, since the metabolism of lipoproteins is disturbed during the convalescent period and analytical results may be misleading.

The combination of increasing awareness of the importance of hyperlipidaemia as a risk factor for CHD, the trend towards preventative medicine and the introduction of effective agents for treating hyperlipidaemia has resulted in a considerable increase in the number of requests for lipid analysis. Lipid studies are *mandatory* in individuals with:

- CHD
- A family history of premature CHD (that is, occurring at less than 60 years of age)
- Stigmata of hyperlipidaemia (e.g., tendon xanthomata, corneal arcus if below 50 years of age)
- Lipaemic plasma.

They are *advisable* in patients with conditions such as diabetes mellitus and hypertension, which are themselves risk factors for CHD. And given the high prevalence of hyperlipidaemia, there is an increasing tendency to screen for the condition in the adult population at large, particularly in males in the 20–60 age group.

| WHO classification of hyperlipoproteinaemias | | | | | |
|---|---|---|---|---|---|
| **Type** | **CM** | **VLDL** | **LDL** | **Cholesterol** | **Triglyceride** |
| I | ↑ | N | N | N | ↑↑ |
| IIa | – | N | ↑↑ | ↑↑ | N |
| IIb | – | ↑ | ↑ | ↑ | ↑ |
| III | – | 'broad β band' | | ↑ | ↑ |
| IV | – | ↑ | N | N (↑) | ↑ |
| V | ↑ | ↑ | N | N (↑) | ↑↑ |

**Fig. 14.13** WHO classification of hyperlipidaemias. An indication of the concentrations of cholesterol and triglyceride characteristic of these types (N = normal, ↑ = raised) is shown but is not part of the basis of the classification. HDL levels, though usually normal, may be reduced in Types I, IV and V; total cholesterol may be slightly increased in Types IV and V due to the cholesterol in VLDL. Chylomicrons (CM) are not usually present in fasting plasma.

| Condition | WHO Type | Lipid abnormality cholesterol | triglyceride | HDL |
|---|---|---|---|---|
| obesity | IV | N or sl ↑ | ↑ | ↓ |
| excessive alcohol intake | IV, V | N | ↑ | ↑ |
| diabetes mellitus | IIb, IV, V | N or sl ↑ | ↑↑ | ↓ |
| hypothyroidism | IIa, IIb, III | ↑ | N or ↑ | N |
| nephrotic syndrome | IIa, IIb, IV, V | ↑↑ | ↑↑ | ↓ |
| chronic renal failure | IV | N or ↑ | ↑ | ↓ |
| cholestasis | see caption | ↑ | N | N |

**Fig. 14.14** Common causes of secondary hyperlipidaemia. In cholestasis, hypercholesterolaemia is due to the accumulation of lipoprotein X, an aggregate of free cholesterol, lecithin, albumin and apo C. The changes shown for diabetes are for untreated disease. Abnormalities can persist with treatment and are discussed further in *Chapter 11* (sl, slight).

## DISORDERS OF LIPID METABOLISM

There are several rare, inherited metabolic diseases associated with the accumulation of lipids in tissues and others in which plasma lipoprotein concentrations are reduced. By far the commonest disorders, however, are the hyperlipidaemias and it is to these conditions that the rest of this chapter is devoted.

## Classification

The WHO classification of hyperlipidaemias, based on the work of Fredrickson, is essentially a phenotypic classification, being based on the type of lipoprotein involved (*Fig. 14.13*). These WHO types do not correspond to specific disease entities; hyperlipidaemias may be secondary to other conditions (*see below*) and different patients with the same condition may manifest different WHO types: for example, both Types IIa and IIb may be seen in hypothyroidism. Further, even with primary, inherited hyperlipidaemia, individuals with the same condition may show different WHO types, while the same pattern of lipoprotein excess may occur in more than one distinct inherited condition, for instance Type IIa in both familial (monogenic) and 'common' (polygenic) hypercholesterolaemia. The WHO classification has another drawback in that the WHO type of an individual patient may change in response to dietary or drug treatment. Finally, this classification takes no account of HDL cholesterol.

## Secondary hyperlipidaemias

These are common (*see Fig. 14.14*) and, since resolution of the lipid abnormality should follow successful treatment of the underlying condition, management should be directed towards the cause. Although the presence of a primary disorder may be inferred from a relevant family history, it is always important to exclude secondary causes in the investigation of patients with hyperlipidaemias. Occasionally, such a cause may coexist with a primary hyperlipidaemia and exacerbate its manifestations.

Several drugs can also cause or exacerbate hyperlipidaemia, including thiazides, β-blockers lacking intrinsic sympathomimetic activity (ISA) and corticosteroids. Ideally, calcium antagonists, angiotensin-converting enzyme (ACE) inhibitors, β-blockers with ISA or α-blockers should be used for treating hypertension in patients with hyperlipidaemia. Oestrogens, especially when given to post-menopausal women, often lower plasma cholesterol concentrations but may cause, or exacerbate, hypertriglyceridaemia. Certain progestogens used in oral contraceptives also have an adverse effect on plasma lipids.

---

### CASE HISTORY 14.1

A 55-year-old man presented with a history of lethargy, loss of concentration and constipation. He had suffered from angina for two years, but this had become less of a problem recently, since he had become much less active. On examination, he appeared myxoedematous.

#### Investigations

serum: TSH       more than 100 mU/L
      cholesterol       12.2 mmol/L
      triglyceride       1.5 mmol/L

He was treated cautiously with tri-iodothyronine; his

angina was controlled effectively with nitrates and a calcium antagonist. His serum cholesterol fell to 8.2 mmol/L on treatment, with an LDL cholesterol of 6.4 mmol/L.

#### Comment

Hypothyroidism is commonly associated with hypercholesterolaemia, due to decreased removal of LDL from the circulation. The persistence of a raised cholesterol despite adequate treatment of the hypothyroidism is suggestive, in this case, of the presence of an additional, genetically determined, predisposition to hypercholesterolaemia.

---

### CASE HISTORY 14.2

A 45-year-old obese barman who complained of recurrent epigastric pain underwent gastroscopy. Because he admitted to heavy alcohol ingestion, blood was taken for liver function tests prior to the procedure. Gastroscopy revealed a duodenal ulcer.

In the laboratory, the technician noticed that the serum looked opalescent and analyzed it for lipids.

#### Investigations

serum: cholesterol       7.5 mmol/L
      triglyceride       8.4 mmol/L

lipid electrophoresis:
      excess pre-β-lipoprotein
      slight excess of α-lipoprotein
      normal β-lipoprotein

#### Comment

Alcohol causes hypertriglyceridaemia by increasing triglyceride synthesis and the insulin resistance seen in obesity has a similar effect. Massive hypertriglyceridaemia (more than 20 mmol/L) may occur in patients with a high alcohol intake when there is an additional, inherited tendency to hypertriglyceridaemia. Alcohol increases HDL cholesterol concentration (accounting for the slight excess of α-lipoprotein in this case), although HDL cholesterol is often reduced when the high triglyceride level has another cause.

## CASE HISTORY 14.3

An obese 44-year-old woman with insulin-dependent diabetes was found to have a blood glucose level of 32 mmol/L at the out-patient clinic and was admitted to hospital. Blood was taken for further biochemical analysis and the serum was seen to be grossly lipaemic.

### Investigations
serum:  cholesterol        53 mmol/L
        triglyceride      150 mmol/L

The sample was inspected after standing overnight and had a creamy, supernatant layer, though the infranatant remained lipaemic.

### Comment
The appearance of the serum is characteristic of the WHO Type V phenotype. Hyperlipidaemia can complicate uncontrolled insulin-dependent diabetes and is due to a combination of decreased lipoprotein lipase activity and increased hepatic triglyceride synthesis. It may exacerbate a co-existing familial hyperlipidaemia. This patient was treated with an intravenous insulin infusion. Her blood glucose concentration fell rapidly and she was restabilized on an appropriate regimen of subcutaneous insulin injections. After a week her serum cholesterol and triglycerides were 8.0 and 11 mmol/L, respectively. Thereafter diabetes remained well controlled and follow-up lipid analysis showed cholesterol 6.0 mmol/L and triglycerides 5.3 mmol/L. Her immediate family had normal serum lipids and it was concluded that her persistently elevated triglyceride was related at least in part to her obesity.

## Primary hyperlipidaemias
### *Familial hypercholesterolaemia (FH)*
This condition is characterized by very high plasma cholesterol levels which are present from early childhood and do not depend upon the presence of environmental factors (*see polygenic hypercholesterolaemia, p.225*). It is inherited as an autosomal dominant characteristic, with a frequency in the population of about 1 in 500. Different mutations affect LDL synthesis, transport, ligand binding and clustering in coated pits but all cause a similar phenotype. A mutant apo B-100, which does not bind normally to the LDL receptor, has also been described and produces a phenotype similar to FH. In all cases, there is a defect in the uptake and catabolism of LDL, and its plasma concentration is increased. In heterozygotes, total cholesterol is typically in the range 7.8–12 mmol/L.

In the very rare homozygotes (1 in 1,000,000), no receptors are present. Plasma cholesterol concentrations can be as high as 20 mmol/L. These individuals develop coronary artery disease in childhood and, if untreated, rarely survive into adult life; heterozygotes tend to develop coronary artery disease some 20 years earlier than the general population; more than half of those untreated die before the age of 60.

## CASE HISTORY 14.4

A 36-year-old man consulted an optician to obtain a prescription for reading glasses. The optician noticed that the patient had bilateral arcus senilis, and recommended that he consult his general medical practitioner. The GP found that he also had tendon xanthomata, arising from the Achilles tendons. Blood pressure was normal; he was a non-smoker and not overweight. His father had died of a heart attack at the age of 40. An ECG taken at rest was normal but ischaemic changes developed on exercise. Analysis of fasting blood for lipids showed the following.

### Investigations
serum:  cholesterol        13.2 mmol/L
        triglyceride        1.3 mmol/L
        LDL cholesterol    11.4  mmol/L
        HDL cholesterol     1.2 mmol/L

### Comment
This is a characteristic picture of familial hypercholesterolaemia. Tendon xanthomata, though not an invariable finding, are virtually pathognomic of FH. Their development is age-related. They are accumulations of cholesterol, but deep-seated with the result that the overlying skin has a normal colour. Arcus senilis and xanthelasmata are frequently present, but unlike tendon xanthomata, may occur in the absence of an obvious disturbance of lipid metabolism, though usually only in older people (>60 years). Even though this patient is normotensive and a non-smoker the hypercholesterolaemia alone

considerably increases his risk of dying of ischaemic heart disease and indeed he has an abnormal exercise ECG. Familial hypercholesterolaemia is 10 times more common in victims of myocardial infarctions than in the rest of the population. Patients with FH require rigorous treatment, usually with lipid-lowering drugs as well as diet (*see below*) and if other risk factors are present these, of course, must also be tackled. Children and most adults with FH show a Type IIa phenotype, but in some adults the phenotype is IIb.

### 'Common' (polygenic) hypercholesterolaemia

In FH, the distribution of plasma cholesterol concentrations in relatives of the proband is bimodal, with a clear distinction between heterozygotes and normals. More frequently, when the family of an individual with hypercholesterolaemia is studied, a continuous distribution is found, consistent with the plasma cholesterol being influenced by several genes. This entity has been termed 'common' or polygenic hypercholesterolaemia. Plasma cholesterol is not as high as in FH, and is influenced to a greater extent by environmental factors, e.g., diet.

The significance of this condition again lies in its relationship to the risk of coronary artery disease and the principles of management are similar to those for FH; in polygenic hypercholesterolaemia, however, dietary treatment alone is often successful with the result that the use of lipid-lowering drugs may not be required.

### Familial dysbetalipoproteinaemia (broad β disease)

This condition is characterized clinically by the presence of fat deposits in the palmar creases and by tuberous xanthomata; the latter tend to occur over bony prominences and, unlike tendon xanthomata, are reddish in colour. However, neither of these cutaneous stigmata is invariably present. In some patients eruptive xanthomata are present. Biochemically, the condition is characterized by the presence of a broad β band on electrophoresis of serum, due to the presence of an excess of IDL and chylomicron remnants; chylomicrons are sometimes also present. An alternative name is remnant hyperlipoproteinaemia. Total cholesterol and triglyceride levels are elevated and the molar ratio VLDL-cholesterol/total triglyceride characteristically exceeds 0.68 (although this cannot be determined routinely since an ultracentrifuge is required to separate out VLDL). Patients with remnant hyperlipoproteinaemia have an increased risk not only of coronary artery disease but also of peripheral and cerebral vascular disease.

Apo E shows polymorphism. The commonest phenotype is termed E3/3. Familial dysbetalipoproteinaemia is associated with the E2/2 phenotype, which can result in impaired IDL uptake by the liver. However, the fact that this phenotype is present in 1 in 100 of the normal population, while dysbetalipoproteinaemia is an uncommon disorder (prevalence approximately 1 in 10,000), implies a role for other factors in its expression, and in this context it is noteworthy that although the variant apoprotein is present from birth, the condition does not appear clinically until adult life. Such factors include obesity, alcohol, hypothyroidism and diabetes.

Although the diagnosis can be inferred from the clinical and biochemical findings, it should ideally be confirmed by apo E phenotyping.

The significance of apo E polymorphism is not limited to lipid metabolism. Increased frequency of the e4 allele has been demonstrated in patients with familial Alzheimer's disease.

---

### CASE HISTORY 14.5

A middle-aged man was referred by his family doctor to a dermatologist because of extensive yellowish papules, with erythematous bases, on his buttocks and elbows. The dermatologist recognized these as eruptive xanthomata and noticed that there were yellow, fatty streaks in the palmar creases. Blood was drawn after an overnight fast for lipid analysis and the serum was seen to be slightly turbid.

### Investigations
serum:  cholesterol       8.5 mmol/L
       triglyceride     6.4 mmol/L

Serum protein electrophoresis showed a broad β band and a trace of chylomicrons.

### Comment
This patient was treated with a low-fat diet and bezafibrate and after three months serum lipid concentrations had become normal as had the electrophoretic appearance. There was also considerable regression of the xanthomata. When the bezafibrate was stopped, the abnormality returned but resolved again on restarting the drug. Familial dysbetalipoproteinaemia characteristically responds very well to treatment.

### Familial chylomicronaemia

Fasting chylomicronaemia is a feature of two rare hyperlipidaemias both having an autosomal recessive inheritance; in one there is a deficiency of the enzyme lipoprotein lipase and in the other a deficiency of apo C-II which is required for activation of this enzyme. The result in each case is a failure of chylomicron clearance from the blood stream. Presentation is usually in childhood, with eruptive xanthomata, recurrent abdominal pain due to pancreatitis and sometimes hepatosplenomegaly.

Chylomicronaemia may also be seen in other patients with a genetic predisposition to hypertriglyceridaemia when this is exacerbated by obesity, diabetes mellitus, hyperuricaemia or alcohol ingestion; some drugs, for example thiazides, may also have this effect.

Management involves giving a low fat diet, with substitution of some fat by triglycerides based on medium-chain fatty acids; these are absorbed directly from the gut into the blood stream and therefore do not produce chylomicrons. The major complication of the chylomicronaemic syndromes is recurrent pancreatitis and since this is uncommon with triglyceride concentrations below 10 mmol/L, it is not usually considered necessary to achieve normalization of plasma triglyceride concentration.

### Familial hypertriglyceridaemia

This condition, which has a prevalence of approximately 1 in 600, is usually associated with a Type IV phenotype, i.e., there is an excess of VLDL in plasma. The molecular basis is uncertain; there is increased hepatic synthesis of VLDL. Inheritance is autosomal dominant. In severe cases, in which other factors, e.g., obesity and alcohol, are often implicated, chylomicronaemia is present (WHO Type V) and only then are physical signs, e.g., eruptive xanthomata and lipaemia retinalis, usually present.

It is uncertain whether there is an increased risk of CHD in patients with familial hypertriglyceridaemia, though HDL concentration is often reduced; in severe cases, there is a risk of pancreatitis.

### Familial combined hyperlipidaemia

This is due to hepatic overproduction of apo B leading to increased VLDL secretion and increased production of LDL from VLDL. Either plasma cholesterol or triglyceride, or both, may be elevated; typically, in affected relatives, one-third have an increase in LDL, one-third in VLDL and one-third have an excess of both lipoproteins; phenotypic expression may be IIa, IIb or IV. Cutaneous manifestations of hyperlipidaemia may be present and in all cases there is an increased risk of coronary artery disease.

The prevalence is approximately 1 in 300; inheritance is probably autosomal dominant. There are no distinctive clinical features and the diagnosis is often presumptive, based on the presence of a IIb phenotype in the absence of tendon xanthomata or a secondary cause of hyperlipidaemia.

### Familial hyperalphalipoproteinaemia

In this condition there is hypercholesterolaemia due to an increase in only the HDL fraction, which may be present in other members of the family. Coronary heart disease risk is decreased, and no treatment is required. The existence of this condition underlines the need to measure HDL cholesterol in patients with hypercholesterolaemia. Generally, if total cholesterol is greater than 7 mmol/L, there will always be an increase in LDL, but even then, measurement of HDL helps in the assessment of CHD risk.

## MANAGEMENT OF LIPID DISORDERS

The decision as to whether to treat a patient with a hyperlipidaemia may not be straightforward. There is no doubt that treatment is vital for patients with FH, but in those with mild hyperlipidaemia, the possible risks of the use of drugs for treatment may outweigh those associated with the disease *per se*. In general, hypercholesterolaemia is more sinister than hypertriglyceridaemia alone.

It is important to treat any condition known to exacerbate hyperlipidaemia and in the context of coronary artery disease, attention to other risk factors such as smoking, hypertension and lack of exercise is vital. All patients should be encouraged to achieve their ideal body weight. In general, management should be more aggressive in younger patients, when other risk factors are present, when there is a personal or family history of arterial disease and when HDL cholesterol is low.

### Hypercholesterolaemia

In hypercholesterolaemia, a diet low in cholesterol and saturated fat should be prescribed; unsaturated fats may be substituted for saturated. In FH, dietary treatment alone is seldom sufficient to normalize cholesterol levels. A total cholesterol concentration of >7.8 mmol/L or a ratio HDL CHOL/(TOTAL CHOL – HDL) of less than 0.2 is often taken as an indication for drug treatment even in the absence of other risk factors. If unmodifiable risk factors are present, and in patients known to have CHD, drug treatment is often indicated at lower cholesterol levels. There is now compelling evidence that cholesterol-lowering reduces both the incidence of further coronary events and overall mortality in patients with CHD.

Drugs used for the treatment of hypercholesterolaemia include statins and bile acid sequestrants. The former are inhibitors of HMG-CoA reductase; they decrease intracellular cholesterol synthesis and thus increase LDL receptor expression and decrease plasma LDL concentration. Bile acid sequestrants bind bile acids in the gut and prevent their reabsorption; this depletes the hepatic bile acid pool and stimulates their formation from cholesterol. These agents may be used in combination in severe hypercholesterolaemia. Bile acid sequestrants may increase triglyceride concentrations and should not be used in familial dysbetalipoproteinaemia. The fibrates increase VLDL catabolism and are effective in mild hypercholesterolaemia, particularly if accompanied by hypertriglyceridaemia. They increase HDL concentration and may lower fibrinogen, another CHD risk factor.

Options for the treatment of FH homozygotes, who may not respond adequately to drug treatment, include physical removal of LDL by LDL apheresis, partial ileal by-pass and liver transplantation.

## Hypertriglyceridaemia

Hypertriglyceridaemia may respond well to control of body weight and any coexistent exacerbating factors, such as diabetes, excessive alcohol intake , obesity or hyperuricaemia. The main classes of drug used for treating hypertriglyceridaemia are the fibrates, nicotinic acid derivatives and fish oils. Nicotinic acid derivatives decrease VLDL synthesis and may also decrease LDL and increase HDL. Fish oils, rich in $\omega$-3 polyunsaturated fatty acids, also decrease VLDL synthesis.

## LIPOPROTEIN DEFICIENCY

There are three rare inherited lipoprotein deficiencies.

## Abetalipoproteinaemia

In abetalipoproteinaemia, there is a defect in the synthesis of apo B; CM, VLDL and LDL are absent from the plasma. Clinically, there is malabsorption of fat, acanthocytosis, retinitis pigmentosa and an ataxic neuropathy.

## Hypobetalipoproteinaemia

In this condition, there is partial deficiency of apo B; CM, VLDL and LDL are present, but in low concentrations.

## Tangier disease

In Tangier disease, HDL levels are reduced; clinically, the condition is characterized by hyperplastic, orange tonsils and the accumulation of cholesteryl esters in other reticuloendothelial tissues. The condition is due to accelerated catabolism of apo A-I.

## SUMMARY

The main lipids in the blood are triglyceride, an important energy substrate, and cholesterol, a component of the membranes of cells and their organelles. Cholesterol and triglycerides are insoluble in water and are transported in the blood in lipoproteins, complexes of lipids with specific proteins known as apolipoproteins. There are four major classes of lipoprotein; (i) chylomicrons, which carry exogenous, that is, dietary, fat (mainly triglyceride) from the gut to peripheral tissues; (ii) very low density lipoproteins (VLDL), which carry endogenous triglyceride from the liver to those tissues; (iii) low density lipoproteins, which transport cholesterol from the liver to peripheral tissues; and (iv) high density lipoproteins (HDL), involved in reverse cholesterol transport from peripheral tissues to the liver whence it can be excreted. These particles are in a dynamic state and there is considerable exchange of lipid and proteins between them.

Hypercholesterolaemia, when due to an increase in LDL, is an important risk factor for coronary heart disease; an excess of cholesterol in HDL confers some protection against this condition. Hypertriglyceridaemia is a less important risk factor for coronary heart disease but, when very severe, can cause pancreatitis. Both hypercholesterolaemia and hypertriglyceridaemia are associated with various types of cutaneous fat deposition, or xanthomata.

Hyperlipidaemia may be classified into six distinct phenotypes (the WHO classification) according to which lipoprotein particles are present in excess. They may be either primary, that is, genetically determined, or occur secondarily to a variety of other conditions, including diabetes mellitus, hypothyroidism, obesity, alcoholism, renal disease and certain drugs. The diagnosis of a primary hyperlipidaemia is supported when such conditions can be excluded, especially if there is a family history; often, however, an underlying genetic tendency to hyperlipoproteinaemia is exacerbated by the presence of one of these conditions.

The most important primary hyperlipidaemia is familial hypercholesterolaemia. The molecular basis of this condition is a functional defect in, or a decrease in the number of, LDL receptors which leads to decreased clearance of these lipoproteins from the blood and an increase in cholesterol synthesis. Heterozygotes for the condition occur with a frequency of approximately 0.2% and have a greatly increased risk of coronary heart disease. Homozygotes are fortunately very rare; affected patients develop coronary heart disease in their teens. Other inherited hyperlipidaemias include familial hypertriglyceridaemia, familial combined hyperlipidaemia and dysbetalipoproteinaemia, in which particles with a density intermediate between the low and very low density lipoproteins accumulate.

A case can be made for screening all adults for hyper-cholesterolaemia but this is essential in those with coronary heart disease or a family history of this condition or of a hyperlipoproteinaemia; in patients with xanthomata, and in patients whose plasma is observed to be lipaemic.

The management of secondary hyperlipidaemias is to treat the underlying condition; primary disorders are treated with diet, although drugs may be required as well. Drugs that can be used include HMG-CoA reductase-inhibitors and bile acid sequestrants for hypercholesterolaemia; fibrates and nicotinic acid derivatives are effective in hypertrigly-ceridaemia and may have beneficial effects on cholesterol in addition. In patients with hypercholesterolaemia, it is essential to identify, and if possible eliminate, any other risk factors for coronary heart disease, such as smoking and hypertension.

## FURTHER READING

Feher M & Richmond W (1991) *Lipids and Lipid Disorders.* London: Gower Medical Publishing.

Hunningshake D B (ed.) (1994) Lipid disorders. *The Medical Clinics of North America,* **78**, 1–266.

Thompson G R (1989) *A Handbook of Hyperlipidaemia.* London: Current Science.

# 15. Clinical Enzymology

## INTRODUCTION

Measurements of enzyme activity are of value in the diagnosis and management of a wide variety of diseases. Genetically determined abnormalities of enzymes are the cause of many inherited metabolic diseases (*Chapter 16*), but this chapter is devoted mainly to the use of enzyme assays in conditions where a change in the concentration of an enzyme is a reflection, rather than the cause, of a disease process. Such measurements are usually made in plasma, although enzyme assays in other body fluids, such as urine and pancreatic juice, can also provide useful information. Most enzymes measured in plasma are primarily intracellular, being released into the blood when there is damage to cell membranes, but many enzymes, for example renin, complement factors and coagulation factors, are actively secreted into the blood, where they fulfil their physiological function.

Small amounts of intracellular enzymes are present in the blood as a result of normal cell turnover. When damage to cells occurs, increased amounts of enzymes will be released and their concentrations in the blood will rise. However, such increases are not always due to tissue damage. Other possible causes include:

- Increased cell turnover;
- Cellular proliferation (e.g., neoplasia);
- Increased enzyme synthesis (enzyme induction);
- Obstruction to secretion;
- Decreased clearance.

Little is known about the mechanisms by which enzymes are removed from the circulation. Small molecules, such as amylase, are filtered at the glomerulus but most enzymes are probably removed by reticuloendothelial cells. Plasma amylase activity rises in acute renal failure but, in general, changes in clearance rates are not known to be important as causes of changes in plasma enzyme levels.

## Enzyme activity

Enzyme assays usually depend on the measurement of the catalytic *activity* of the enzyme, rather than the *concentration* of the enzyme protein itself. Since each enzyme molecule can catalyze the reaction of many molecules of substrate, measurement of activity provides great sensitivity. It is, however, important that the conditions of the assay are optimized and standardized to give reliable and reproducible results.

Reference ranges for plasma enzymes are dependent on assay conditions, for example, temperature, and may also be subject to physiological influences. It is thus important to be aware of both the reference range for the laboratory in question and the physiological circumstances when interpreting the data provided. Ranges quoted in this book (*see p. 311*) are from the author's own laboratory and may not necessarily be the same as those of the reader's.

## Disadvantages of enzyme assays

A major disadvantage in the use of enzymes for the diagnosis of tissue damage is their lack of specificity to a particular tissue or cell type. Many enzymes are common to more than one tissue, with the result that an increase in the plasma activity of a particular enzyme could reflect damage to any one of these tissues. This problem may be obviated to some extent in two ways: first, different tissues may contain (and thus release when they are damaged) two or more enzymes in different proportions; thus alanine and aspartate transaminase are both present in cardiac muscle and hepatocytes, but there is relatively more alanine transaminase in the liver; secondly, some enzymes exist in different forms (isoforms), colloquially termed isoenzymes (although, strictly, the term 'isoenzyme' refers only to a genetically determined isoform). Individual isoforms are often characteristic of a particular tissue; although they may have similar catalytic activities, they often differ in some other measurable property, such as heat stability or sensitivity to inhibitors.

After a single insult to a tissue, the activity of intracellular enzymes in the plasma rises as they are released from the damaged cells, and then falls as the enzymes are cleared. It is thus important to consider the time at which the blood sample is taken in relation to the insult. If taken too soon, there may have been insufficient time for the enzyme to reach the blood stream and if too late, it may have been completely cleared (see *Case History 15.2*). As with all diagnostic techniques, data acquired from measurements of enzymes in plasma must always be assessed in the light of whatever clinical and other information is available, and their limitations borne in mind.

In the tables that follow, typical ranges for the plasma concentrations of enzymes in various conditions are given. Higher (or lower) levels may of course occur in more (or less) severe cases

# ENZYMES OF DIAGNOSTIC VALUE

## Alkaline phosphatase (ALP)

This enzyme is present in high concentrations in the liver, bone (osteoblasts), placenta and intestinal epithelium. These tissues each contain specific isoenzymes of ALP. Pathological increases in ALP activity are most frequently seen in cholestatic liver disease and in certain diseases of bone. In the liver, cholestasis stimulates ALP synthesis (an example of enzyme induction); in bone, the enzyme is actively secreted by osteoblasts (cells responsible for bone formation) and the amount of the enzyme in plasma can be increased by increased osteoblastic activity.

The causes of an increase in plasma ALP activity are summarized in *Fig. 15.1*. Physiological increases are seen in pregnancy, due to the placental isoenzyme, and in childhood (when bones are growing), due to the bone isoenzyme. The plasma level is high at birth but falls rapidly thereafter. However, it remains two to three times the normal adult level and rises again during the adolescent growth spurt before falling to the adult level as bone growth ceases (*Fig. 15.2*).

Plasma ALP activity is slightly higher than normal in apparently healthy elderly people. This may reflect the high incidence of mild, subclinical Paget's disease in the elderly. Levels of ALP as high as ten times the upper limit of normal (10 × ULN) may be seen in severe Paget's disease

| Causes of an increased plasma alkaline phosphatase |
|---|
| **Physiological** |
| pregnancy (last trimester) |
| childhood |
| |
| **Pathological** |
| often >5 × ULN |
|   Paget's disease of bone |
|   osteomalacia and rickets |
|   cholestasis (intra- and extra-hepatic) |
|   cirrhosis |
| |
| usually <5 × ULN |
|   bone tumours (primary and secondary) |
|   renal bone disease |
|   primary hyperparathyroidism with bone involvement |
|   healing fractures |
|   osteomyelitis |
|   hepatic space-occupying lesions (tumour, abscess) |
|   infiltrative hepatic disease |
|   hepatitis |
|   inflammatory bowel disease |

**Fig. 15.1** Causes of an increased plasma alkaline phosphatase activity.

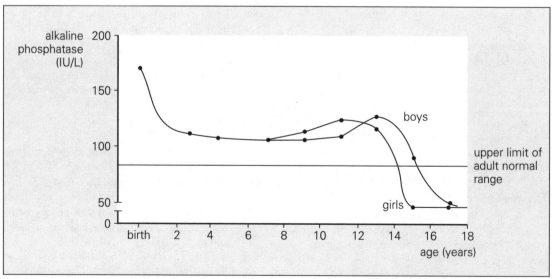

**Fig. 15.2** Serum alkaline phosphatase activity as a function of age in childhood. Mean values are shown; the peaks between 10 and 16 years correspond to the pubertal growth spurt, and levels of up to three times the upper limit of the adult normal range may be seen at this time.

of bone, rickets and osteomalacia and occasionally in cholestatic liver disease. Lesser increases are, however, more common in these conditions (*see Fig. 15.1*). ALP activity is not increased in uncomplicated osteoporosis, unless the condition has been complicated by collapse or fracture of bone.

Plasma ALP is commonly elevated in malignant disease; it may be of bony or hepatic origin and associated with the presence of both primary and secondary tumours in these tissues. A number of apparently tumour-specific ALPs, secreted by tumour cells themselves, have also been described. The best known of these is the Regan isoenzyme, which has similar heat stability to placental ALP and is found in some patients with bronchial carcinoma.

ALP is frequently measured as part of a biochemical profile and it is not uncommon to find a raised level in the absence of clinical evidence of bone or liver disease, and in the absence of other biochemical abnormalities. In establishing the cause of such an increase it is clearly helpful to determine the tissue of origin. This can be done by measuring tissue-specific isoenzymes of ALP. These can be separated and quantitated using various techniques, including electrophoresis and differential heat inactivation. A simpler but less reliable alternative is to measure plasma γ-glutamyl transferase. This enzyme is found in the liver but not bone. Its plasma activity is often (but not always) increased when there is an excess of hepatic ALP in the plasma.

## Acid phosphatase

This enzyme is present in high concentrations in the prostate gland and is elevated in the plasma of some patients with prostatic cancer. It is of little value in the diagnosis of this condition, plasma activity being raised in only about 20% of patients in whom the tumour is confined to the gland. It is, however, raised in up to 80% of cases when there are metastases and its use as a tumour marker in such patients is discussed in *Chapter 19*. Acid phosphatase is also increased in some cases of prostatitis and occasionally in benign prostatic hypertrophy.

The prostate is examined clinically *per rectum*, a procedure that may cause some release of acid phosphatase into the circulation, producing a transient increase in its activity. Although this happens much less frequently than was once thought, it is wise to take a blood sample for acid phosphatase determination before, rather than after, clinical examination. The enzyme is labile and blood for analysis must be transported to the laboratory rapidly and the serum deep-frozen until the assay is performed. Since the enzyme is present in red blood cells, haemolysis invalidates acid phosphatase measurements.

In addition to the prostate and red blood cells, acid phosphatase is also present in platelets, bone, liver and spleen. The prostatic isoenzyme is characteristically inhibited by tartrate but not formaldehyde. In most laboratories, acid phosphatase is measured as the prostate-specific 'tartrate-labile' or 'formol-stable' isoenzyme. High levels of non-prostatic acid phosphatase may be seen in bone diseases (particularly Paget's disease), in thrombocythaemia and in Gaucher's disease, an inherited disorder of lipid storage.

## Transaminases

Two transaminases (strictly, aminotransferases) are of use in diagnostic enzymology. These are aspartate transaminase (AST, also known as glutamate-oxaloacetate transaminase, GOT) and alanine transaminase (ALT, or glutamate-pyruvate transaminase, GPT). Both enzymes are widely distributed in body tissues, the concentration of AST being lower in all tissues except the liver where they are present in approximately equal amounts.

The causes of increased plasma AST are shown in *Fig. 15.3*. Very high levels, sometimes in excess of $100 \times$ ULN, are seen with severe tissue damage, such as in acute hepatitis, crush injuries and tissue hypoxia. More usually in hepatitis

---

**Causes of an increased plasma aspartate transaminase**

often >10 × ULN
   acute hepatitis and liver necrosis
   major crush injuries
   severe tissue hypoxaemia
   (levels may sometimes exceed
   100 × ULN in these conditions)

5–10 × ULN
   myocardial infarction
   following surgery or trauma
   skeletal muscle disease
   cholestasis
   chronic hepatitis

usually <5 × ULN
   physiological (neonates)
   other liver diseases
   pancreatitis
   haemolysis (*in vivo* and *in vitro*)

**Fig. 15.3** Causes of an increased plasma aspartate transaminase activity. Plasma alanine transaminase is raised to a similar extent in liver diseases but to a lesser degree, if at all, in the other conditions.

the peak level is only 10–20 × ULN; this peak may occur in the prodromal stage before the patient is jaundiced or at the time of onset. In myocardial infarction, plasma AST begins to rise some 12 h after the infarct, reaching a peak of up to 10 × ULN at 24–36 h and then declining over two to three days providing that there is no further cardiac damage (*see p. 235*).

In most conditions where AST is elevated there is a concurrent, though proportionally smaller, rise in ALT. In hepatitis, however, plasma levels of ALT may exceed those of AST. If, as in many laboratories, only one transaminase assay is available, this should be for AST. Its major use is in the management of liver disease, where a raised level suggests hepatocellular damage and the results of serial estimation can indicate persistence of, or recovery from, such damage (*see p. 78*). AST is often measured as part of a biochemical profile in multichannel autoanalyzers. It is very uncommon to find levels greater than 20 × ULN unexpectedly; this is most likely to occur in the prodromal phase of viral hepatitis. Levels of up to 2 × ULN are sometimes found in patients who have no clinical evidence of tissue damage. Alcohol abuse should be considered as a possible cause in such cases. There are no tissue-specific isoenzymes of AST and if there are no other biochemical changes, nor any readily apparent cause of the raised level, the wisest procedure is to repeat the analysis after an interval of one or two weeks.

An increase in plasma AST activity is a sensitive indication of graft rejection following liver transplantation.

## γ-Glutamyl transferase (GGT)

This enzyme is present in high concentrations in the liver, kidney and pancreas. Measurement of its plasma activity provides a sensitive indicator of hepatobiliary disease although it is of no value in distinguishing *between* cholestatic or hepatocellular disease. In biliary obstruction, plasma GGT activity may increase before that of alkaline phosphatase.

Plasma GGT is raised in the absence of liver disease in many patients taking the anticonvulsant drugs, phenytoin and phenobarbitone; rifampicin, used in the treatment of tuberculosis, can have a similar effect. This is an example of enzyme induction. The increased plasma GGT is not due to cell damage but to an increase in enzyme production within cells with the result that an increased amount is released during normal cell turnover.

Plasma GGT activity is frequently very high in patients with alcoholic liver disease but can be elevated, due to enzyme induction, in heavy alcohol drinkers in the absence of other evidence of liver damage. Up to 70% of

| Some causes of an increased plasma γ-glutamyl transferase |
| --- |
| often >10 × ULN<br>  cholestasis<br>  alcoholic liver disease |
| 5–10 × ULN<br>  hepatitis (acute and chronic)<br>  cirrhosis (without cholestasis)<br>  other liver diseases<br>  pancreatitis |
| usually <5 × ULN<br>  excessive alcohol ingestion<br>  enzyme-inducing drugs<br>  congestive cardiac failure |

**Fig.15.4** Causes of an increased plasma g-glutamyl transferase activity. Increases of less than 5 × ULN are seen in many conditions and probably reflect secondary effects on the liver. γ-Glutamyl transferase is not usually increased with hepatic space-occupying lesions provided that liver function is normal.

such people may have elevated levels of the enzyme but it should be appreciated both that similar increases may be seen in other conditions (*see Fig. 15.4*) and that a significant number of people who abuse alcohol have a normal plasma enzyme activity. Plasma GGT activity can remain elevated for up to 3–4 weeks following abstinence from alcohol, even in the absence of liver damage.

## Lactate dehydrogenase (LD)

This enzyme exists in body tissues as a tetramer. Two monomers, H and M, can combine in various proportions with the result that five isoenzymes of LD are known. The isoenzymes can be distinguished on the basis of several properties, including their sensitivity to heat and various inhibitors, and their electrophoretic mobility.

Few laboratories in the United Kingdom now measure total LD, because of its lack of tissue specificity. Increases are seen in a wide variety of conditions including acute damage to the liver, skeletal muscle and kidneys, and also in megaloblastic and haemolytic anaemias. In patients with lymphoma, a high plasma LD activity indicates a poor prognosis. There is a correlation between enzyme activity and tumour bulk and so serial measurements may be useful in following response to treatment.

## Causes of an increased plasma creatine kinase

often >10 × ULN
  myocardial infarction
  rhabdomyolysis
  malignant hyperpyrexia

5–10 × ULN
  following surgery
  skeletal muscle trauma
  severe exercise
  grand mal convulsions
  myositis
  muscular dystrophy

usually <5 × ULN
  physiological (neonates)
  hypothyroidism

**Fig. 15.5** Causes of an increased plasma creatine kinase activity. Concentrations as high as 100 × ULN may be seen in rhabdomyolysis and malignant hyperpyrexia.

Lactate dehydrogenase isoenzyme measurements can be of use in suspected myocardial infarction and in the diagnosis of haemolytic crises in sickle cell disease. In both cardiac muscle and red blood cells $LD_1$ ($H_4$) is the predominant isoenzyme. This shows much greater catalytic activity with α-hydroxybutyrate (rather than lactate) as a substrate than the other isoenzymes. Consequently, $LD_1$ is usually measured by means of a reaction using this substrate and has the alternative name, α-hydroxybutyrate dehydrogenase (HBD).

α-Hydroxybutyrate dehydrogenase has a long half-life in the plasma; after myocardial infarction its activity rises slowly to reach a peak at 2–3 days, declining thereafter over a period of one week or more. Since it is present in red blood cells, levels increase after pulmonary embolism which may resemble myocardial infarction clinically. The presence of haemolysis invalidates the use of HBD in diagnosis.

## Creatine kinase (CK)

The enzymatically active CK molecule is a dimer; there are two monomers, M and B. Three isoenzymes, BB, MM and MB, are found. BB is confined mainly to the brain. There is little of the BB isoenzyme in the plasma normally, and even with severe brain damage (due, for example, to a stroke) the concentration barely rises. Most of the CK normally present in the plasma is the MM isoenzyme which originates from skeletal muscle. An increase in concentration is seen with skeletal muscle damage and with severe prolonged exercise (*Fig. 15.5*).

Creatine kinase present in cardiac muscle contains a considerably higher proportion of the MB isoenzyme (approximately 30%) than does skeletal muscle (less than 1%). A raised plasma CK is characteristic of myocardial infarction and, in the absence of a possible contribution from skeletal muscle, separate measurement of the MB isoenzyme is not necessary. However, in a patient in whom suspected myocardial infarction has occurred following exercise, trauma or the administration of an intramuscular injection (all of which can increase CK), the finding that more than 5% of the total creatine kinase is due to the MB isoenzyme suggests that myocardial damage has been sustained.

CK-MB can be measured either by measurement of enzyme activity in the presence of an antibody which inhibits the M subunit, or by measurement of enzyme mass using an immunoassay. In the plasma, the terminal lysine residue of the CK-M polypeptide is removed by a carboxypeptidase. This does not affect enzyme activity but alters the charge on the polypeptide and hence the electrophoretic mobility of the enzyme. The three possible forms of CK-MM are termed isoforms: CK-MM3 is composed of two intact CK-M polypeptides; in CK-MM1, both polypeptides have had their terminal lysines removed; CK-MM2 has one polypeptide of each type. An increase in the ratio CK-MM3:CK-MM1 occurs earlier than other enzyme changes following myocardial infarction (2–5 h after the onset of chest pain). However, the measurement of CK isoforms is technically demanding and few laboratories presently offer it routinely.

## Amylase

This enzyme is found in the salivary glands and exocrine pancreas and tissue-specific isoenzymes can be distinguished by means of electrophoresis or the use of inhibitors.

Causes of a high plasma amylase are shown in *Fig. 15.6*. The most important use of this enzyme is in the differential diagnosis of the acute abdomen. Its plasma activity is usually raised in acute pancreatitis, and levels greater than 10 × ULN are virtually diagnostic, being only very occasionally seen in other conditions. However, levels are not as high as this in all cases of pancreatitis and may be 5 × ULN or more in other abdominal emergencies, particularly perforation of a duodenal ulcer. Acute pancreatitis is usually managed conservatively, while urgent laparotomy and exploration is indicated for most other abdominal emergencies.

Extra-abdominal causes of a raised plasma amylase activity rarely cause increases of more than 5 × ULN.

| Causes of an increased plasma amylase |
|---|
| > 10 × ULN<br>acute pancreatitis<br><br>> 5 × ULN<br>perforated duodenal ulcer<br>intestinal obstruction<br>other acute abdominal disorders<br>acute oliguric renal failure<br>diabetic ketoacidosis<br><br>usually < 5 × ULN<br>salivary gland disorders, e.g., calculi<br>and inflammation (including mumps)<br>chronic renal failure<br>macroamylasaemia<br>morphine administration (spasm of<br>sphincter of Oddi) |

**Fig. 15.6** Causes of an increased plasma amylase activity.

Macroamylasaemia is an example of a high plasma enzyme activity being due to reduced clearance. In this condition, amylase becomes complexed with another protein (in some cases, an immunoglobulin) to form an entity of much greater apparent molecular weight; renal clearance is reduced as a result. This has no direct clinical sequelae but can misleadingly suggest the presence of pancreatic damage.

Measurement of the pancreas-specific amylase can improve the diagnostic specificity of plasma amylase determinations.

## Cholinesterase

This enzyme is secreted by the liver into the blood stream and low plasma activities occur in chronic hepatic dysfunction. It is, however, rarely measured for this reason.

Interest in this enzyme derives from the fact that it hydrolyzes a muscle-relaxant drug, widely used in anaesthesia, called succinylcholine (scoline). Occasionally, patients are found in whom the effect of this drug, which paralyzes respiration, persists for several hours after it has been administered (scoline apnoea). Many of these patients have an abnormal cholinesterase activity.

Four enzyme variants have been recognized on the basis of the activity of the enzyme in the presence of inhibitors: normal, dibucaine-resistant, fluoride-resistant and inactive. Normal homozygotes (genotype $E_1^u E_1^u$) account for 95% of the population, and heterozygotes for dibucaine resistance

$(E_1^u E_1^a)$ 4%. Such individuals do not usually react abnormally to succinylcholine, but homozygotes for dibucaine resistance $(E_1^a E_1^a)$ (0.05%), are at risk of developing scoline apnoea as are patients who produce an inactive enzyme $(E_1^s E_1^s)$. Individuals having an adverse reaction to scoline, and their relatives, should be screened to identify those who have an abnormal cholinesterase so that scoline can be avoided should they need to undergo anaesthesia.

# ENZYME MEASUREMENTS IN DISEASE

## Liver disease

The use of plasma enzyme measurements in liver disease is discussed in detail in *Chapter 5*. In a patient with jaundice, an increase in aspartate or alanine transaminase levels, often to 10 × ULN or more, suggests that the jaundice is due to hepatocellular damage. An increase in ALP of 2–3 × ULN or more is characteristic of cholestasis. Transaminases may be slightly increased with cholestasis, but usually not to more than 2–3 × ULN, while the ALP is not usually more than 2 × ULN in predominantly hepatocellular disease.

A high transaminase activity generally precedes any other biochemical change in early hepatitis, including the increase in plasma bilirubin. An increase in liver-specific ALP is often the only biochemical abnormality in patients with compensated cirrhosis and with space-occupying lesions of the liver, such as secondary tumour deposits. The value of serial enzyme measurements in monitoring patients with liver disease is emphasized in *Chapter 5*.

γ-Glutamyl transferase has become widely adopted as a useful 'liver enzyme', but in the jaundiced patient it provides little information in addition to that obtained from other enzyme and liver function tests.

## Heart disease

Plasma enzyme measurements are often requested routinely in patients with suspected myocardial infarction, although it has been estimated that biochemical confirmation of the diagnosis is required in only 15–30% of patients. Many patients with myocardial infarction will have a classical history of crushing central chest pain, perhaps radiating to the arm or jaw, and typical electrocardiograph (ECG) changes. Myocardial infarction can present atypically, however, or may even be clinically silent, particularly in the elderly (see *Case History 22.1*). The ECG changes may not always be typical, particularly with partial thickness infarcts, when there has been a previous infarction, or in left bundle branch block.

Significant changes in the plasma activities of CK, AST and HBD occur following myocardial infarction. The typical time course of these changes is shown in *Fig. 15.7*. Also

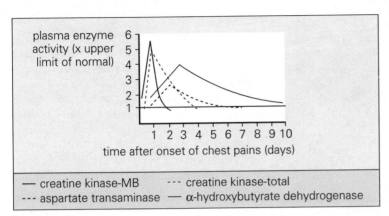

**Fig. 15.7** Plasma enzyme activities after myocardial infarction.

shown is the time course of the change in the MB iso-enzyme of CK; this enzyme appears first and is rapidly cleared from the plasma after myocardial infarction. It is obviously vital when interpreting plasma enzyme changes that the time of the samples relative to the time of the suspected infarct is known and is appropriate. Thus the 'time-window' for CK is between 12 and 36 h but little change in HBD would be expected during this time.

## Diagnosis

Given the lack of specificity of AST, the most useful enzymes for diagnostic purposes in a patient with suspected myocardial infarction are CK (or CK-MB), for early confirmation of the diagnosis, and HBD for the few patients who present (often with atypical clinical features) several days after the suspected infarct.

In patients with a typical history and ECG changes of myocardial infarction, enzyme measurements do not contribute to the initial management. Thrombolytic therapy is usually given unless there is a contraindication to do so. Enzyme measurements may help in patients with chest pain who do not have typical ECG changes. High levels of either total CK (provided that there is no skeletal muscle damage) or CK-MB suggest myocardial infarction. So, too, does the demonstration of an increase of more than 15% in CK-MB or total CK over a four hour period even if both concentrations are within the reference range. However, the ability to demonstrate this for all patients where appropriate requires the provision of a rapid, 24 h analytical service, which may not be practicable.

If no increase in CK occurs in a patient with chest pain, myocardial infarction is unlikely. A failure of CK to fall within the normal time course (*see Fig. 15.7*) suggests that extension of the infarct or a second infarct has occurred. Measurements of other proteins present in cardiac muscle,

e.g., myoglobin, troponins or myosin light chains, have not been shown to be superior to measurements of CK in the management of myocardial infarction. Unlike CK, however, troponin T may be released into the plasma before irreversible damage has occurred (e.g., in unstable angina).

Both myoglobin and CK levels correlate with infarct size and so with prognosis, although this information is rarely of practical value.

If thrombolytic therapy is successful in establishing reperfusion, there is a rapid rise in the plasma concentration of markers of cardiac damage (wash-out phenomenon). Slower rises occur if perfusion remains compromised. Serial measurements of CK-MB or myoglobin appear to provide the earliest biochemical evidence of reperfusion.

### CASE HISTORY 15.1

A recently retired lawyer was admitted to hospital with chest pain which had developed during the evening after a day spent digging in the garden.

There were no specific signs of myocardial infarction on the ECG. He was monitored in the acute coronary unit for 24 h and then transferred to a general ward. His pain subsided rapidly and he was discharged after five days.

### Investigations

| | on admission | 48 h | 72 h |
|---|---|---|---|
| serum: | | | |
| creatine kinase (total) | 300 IU/L | 80 IU/L | 40 IU/L |
| creatine kinase (CK-MB) | 5 IU/L | – | – |

| hydroxybutyrate dehydrogenase | – | – | 70 IU/L |

### Comment

Although the total CK activity was raised, the MB isoenzyme was normal. It was concluded that no myocardial infarction had taken place and that the chest pain was musculoskeletal in origin, related to the unaccustomed exercise. Total CK may reach a peak of greater than 20 × ULN after severe exercise, especially if the individual is unaccustomed to this. The normal HBD supported these conclusions.

### CASE HISTORY 15.2

Two days after sustaining myocardial infarction, confirmed by ECG changes and the finding of a raised total CK, a 54-year-old social worker complained of discomfort in the right epigastrum. On examination, the jugular venous pressure was elevated and the liver was slightly enlarged and tender.

### Investigations

| serum: | bilirubin | 60 μmol/L |
| | alkaline phosphatase | 130 IU/L |
| | aspartate phosphatase | 125 IU/L |
| | creatine kinase | 80 IU/L |
| | | (280 IU/L on admission) |

### Comment

The serum ALP is not usually increased after uncomplicated myocardial infarction but this patient has clinical evidence of right heart failure. Hepatic venous congestion is a consequence of this and can cause a mild, usually transient, cholestatic jaundice, reflected here by the increase in ALP and bilirubin. If it is measured, the ALT is often elevated to an extent commensurate with AST, whereas in uncomplicated myocardial infarction, the ALT is usually normal. In pulmonary embolism, which may mimic myocardial infarction clinically, AST (from an infarcted area of lung) and HBD (from lysis of red blood cells in the embolus and infarct) may be elevated, but the CK is not. Note that the CK has become normal by 48 h (*see Fig. 15.7*).

## Bone disease

Alkaline phosphatase is secreted by osteoblasts and an increased plasma activity is seen in many diseases of bone (*see Chapter 12*); osteoporosis is an important exception to this. Unless there is coexisting osteomalacia or a fracture occurs, the ALP is normal. In multiple myeloma, despite extensive tumour deposition in bone, the ALP is not raised since there is no concomitant increase in osteoblastic activity.

Serial measurements of plasma ALP are of particular value in the assessment of healing in osteomalacia, rickets, renal osteodystrophy and in Paget's disease.

## Muscle disease

Enzymes present within striated muscle cells appear in the plasma in certain muscle diseases, including muscular dystrophies (particularly Duchenne type), polymyositis, toxic and other myopathies, and also after trauma and in ischaemia. Enzyme levels tend to be normal in neurogenic muscle disease, that is, syndromes of denervation such as motor neuron disease and lower motor neuron lesions.

The measurement of plasma CK activity provides the most reliable evidence of muscle disease being more sensitive than, for example, AST or aldolase. However, enzyme measurements do not indicate either the cause or nature of the disorder. Serial measurements of CK are valuable in assessing the response to treatment (usually with corticosteroids) of patients with polymyositis.

### Duchenne muscular dystrophy

Duchenne muscular dystrophy is a sex-linked recessive disorder of muscle which usually affects males. Plasma CK activity may be very high in children with this condition even before the onset of symptoms though levels tend to fall in the later stages when most of the muscle has been destroyed. Female carriers of Duchenne muscular dystrophy are asymptomatic but some 75% have raised plasma CK activities. It is helpful to be able to detect carriers to assist genetic counselling. However, in about one-third of cases of this condition there is no family history, nor is maternal plasma CK raised, suggesting that there is a high incidence of spontaneous mutation giving rise to the disorder.

There are several other forms of muscular dystrophy and an increased plasma CK is not always present. Increases that are present tend to be of a lesser magnitude than those seen in Duchenne muscular dystrophy.

## Malignant disease

Changes in plasma enzyme activities are common in patients with malignant disease. They may be tumour-derived, that is, due to the release of normal or variant enzymes from the tumour itself (for example, acid phosphatase in carcinoma of the prostate, Regan isoenzyme of ALP in carcinoma of lung) or tumour-related, that is, due to the response of surrounding tissues to the presence of the tumour (for example, ALP in hepatic and osseous tumours). A raised plasma ALP may be caused by metastases in a patient known to have carcinoma, but the possibility of metastases from a clinically silent tumour should be considered when a raised ALP is discovered incidentally.

## ENZYMES IN OTHER BODY FLUIDS AND TISSUES

### Red blood cells

Many inherited defects of red cell enzymes have been described, most of which cause a haemolytic anaemia. Glucose 6-phosphate dehydrogenase (G6PD) deficiency is the commonest of these. This enzyme protects red cells against oxidative damage through catalyzing the generation of reduced NADP in the first reaction of the hexose monophosphate shunt. The gene for the enzyme is on the X-chromosome with the result that most affected patients are males. There is a particularly high incidence in tropical Africa and the Middle- and Far-East. G6PD deficiency provides some protection against *Plasmodium falciparum* malaria, which is endemic in these areas.

There is considerable variability in the clinical presentation, due to the existance of a large number of different abnormal enzymes. Many individuals bearing an abnormal enzyme are unaffected; the most frequent manifestation is acute haemolysis, which may be precipitated by infection, drugs such as primaquine and sulphonamides, or a substance in fava beans (favism). Erythrocyte pyruvate kinase deficiency can also cause a haemolytic anaemia, and be a cause of neonatal jaundice. In many hospitals, the responsibility for the measurement of these and other red cell enzymes falls to the haematology rather than the clinical chemistry laboratory.

Measurements of red cell enzymes can be used in the diagnosis of certain vitamin deficiencies (*see Chapter 21*) and in the diagnosis of some inherited metabolic diseases (*see Chapter 16*). Unfortunately, however, the definitive diagnosis of many inherited metabolic diseases requires the measurement of an enzyme in less readily available material, for example, liver or muscle. The measurement of enzymes in cultured amniotic cells and fetal blood for the antenatal diagnosis of inherited metabolic disease is also discussed in *Chapter 16*.

### Urine

The measurement of enzymes in urine is technically difficult because of the presence of inhibitors, but some can usefully be measured, for example, amylase. The latter is excreted in urine and the presence of a high urinary amylase reflects an increase of its activity in the plasma. Measurement of urinary amylase may occasionally be of value in the diagnosis of short-lived episodes of pancreatitis, when the plasma amylase is increased only transiently. In the majority of cases of acute pancreatitis, however, the plasma amylase remains elevated for several days.

Enzymes derived from renal tubular cells can also be detected in the urine and many have been investigated for a possible role in the diagnosis of tubular dysfunction (due, for example, to drugs) and renal graft rejection. The enzyme β-N-acetylglucosaminidase has been used for this purpose.

### Intestinal secretions

The measurement of digestive enzymes in the investigation of malabsorption is considered in *Chapter 6*.

## SUMMARY

The enzymes present in the plasma include those that have a physiological function there, for example, renin and the blood clotting factors, and those that have been released from cells as a result of damage or normal cell turnover. Diagnostic enzymology is principally concerned with the latter and the measurement of enzyme activity in the plasma can give useful diagnostic information concerning the site and extent of tissue damage. Examples of such enzymes include creatine kinase, which is released from cardiac muscle following myocardial infarction and damage to skeletal muscle, and the transaminases, which are widely distributed and are released into the blood in a variety of conditions, including hepatitis, myocardial infarction and skeletal muscle injury.

Alkaline phosphatase (ALP) is present in osteoblasts and an increase in its plasma activity occurs in conditions in which osteoblastic activity is increased, such as osteomalacia and Paget's disease of bone. Plasma ALP activity is also increased in patients with cholestatic jaundice.

Few enzymes that are measured for diagnostic purposes in plasma are tissue specific, but when the origin of increased plasma activity is not obvious either clinically or for other reasons, measurement of the isoenzymes (molecular variants of the enzymes which have similar catalytic activity but a different chemical structure rendering them distinguishable, for example, immunochemically or by electrophoresis) can often provide this information. Thus the measurement of ALP isoenzymes will distinguish between a hepatic, bony or other source for increased plasma activity of this enzyme, and the measurement of isoenzymes of creatine kinase will distinguish between a cardiac or skeletal muscle origin. Another method to improve specificity involves measuring more than one enzyme, since the concentration of different enzymes, and thus the amount released when cells are damaged, varies between different tissues.

Though tending to lack specificity, the measurement of plasma enzyme activity can provide a very sensitive means of detecting tissue damage and can be invaluable in following the course of an illness such as hepatitis or Paget's disease of bone, even though the diagnosis may have been established using another technique.

Other enzymes that are frequently measured for diagnostic purposes include transaminases (released into the plasma in hepatitis and from damaged muscle cells), amylase (elevated in acute pancreatitis) and γ-glutamyl transferase (a sensitive, but non-specific indicator of hepatobiliary disease, also of use in detecting alcohol abuse).

The measurement of enzymes in other body fluids can also provide useful diagnostic information and the measurement of enzymes in tissue samples may provide the definitive diagnosis in certain inherited metabolic diseases; for example, the enzyme galactose 1-phosphate uridyl transferase is deficient from red blood cells in classical galactosaemia. The measurement of enzymes in cultured amniotic cells, obtained by amniocentesis, and in fetal tissue, obtained at fetoscopy, can be used for the antenatal diagnosis of some inherited metabolic diseases and, if acceptable, for termination of pregnancy when an infant is likely to be seriously affected.

## FURTHER READING

Goldberg D M, Werner M & Zaidman J L (eds) (1987) Enzymes and isoenzymes in pathogenesis and diagnosis. *Advances in Clinical Enzymology*, vol. 5. Basel: Karger.

Moss D W (1982) *Isoenzymes*. London: Chapman & Hall.

Adams J E, Abendscein D R Jaffe D S (1993) Biochemical markers of myocardial injury: is MB creatine kinase the choice for the 1990s? *Circulation*, **88**, 750–763.

# 16. Inherited Metabolic Diseases

## INTRODUCTION

Many inherited diseases are known to be due to the genetically determined absence or modification of specific proteins. For example, in sickle cell anaemia, the protein is haemoglobin; in agammaglobulinaemia, antibody production is defective. However, in the majority of such diseases, the protein in question is an enzyme and the effect is to cause a metabolic disorder. Other inherited metabolic diseases may be due to defective receptor synthesis (for exam-

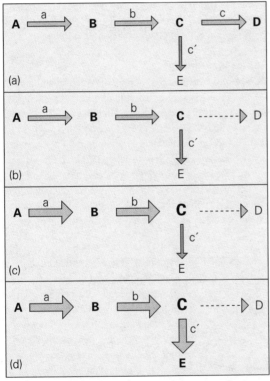

(a)

(b)

(c)

(d)

**Fig. 16.1** Effects of enzyme defects: (a) Product D is synthesized from A by a series of reactions catalyzed by enzymes a, b and c. Enzyme c' catalyzes the formation of a small amount of product E in a minor pathway. (b) In the absence of the enzyme c, no D is synthesized. (c) If the conversion of C to D is blocked, the concentration of the intermediate C, and possibly other precursors, may increase. (d) Increased formation of E may occur if the concentration of C increases and conversion of C to D is blocked.

ple, familial hypercholesterolaemia, which affects the receptor for low density lipoprotein), or to defects involving carrier proteins (for example, cystinuria, in which renal tubular reabsorption of cystine is impaired). Whatever the cause, the clinical features of inherited metabolic diseases stem directly from the metabolic abnormalities to which they give rise. Although individually these conditions are rare, they are of considerable significance; the consequences of many of them are potentially severe but may in some cases be ameliorated if an early diagnosis is made and the appropriate treatment instituted.

The majority of these conditions have an autosomal recessive mode of inheritance, and heterozygotes are usually phenotypically normal. Familial hypercholesterolaemia and most of the porphyrias are important exceptions, being inherited as autosomal dominants.

In a book of this size, it is only possible to discuss a selection of the more common inherited metabolic diseases, together with some that illustrate important general principles.

The recently developed techniques of molecular genetics that are increasingly being used for the diagnosis of inherited metabolic diseases are also throwing considerable light on genetic susceptibility to disease in general. This matter is discussed in more detail later in this chapter.

## EFFECTS OF ENZYME DEFECTS

*Fig. 16.1a* shows a hypothetical metabolic pathway involving the synthesis of product D from substrate A by successive, enzyme-catalyzed reactions through intermediates B and C. If the formation of B from A, catalyzed by enzyme a, is rate-limiting, as the first step unique to a metabolic pathway commonly is, then the concentrations of intermediates B and C will normally be low. The formation of product E from C, catalyzed by enzyme c' is normally a minor pathway, only a small amount of E being formed.

Three distinct sequelae of a lack of enzyme c, that could occur alone or in combination, can be envisaged.

### Decreased formation of the product

Decreased formation of the product of a reaction is the most obvious consequence of a lack of enzyme c (*Fig. 16.1b*). If enzyme c is defective, D cannot be synthesized. Clinical features will arise due to a lack of D if it is an essential product with no alternative pathway for its synthesis.

## Accumulation of the substrate

Accumulation of the substrate (C) of the missing enzyme would also be expected (*Fig. 16.1c*). If this is toxic, clinical manifestations will result. Other, earlier substrates may also accumulate if the reactions prior to the one blocked are reversible. This will occur particularly if there is negative feedback by the product on an early reaction in the pathway, with the result that, with decreased formation of the product, the feedback is lost, thus releasing the inhibition and stimulating the formation of the intermediate substrates.

## Increased formation of other metabolites

Increased formation of E, the product of a minor pathway, may occur if the concentration of C is increased as a result of the enzyme deficiency, the reaction being promoted by a mass action effect (*Fig. 16.1d*). Again, if E is toxic, a clinical syndrome will result.

## INHERITED METABOLIC DISORDERS

### Glucose 6-phosphatase deficiency

Glucose 6-phosphatase deficiency (glycogen storage disease Type 1) exemplifies the production of a clinical syndrome due to lack of formation of the product of an enzyme-catalyzed reaction. Glucose synthesis from glycogen or by gluconeogenesis is blocked (*Fig. 16.2*). Children with this disorder are prone to severe fasting hypoglycaemia since their only source of glucose is dietary carbohydrate.

In this condition, blood glucose must be maintained by constant intragastric infusion of glucose or frequent ingestion of glucose and starch. Glucose 6-phosphatase deficiency also exemplifies the consequences of accumulation of a precursor other than the immediate substrate of the defective enzyme. Glycogen accumulates in the liver causing hepatomegaly. The block in gluconeogenesis results in an accumulation of lactate, and lactic acidosis is a common finding. Hyperlipidaemia results from increased fat synthesis and hyperuricaemia is also frequently present. Accumulation of glycogen in platelets leads to disordered platelet function and a bleeding tendency. Due to the enzyme block, neither glucagon nor adrenaline increase the blood glucose in glucose 6-phosphatase deficiency but the definitive diagnosis is made by demonstrating lack of enzyme activity in a sample of liver obtained by biopsy. At least eight other glycogen storage diseases related to defects in glycogen metabolism are known.

### Galactosaemia

Three enzyme defects can cause galactosaemia, and exemplify the production of a clinical syndrome due to the accumulation of a substrate of the missing enzyme. In classical galactosaemia, the absence of the enzyme galactose 1-phosphate uridyl transferase, which is required for the conversion of galactose to glucose (*Fig. 16.3*), results in the accumulation of galactose 1-phosphate, and the clinical features of the condition are thought to be due directly to the toxicity of this metabolite. In addition, the plasma concentration of galactose is increased and galactose is excreted

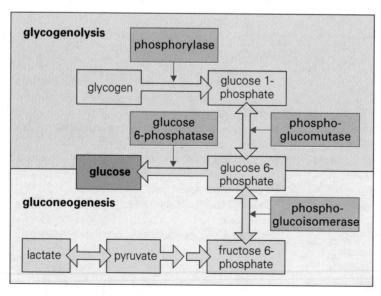

**Fig. 16.2** Glucose production by glycogenolysis and gluconeogenesis. Glucose 6-phosphate is an essential intermediate in the production of glucose by either glycogenolysis or gluconeogenesis. In the absence of glucose 6-phosphatase, glucose cannot be formed from glucose 6-phosphate.

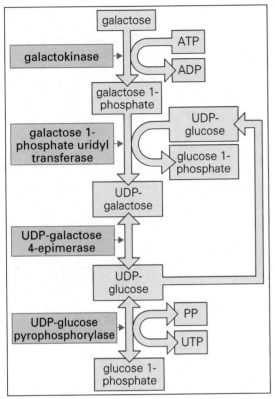

**Fig. 16.3** Metabolic pathway for the conversion of galactose to glucose. UDP = uridine diphosphate.

in the urine. Infants with galactosaemia present with failure to thrive, vomiting, hepatomegaly and jaundice. Septicaemia, particularly due to *E. coli*, is also common. Cataracts may be present as a result of the conversion of excess galactose to galacticol in the lens. There may also be hypoglycaemia and impairment of renal tubular function. Galactose is a reducing sugar and a positive Clinitest in a child, diagnosed as galactosaemic on clinical grounds, merits withdrawal of galactose (and lactose) from the diet pending a definitive diagnosis, based on measurements of galactose 1-phosphate uridyl transferase in erythrocytes. A case of classical galactosaemia is presented in *Case History 22.5*. Deficiency of the enzyme UDP-galactose 4-epimerase causes a similar clinical syndrome, but is much less common. Deficiency of the enzyme galactokinase prevents the phosphorylation of galactose and leads to an increase in the plasma concentration of galactose and thus to galactosuria. Because galactose 1-phosphate formation is blocked, this metabolite does not accumulate and although cataracts may occur, the other clinical features of classical galactosaemia are not seen in galactokinase deficiency.

## Phenylketonuria

Phenylketonuria (PKU) is another condition in which the accumulation of the substrate of the missing enzyme gives rise to a clinical syndrome. The enzyme concerned is phenylalanine hydroxylase, which hydroxylates phenylalanine to form tyrosine (*Fig. 16.4*).

Phenylalanine accumulates in the blood and if the condition is untreated it results in severe learning difficulties, thought to be due directly to the effect of excess phenylalanine on the developing brain. The name of the condition derives from the urinary excretion of phenylpyruvic acid, a phenylketone. This is normally a minor metabolite of phenylalanine but is produced in excess when the normal, major metabolic pathway is blocked. Many children with PKU have fair hair and blue eyes, due to defective melanin synthesis; tyrosine, the formation of which is blocked, is a precursor of this pigment. The diagnosis depends on the demonstration of an abnormally high concentration of phenylalanine in the blood; neonatal screening for the condition is discussed below.

The management involves restricting the dietary intake of phenylalanine using diets based on special proteins and pure amino acids. The plasma concentration of phenylalanine should not be allowed to exceed 0.3 mmol/L in the first year of life when there is rapid brain development, but may, without detriment, be allowed to rise to 0.5 mmol/L by the age of four. The diet is unpalatable, and compliance can be a major problem. Although there has been a tendency to allow less rigorous dietary restriction after the age of ten, many paediatricians now advocate a policy of 'diet for life'. Strict dietary control is essential when a woman with PKU becomes pregnant, since maternal hyperphenylalaninaemia has been shown to affect the fetus *in utero* even if it does not itself have PKU.

Since phenylalanine is an essential amino acid, a certain amount must be provided in the diet and while tyrosine is not normally an essential amino acid, it becomes so when the intake of phenylalanine is limited; adequate quantities must therefore be provided. Thus treated, children in whom a diagnosis of PKU is made shortly after birth will grow and develop normally. Untreated, they rarely achieve an IQ of above 70, and may have to be cared for in institutions for the mentally handicapped for life.

### *Variants*

The enzyme phenylalanine hydroxylase has tetrahydrobiopterin as a coenzyme. A number of variant forms of PKU have been described, some involving a defect in the metabolism of this coenzyme. Several other inherited

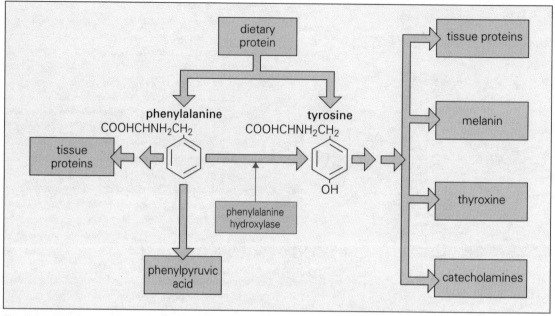

**Fig. 16.4** Metabolic pathway for the conversion of phenylalanine to tyrosine. The site of action of phenylalanine hydroxylase, the enzyme deficient in PKU, is shown.

metabolic diseases are associated with abnormalities of phenylalanine and tyrosine metabolism, including tyrosinosis and alcaptonuria.

### Steroid 21-hydroxylase deficiency

Steroid 21-hydroxylase deficiency, the commonest cause of congenital adrenal hyperplasia, exemplifies the effects of increased activity of a normally minor metabolic pathway, in this case, the synthesis of adrenal androgens (*Fig. 16.5*). Due to the defective synthesis of cortisol, there is a decreased negative feedback to the pituitary and thus increased secretion of ACTH which stimulates the synthesis of adrenal androgens.

### Cystic fibrosis

Cystic fibrosis is a common inherited metabolic disease, with an incidence of approximately 1 in 2500 live births in the United Kingdom. It is a generalized disorder of exocrine secretion, in which the secretions have greatly increased viscosity. The functional defect is impaired chloride transport. Affected children develop recurrent respiratory infections leading to irreversible lung disease, and pancreatic insufficiency leading to malabsorption. Intestinal obstruction may occur in the neonatal period ('meconium ileus'), due to the increased viscosity of faecal material.

In contrast to most inherited metabolic diseases, the basis of the functional defect in cystic fibrosis was not understood until the gene responsible had been identified, cloned and sequenced. This allowed the amino acid sequence and hence the three-dimensional structure of the gene product to be predicted. This protein, known as the 'cystic fibrosis transmembrane conductance regulator' is, as its name implies, involved in the control of transmembrane chloride transport.

Sweat sodium concentration is increased in cystic fibrosis and its measurement provides the definitive test for the condition (a concentration of >80 mmol/L or more being diagnostic). This is too time-consuming to be a practical screening test. Infants with cystic fibrosis have a high concentration of immunoreactive trypsin in their plasma, and this is the basis of a neonatal screening test for the condition in some centres.

Management is directed towards the prevention of respiratory infections by regular physiotherapy and prophylactic antibiotic treatment, and maintenance of adequate nutrition with a good diet; pancreatic enzymes can be added to food to counter the effects of pancreatic insufficiency.

Although the prognosis for children with cystic fibrosis has greatly improved with modern methods of treatment,

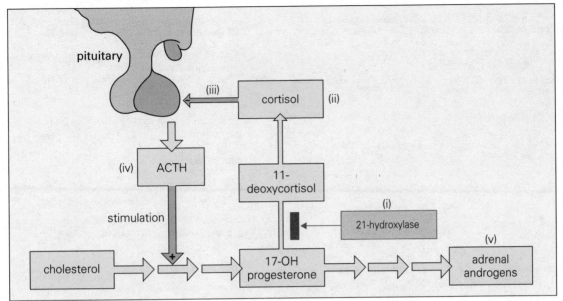

**Fig. 16.5** Adrenal steroid hormone synthesis, showing the increased synthesis of androgens when cortisol synthesis is blocked. Decreased 21-hydroxylase activity (i) leads to decreased cortisol synthesis (ii). Negative feedback to the pituitary (iii) is decreased leading to increased secretion of ACTH (iv). The conversion of cholesterol to 17-hydroxyprogesterone is stimulated, leading to increased synthesis of androgens (v).

this is not achieved without cost to patient and parents. Many patients still die in early adult life.

It is debatable whether the prognosis in cystic fibrosis is significantly improved if the diagnosis is made before the condition presents clinically. For these reasons, the prospect of prenatal (rather than neonatal) screening for cystic fibrosis is an attractive one; this topic is discussed further in a later part of this chapter.

## DIAGNOSIS

The diagnosis of an inherited metabolic disease may be suggested by clinical features and the results of simple tests. However, the diagnosis will not be made if a possible metabolic origin of the symptoms is not considered. Although most inherited metabolic diseases are rare, as a group they are an important cause of failure to thrive in neonates and infants. Effective treatment is now available for many of these conditions and thus it would be tragic if treatment were not given because of a missed diagnosis.

The definitive diagnosis usually depends on the demonstration of decreased activity of the enzyme or concentration of the protein responsible in an appropriate tissue. This may involve biopsy of an affected organ but in some cases the enzyme can be assayed in red or white blood cells. The identification of probable cases by neonatal or prenatal screening merits special consideration. Contrasting examples of the clinical presentation and management of two inherited metabolic diseases are provided by *Case Histories 11.8* and *22.5.*

## NEONATAL SCREENING

Screening is designed to detect individuals affected with a condition before it is apparent clinically. This may be done prenatally, during the neonatal period or later, according to the nature of the condition. The criteria for an effective neonatal screening programme are indicated in *Fig. 16.6.* Neonatal screening is exemplified by the programme for the detection of phenylketonuria.

### Phenylketonuria (PKU)

In many countries, including the United Kingdom and the United States, all babies are screened at birth for PKU (*see also p. 9*) which has an incidence of approximately 1 in 10,000. The screening test involves measurement of the concentration of phenylalanine in a sample of capillary blood taken from a heel-prick six to ten days after birth. The delay after birth is to allow sufficient time for feeding (and hence protein intake) to become established, and for the effect of

| Indications for neonatal screening tests |
|---|
| condition is fatal or leads to severe disability if untreated |
| condition is treatable |
| condition is relatively common |
| reliable, cheap screening test available (no false negatives; some false positives acceptable) |

**Fig.16.6** Indicators for neonatal screening tests.

| Indications for prenatal diagnosis |
|---|
| disease sufficiently serious to justify termination of pregnancy if present |
| disease not amenable to treatment |
| reliable, safe diagnostic test available for use in early pregnancy |
| significant risk of disease occurring |
| parents are willing that pregnancy should be terminated if fetus is shown to be affected |

**Fig. 16.7** Indications for prenatal diagnosis.

maternal metabolism on fetal metabolism to subside. Formerly, the Guthrie test, a microbiological test using a strain of *Bacillus subtilis* in conditions such that growth is only seen if excess phenylalanine is present, was used to detect high concentrations of phenylalanine, but most laboratories now use a chromatographic technique. If the screening test is found to be positive, further, definitive tests are then performed. Many babies are now also screened for congenital hypothyroidism (incidence of 1 in 4500). Economic considerations dictate that a screening test should be cost-effective. Even though it may be technically feasible, it is not economic to screen whole populations for very rare diseases.

In screening for PKU, the concentration of phenylalanine taken as positive is set such that the sensitivity of the test is virtually 100% (all cases are detected). The specificity is greater than 99% (there are very few false positives). However, because the condition is rare, the predictive value of a positive test is low (*see p. 9*); thus most positive screening tests are found not to be due to PKU. This means that some children will be subjected to further investigation and subsequently shown not to have the disease, but this is acceptable if it ensures that genuine cases are not missed.

## PRENATAL DIAGNOSIS

When an inherited disease cannot be successfully treated, or the treatment imposes harsh restrictions on the patient, early prenatal diagnosis will allow parents the option of having the pregnancy terminated. The indications for undertaking prenatal diagnosis are set out in *Fig. 16.7*.

Satisfactory diagnostic tests are available for many inherited metabolic diseases but whether an attempt at prenatal diagnosis is justified depends upon the risk of the procedure. Most of these conditions have a recessive mode of inheritance, and thus prenatal diagnosis should usually be considered only if there is an affected child from a previous pregnancy, if one parent is affected, or if there is a strong family history of the disease. Screening of selected populations may be justified if a disease has a high incidence in a particular population, for example, the lipid storage disorder Tay–Sachs disease in Ashkenazi Jews.

## Maternal and fetal screening

The introduction of the technique of chorionic villus biopsy, to obtain samples of fetal tissue very early in pregnancy, together with the development of techniques of molecular genetic analysis, has revolutionized prenatal diagnosis. The number of inherited disorders which can be diagnosed using these techniques is likely to grow considerably in the next few years.

The techniques available for prenatal diagnosis are summarized in *Fig. 16.8*.

Maternal screening is not diagnostic, but may point to the need to proceed to a more invasive, but definitive test. Although the diseases are not metabolic in origin, a method of screening for open neural tube defects (spina bifida and anencephaly) exemplifies this type of procedure. The screening test involves measurement of α-fetoprotein in maternal blood. If the concentration is raised in relation to the expected value for gestational age and no other cause is found, for example, wrong dates, twins, or spurious results, the woman is then offered amniocentesis for measurement of the protein in amniotic fluid, a more accurate predictor of the presence of a neural tube defect.

| Techniques available for prenatal diagnosis |
| --- |
| maternal plasma screening |
| ultrasonography |
| amniocentesis |
| fetoscopy |
| chorionic villus sampling |
| cordocentesis |

**Fig. 16.8** Techniques available for prenatal diagnosis.

Ultrasound examination is also a valuable diagnostic technique in this context and has replaced measurement of α-fetoprotein in many centres. It is also valuable for the detection of other structural abnormalities. In Down's syndrome, a chromosomal disorder, maternal α-fetoprotein concentration is decreased in relation to gestational age; unconjugated estriol concentrations also tend to be decreased, and those of chorionic gonadotrophin, increased. Measurements of these substances can be used to predict the risk of Down's syndrome, and indicate a need for definitive diagnosis by amniocentesis and chromosomal analysis of cultured amniotic cells.

An inherited metabolic defect may be reflected by the presence of an abnormally high concentration of a metabolite in maternal blood as, for example, in some organic acidaemias, but such metabolites, derived from the fetus, would normally be cleared by maternal enzymes. However, analysis of amniotic fluid, or cultures of amniotic cells obtained by amniocentesis, will give a more accurate reflection of fetal metabolism.

Direct inspection of the fetus is possible by fetoscopy, using a fibreoptic endoscope, during the second trimester of pregnancy. At the same time, a fetal blood sample can be obtained for analysis. If only a fetal blood sample is required, this can be obtained by cordocentesis – transabdominal aspiration from the umbilical cord under ultrasound control.

Chorionic villus sampling allows the collection of fetal tissue earlier in pregnancy, at 11–12 weeks of gestation. Placental tissue, which is of fetal origin and so contains fetal chromosomes, is removed transabdominally or transcervically and can be used for examination of fetal chromosomes

or analysis of fetal DNA. In experienced hands this is a safe procedure, the excess rate of fetal loss being less than 1%. As is the case with all screening procedures, this risk must be considered in relation to the risk that a severe defect is present and will not be diagnosed.

Some of the issues relating to prenatal diagnosis are exemplified by a consideration of screening for cystic fibrosis.

## Cystic fibrosis

Cystic fibrosis is a serious disorder which, despite considerable improvements in treatment, still has a poor prognosis.

If cystic fibrosis occurs in the family of either partner, prenatal diagnosis would be desirable, while informed genetic counselling could be offered if prospective parents could be screened. Indeed, the frequency of heterozygous carriers in the population is approximately 1 in 25 in the United Kingdom, which is sufficiently high to raise the possibility of offering pre-conception screening to all prospective parents, and not just those in families in which cystic fibrosis has occurred.

Unfortunately, cystic fibrosis is a genetically heterogeneous condition; over 50 mutations in the cystic fibrosis gene have been described in patients with the condition. Many of these are 'private' – that is, they occur only in one family – but 65–70% of mutations causing cystic fibrosis in the United Kingdom involve the deletion of a single codon. This mutation is designated ΔF508. Detection of this mutation would be valuable both in carrier screening and prenatal diagnosis in a family in which it is known to occur, but would be of no use in families in which cystic fibrosis is due to other mutations.

Because the ΔF508 mutation is so common, it would be of some value even if used alone in screening prospective parents from unaffected families. Fortunately, in the United Kingdom, three other mutations are sufficiently common that they, together with ΔF508, account for approximately 85% of cases of cystic fibrosis. It is technically possible to test for the presence of these four mutations simultaneously. Since the rare mutations would not be detected, not all carriers would be identified, but if an individual were to test negative to all four probes, the risk of being a carrier would be reduced from 1 in 25 to approximately 1 in 130, and if a male and female both test negative, the risk of their offspring having cystic fibrosis would be reduced from the normal frequency of the condition (approximately 1 in 2500) to approximately 1 in 60,000. About 72% of carrier couples should be detectable by this technique.

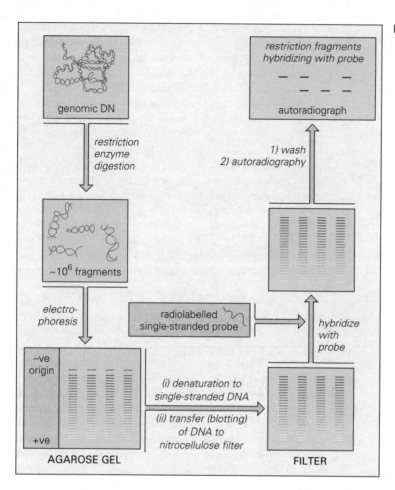

**Fig. 16.9** Restriction analysis.

# DNA ANALYSIS

DNA analysis is now a standard technique for the investigation of an increasing number of inherited disorders. When appropriate, it can be used to genotype fetal tissue for prenatal diagnosis, and to aid genetic counselling by genotyping of individuals, in families in which a particular condition occurs. The index case may have been diagnosed by conventional means, but if the condition is one that is amenable to genetic analysis (*see p. 247*), other members of the family can then be studied. In some cases, notably cystic fibrosis and Duchenne muscular dystrophy, genetic analysis has led to the identification of the gene product.

It is beyond the scope of this book to discuss genetic analysis in detail. The brief descriptions that follow are only examples of the techniques available and the uses to which they may be put. The interested reader is referred to the *Further Reading* for this chapter.

# DNA extraction and processing

Any tissue containing nucleated cells can be used as a source from which DNA can be extracted and purified. This genomic DNA can then be analyzed by amplification of specific sequences using the polymerase chain reaction (PCR, *see p. 248*), or subjected to digestion by restriction enzymes. These bacterial enzymes recognize specific base sequences and cut the double-stranded DNA at sites where they occur to yield a series of 'restriction fragments' (RFs).

The RFs can be separated by electrophoresis, denatured into single strands by heating, and then transferred to a nylon filter or nitrocellulose membrane (Southern blotting). This allows the single-stranded fragments to be transferred without altering their position with respect to each other.

The Southern blot is then analyzed using a DNA probe. This is a piece of single-stranded DNA, labelled usually with $^{32}$P, containing a specific base sequence complementary to the one it is desired to detect. The probe may correspond

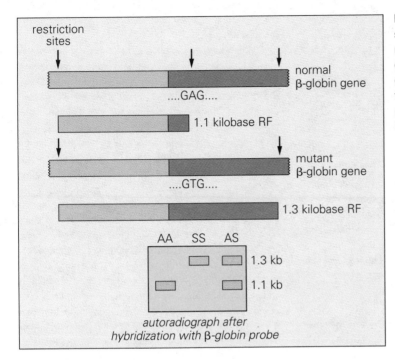

**Fig. 16.10** Restriction analysis for sickle cell haemoglobin (HbS). The mutation responsible for sickle cell disease (GAG to GTG in the β-globin gene) destroys a restriction site. In the presence of the mutation, the gene probe hybridizes with a bigger DNA fragment.

to the gene of interest, to a nearby base sequence ('flanking sequence') or to a more distant sequence. Probes can be native DNA specific to a gene (genomic probes) or synthetic DNA made using the messenger RNA of the gene being studied (complementary, or cDNA). If the sequence recognized by the probe is present in the RFs, the probe will hybridize to it and this can be detected by autoradiography. This technique is illustrated in *Fig. 16.9*.

### Detection of mutations

Some genetic diseases are due to gene deletions. If a suitable probe is available, these can be detected directly by the absence of a specific DNA band on the autoradiograph. Haemophilia A, Duchenne muscular dystrophy and some thalassaemias can be detected in this way.

Occasionally, a point mutation in a gene affects the recognition site of a restriction enzyme. When present, this mutation will alter the size of the RF detected by the probe for that gene. An example is sickle cell disease, in which the point mutation responsible for the amino acid substitution in haemoglobin prevents recognition of a restriction site by the enzyme *MstII*. As a result, a larger RF is produced when the mutation is present (*Fig. 16.10*).

If the base sequence at the site of a mutation is known, oligonucleotide probes (usually about 19 bases) capable of recognizing the normal and mutant sequences ('allele-specific oligonucleotides') can be synthesized. In homozygotes for mutation, only the probe corresponding to the mutant sequence will hybridize with that individual's DNA; only the normal probe will hybridize to DNA from homozygous normal individuals; while both will hybridize to DNA from heterozygotes (*see Fig. 16.13*).

### Genetic analysis by detection of restriction fragment length polymorphism

When the gene responsible for a disease has not been identified, it may be possible to detect the gene if it lies near a DNA sequence that can be detected. Over the entire human genome, about one base in every 150 is polymorphic, that is, varies between individuals. About one in six of these random base changes either creates or destroys a restriction site. Thus, overall, a potential restriction site is present at kilobase intervals along the DNA, and the presence or absence of these in different people will result in restriction enzymes cutting their DNA into RFs of different lengths ('restriction fragment length polymorphism', RFLP). If in family studies it can be shown that a given RFLP is always, or usually, associated with an inherited disease, it can be inferred that the relevant restriction site is located in the vicinity of the gene responsible for the disease. The presence of the RFLP can then be used to predict the presence of the gene in another member of the family and, prenatally,

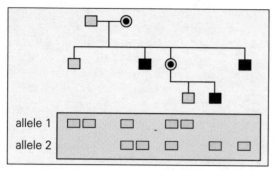

**Fig. 16.11** Polymorphism produces two alleles (1 and 2) which are recognized by an X-chromosomal DNA probe linked to the gene for Becker's muscular dystrophy. The disease segregates with maternal allele 2, which is thus a marker for the disease gene.
Adapted from *ABC of Clinical Genetics* published by the British Medical Journal.

in fetal tissue. The further the restriction site from the gene, the greater the chance of them segregating independently because of recombination. In practice, RFLPs showing less than 5% recombination are useful. It should be stressed that the use of this technique for prenatal diagnosis requires prior study of the family, to find an 'informative' RFLP, that is, one that is linked with the disease gene. An example of the use of this technique, in this case for the detection of Becker's muscular dystrophy, is shown in *Fig. 16.11*. Becker's muscular dystrophy is a less severe condition than Duchenne muscular dystrophy but, like the latter condition, is due to a mutation in the dystrophin gene.

### Gene amplification: the polymerase chain reaction

DNA extraction is a cumbersome process and RFLP analysis as described above requires relatively large amounts of DNA. The polymerase chain reaction (PCR) is a technique that allows selective amplification of a base sequence of interest, in order to make it accessible to analysis. Indeed, it has proved possible to amplify specific base sequences from single molecules of DNA. Since a single cell can be removed from a very early (8–16 cells) embryo without an adverse effect on its later development, this technique makes it possible to ensure that an embryo from an *in vitro* fertilization does not carry a particular mutant gene before it is implanted – i.e., pre-implantation diagnosis.

The technique is illustrated in *Fig. 16.12*. Oligonucleotide primers complementary to unique flanking sequences are used to direct the synthesis of the intervening DNA, and the process is repeated many times to produce sufficient material for analysis.

PCR is an extremely powerful technique which can be applied in several ways. It can be used to amplify a base sequence spanning a restriction site, for RFLP analysis; sufficient material is produced such that it can be visualized directly, by fluorescent staining, without the need for a radioactive probe. PCR can be used to provide sufficient material to test for the presence of a mutant gene using a specific oligonucleotide probe (*Fig. 16.13*), or to identify normal or mutant sequences by the use of appropriate oligonucleotide primers ('competitive oligonucleotide priming PCR'). New techniques, expanding the applicability of PCR in molecular genetic analysis, continue to be introduced.

It should be appreciated that PCR is only possible if suitable primers can be synthesized; for this, it is necessary to know the precise base sequence in the region of DNA of interest. Thus if PCR is to be used for the direct detection of a mutant site, the base sequence at this site must be known. The number of inherited diseases for which this information is available is increasing rapidly and PCR is being increasingly used as a basis for prenatal diagnosis and carrier detection.

### Conclusion

Direct detection of mutant genes is particularly suited to the diagnosis of homogeneous genetic disorders, that is, ones which are always due to the same mutation. As discussed for cystic fibrosis, when a disease can be due to any one of several mutations in the same gene, 100% sensitivity in diagnosis would require the use of a battery of probes, which between them could detect all the mutations. If these are not available, diagnosis and screening must continue to depend at least in part on the detection of the effects of the mutation, usually by measurement of the gene product. And this technique, or, if applicable, the detection of linkage through RFLP analysis, will continue to be used for conditions where the responsible gene has not yet been identified.

It would be wrong to give the impression that these techniques of molecular genetics are applicable only to comparatively rare inherited metabolic diseases due to single gene defects. Genetic factors play an important part in the aetiology of many common conditions, including hypertension, some cancers and coronary heart disease. For example, mutations in the p53 tumour suppressor gene have been detected in more than half of some groups of patients with cancer. Identification of the genes involved in such conditions will make it possible to screen for them, and thus for susceptibility to the conditions. Such knowledge would potentially be a powerful tool in preventative medicine, but its application poses considerable ethical questions.

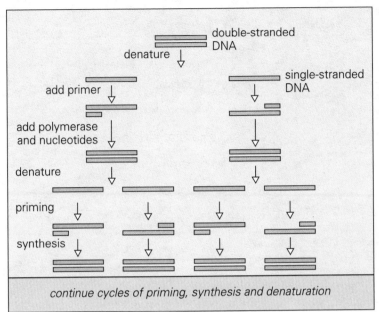

**Fig. 16.12** The polymerase chain reaction. Single-stranded oligonucleotides, complementary to sequences flanking the region of DNA to be amplified, are mixed in solution with the DNA, nucleotides and a DNA polymerase. The temperature is raised to 90°C to denature the DNA, lowered to 50° to allow the oligonucletoides to bind to the DNA ('annealing') and then raised to 70° to allow optimal action of the polymerase enzyme. This cycle is repeated 30–40 times, theoretically resulting in the synthesis of $2^{30-40}$ copies of the DNA template.

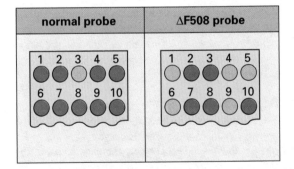

**Fig. 16.13** Gene probing for carriers of cystic fibrosis. Genomic DNA has been amplified using the polymerase chain reaction and the product spotted on to duplicate nylon filters. These have been exposed to $^{32}$P-labelled probes for the normal allele and ΔF508 mutation; autoradiography has been used to detect hybridization. Position 1 is PCR products from a homozygous normal control, position 2 from heterozygous carrier of the ΔF508 mutation, position 3 from a patient with cystic fibrosis (homozygous for the ΔF508 mutation). Positions 4–10 are samples for screening: 4, 5, 6 & 9 are found to be homozygous normal, 7, 8 & 10 are carriers. Adapted from Skogerboe, K J *et al.* (1990) *Clinical Chemistry,* **36**; 1984–1986.

## TREATMENT

Possible approaches to the treatment of inherited metabolic diseases are given in *Fig. 16.4.*

### Restriction of substrate intake

This is exemplified in the treatment of galactosaemia. If all foodstuffs containing galactose and lactose are removed from the diet, clinical symptoms regress. Similarly, hereditary fructose intolerance (*see p. 180*) is asymptomatic if fructose is avoided. The management is less straightforward, however, if the substrate is essential for life. In PKU, the metabolism of phenylalanine to tyrosine is blocked (*see p. 241*), but phenylalanine is an essential amino acid and must therefore be provided in the diet to allow normal growth and development.

### Supply of missing product

Congenital adrenal hyperplasia is managed by giving cortisol, production of which is impaired in this condition. In salt-losing types, a mineralocorticoid must also be given.

### Addition of vitamin cofactors

If the defective enzyme has a vitamin cofactor, the supply of large amounts of the vitamin may, by a mass action

249

| Inherited metabolic disease treatment strategies | |
|---|---|
| **Treatment** | **Example** |
| restriction of substrate intake | galactose in galactosaemia |
| supply of missing product | cortisol in congenital adrenal hyperplasia |
| supply of vitamin cofactors | pyridoxal phosphate in homocystinuria |
| increased excretion of toxic substances | copper in Wilson's disease |
| replacement of missing protein | lysosomal enzyme disorders |
| replacement of mutant gene | organ grafting |

**Fig. 16.14** Treatment strategies for inherited metabolic disease.

effect, increase cofactor binding and thus enzyme activity. Many enzymes have separate catalytic and regulatory sites and amino acid substitution due to a mutant gene may affect either of such sites, or alter the way in which they interact. Homocystinuria is a condition in which the conversion of homocysteine to cystathionine is blocked. The enzyme involved, cystathionine β-synthase, requires pyridoxal phosphate as a cofactor, and giving large amounts of this vitamin may be of therapeutic benefit in some cases. Some organic acidaemias may similarly respond to high-dose vitamin supplementation.

## Increased excretion of toxic substances

This approach is used in the treatment of Wilson's disease (*see p. 84*) to remove the excess copper which is responsible for the tissue damage in this condition. D-Penicillamine forms a soluble complex with copper which is then readily excreted in the urine. This drug is also used in the treatment of cystinuria, an inherited disorder characterized by defective tubular reabsorption of cystine and the dibasic amino acids, lysine, ornithine, and arginine. Cystine is relatively insoluble and there is a marked tendency to urinary stone (calculus) formation. Cystine may be kept in solution if the urine is kept sufficiently dilute and alkaline. If calculi continue to form, penicillamine may be used; the drug complexes with cysteine (from which cystine is derived) and reduces the urinary excretion of cystine.

## Replacement of missing protein

If the replacement of a missing protein were to be a feasible method of treatment it would need to be repeated at regular intervals as there is a continuous turnover of proteins in the body. Replacement of gammaglobulins is the mainstay of treatment of agammaglobulinaemia and, when necessary, factor VIII can be given in haemophilia. With the great majority of inherited metabolic diseases the defective protein is intracellular and thus replacement is not feasible. Attempts have been made to treat some disorders involving lysosomal enzymes by infusing liposomes (lipid droplets) containing the missing enzyme into the blood stream. Unfortunately, the potential of this novel approach to treatment is limited.

## Replacement of the defective gene

This should allow normal synthesis of the product of the gene, for example an enzyme. The technical problems are considerable, including not only the engineering of the gene, but also its insertion into a sufficient number of the appropriate somatic cells in such a way that its activity is subject to normal regulation. Over-expression of a normal gene might be as harmful as the effect of the abnormal gene. Nevertheless, this technique is now the subject of clinical trials.

Organ grafting may be appropriate in some conditions; liver transplantation has been used successfully in patients with Wilson's disease and $\alpha_1$-antitrypsin deficiency who have developed hepatic failure and patients with renal failure due to cystinuria have been treated by kidney transplantation. Organ grafting effectively replaces the missing or mutant gene and the engrafted organ synthesizes the normal gene product.

# SUMMARY

Inherited metabolic diseases are the result of gene mutations, which either prevent the synthesis of a protein or cause the production of an abnormal protein molecule. In the majority of these disorders, the protein is an enzyme and the result is a decrease in catalytic activity. There are several hundred known examples; most of them are rare. Their effects vary in severity from the completely benign (e.g., renal glycosuria) to the invariably fatal (e.g., Tay–Sach's disease). In some inherited metabolic diseases, the defective or missing protein is a receptor (e.g., familial hypercholesterolaemia) or a transport protein (e.g., cystinuria).

Most of these conditions have an autosomal recessive mode of inheritance; heterozygotes are usually phenotypically normal. Some, notably most of the porphyrias (see Chapter 17), are unusual in having a dominant mode of inheritance.

A decrease in catalytic activity can have a number of consequences. In the case of an enzyme involved in a synthetic pathway, there could be decreased synthesis of the product of the enzyme or pathway, accumulation of the substrate and other precursor metabolites, or increased activity in a usually minor pathway which has, as its starting point, one of the intermediates which accumulates. Thus the clinical effects may relate to either decreased levels of a product of the pathway or increased levels of other metabolites (which may be toxic in excess), or to a combination of these.

The definitive diagnosis of an inherited metabolic disorder requires either measurement of the activity of the relevant enzyme, a procedure which may necessitate tissue biopsy unless the enzyme is present in blood cells, or detection of the defective gene. The diagnosis can, however, often be inferred from the clinical features and measurements of the concentrations of metabolites or precursors of the enzyme, and may then be confirmed by the response to treatment.

Many inherited metabolic disorders can be screened for in utero when there is a significant risk of a fetus being affected, for instance when a previous child is known to have had the condition or when there is a strong family history of the disorder. Neonatal screening, though technically feasible for many inherited metabolic disorders, is widely practised in the general population only for phenylketonuria; congenital hypothyroidism is also screened for in the newborn. Screening tests must be highly sensitive and specific; the condition in question should have severe consequences which can be ameliorated by early treatment (or avoided by termination of the pregnancy in the case of prenatal screening); and the condition must occur sufficiently frequently in the population being screened for the exercise to be worthwhile.

Some inherited metabolic disorders can be treated relatively simply. Congenital adrenal hyperplasia, a group of conditions in each of which one of the enzymes involved in the synthesis of cortisol is defective, can be treated by replacing the missing product, cortisol. Others, such as galactosaemia and phenylketonuria, can be treated by dietary modifications which prevent the accumulation of toxic metabolites. A few metabolic disorders are due to decreased ability of the enzyme to bind a coenzyme; giving large amounts of the coenzyme may overcome this by a mass action effect and restore catalytic activity to normal.

The definitive treatment for an inherited metabolic disease would be replacement of the defective protein or gene. Attempts have been made to treat some lysosomal enzyme deficiencies by enzyme replacement but such treatment needs to be repeated frequently and has other disadvantages. Organ transplantation for the renal failure which can occur in cystinuria or the liver failure in Wilson's disease effectively replaces the defective gene, and considerable research is taking place into techniques to allow modification or replacement of specific genes in patients with inherited metabolic diseases.

# FURTHER READING

Davies K E & Read A P (1988) *Molecular Basis of Inherited Disease*. Oxford: IRL Press.

Holton J B (1994) *The Inherited Metabolic Diseases* 2nd edition, Edinburgh: Churchill Livingstone.

Kingston M (1994) *ABC of Clinical Genetics* 2nd edition. London: BMJ Publishing Group.

Scriver C R, Beaudet A L, Sly W S & Valle D (eds) (1994) *The Metabolic Basis of Inherited Disease*. 7th edition. New York: McGraw-Hill Book Company.

Trent R J (1993) *Molecular Medicine: An Introductory Text for Students*. Edinburgh: Churchill Livingstone.

# 17. Haemoproteins, Porphyrins and Iron

## INTRODUCTION

Haemoglobin, the oxygen-carrying pigment of blood, consists of a protein, globin, and four haem molecules (*Fig. 17.1*). Globin comprises two pairs of polypeptide chains (the principal haemoglobin in adults, haemoglobin A, HbA, has two α- and two β-chains) and each polypeptide binds one haem molecule. Haem consists of a tetrapyrrole ring, protoporphyrin IXα, linked to an iron II ion ($Fe^{2+}$) to which oxygen becomes reversibly bound during oxygen transport. Other haemoproteins include myoglobin, which binds oxygen in skeletal muscle, and the cytochromes, enzymes responsible for catalyzing many oxidative processes in the body.

The major part of the body's iron is present in haemoglobin and the major product of porphyrin metabolism is haem. It is thus convenient to discuss the chemical pathology of the haemoproteins, the porphyrins and iron together, although disorders affecting any one of these do not necessarily (indeed do not often) involve the others.

## HAEMOPROTEINS

### Haemoglobin and haemoglobinopathies

Haemoglobin is a very accessible protein and has been extensively studied. The haemoglobinopathies (genetically determined abnormalities of haemoglobin synthesis) fall into two groups: qualitative, involving amino acid substitutions, and quantitative disorders, known as thalassaemias.

#### Amino acid substitutions

Here there is a single amino acid substitution in one of the polypéptide chains. Over 200 such variants have been described. Some of these involve amino acids which are not structurally or functionally vital, and are clinically silent; others have important consequences including effects on haemoglobin solubility (for example, HbS, the haemoglobin of sickle cell disease), stability and oxygen-carrying capacity.

#### Thalassaemias

In the thalassaemias there is an inherited defect in the rate of synthesis of one of the globin chains. This can involve the α-chains (α-thalassaemia), or the β-chains (β-thalassaemia). The consequences include ineffective erythropoiesis, haemolysis and a variable degree of anaemia. The

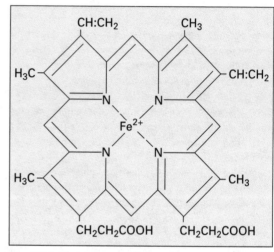

**Fig. 17.1** The structure of haem.

clinical severity varies between the different thalassaemias. Some are clinically silent except during periods of stress such as severe infection or pregnancy when anaemia may develop, while others cause severe, persistent anaemia. When α-chain synthesis is totally absent, affected infants are either stillborn or die shortly after birth.

#### Investigation of haemoglobinopathies

The investigation and management of the haemoglobinopathies are the province of the haematologist, and these disorders are not considered further in this book. It is, however, of relevance to point out that as a result of the amino acid substitution, some abnormal haemoglobins have a different electrophoretic mobility from normal adult haemoglobin (HbA). Indeed, this property is utilized in their identification. Because of this, however, they may co-migrate with $HbA_1$ (the glycated haemoglobin that is present in increased concentration in the blood of patients with diabetes mellitus) when an electrophoretic technique is used for its quantification, and thus give a falsely high result. This also applies to fetal haemoglobin (HbF) which, though normally present in only trace amounts in the blood from a few weeks after birth, is present in significant quantities in some haemoglobinopathies and thalassaemias, and in the benign condition, hereditary persistence of fetal haemoglobin (HPFH).

## Abnormal derivatives of haemoglobin

### *Methaemoglobin*

Methaemoglobin is oxidized haemoglobin, with iron in the $Fe^{3+}$ form. It is incapable of carrying oxygen. A small amount is normally produced spontaneously in red blood cells but can be enzymatically reduced back to haemoglobin. Excessive methaemoglobin (methaemoglobinaemia) can be congenital or acquired. It can occur in some haemoglobinopathies, with an inherited deficiency of the reductase enzyme, and also as a result of the ingestion of large amounts of certain drugs, such as sulphonamides. In toxic methaemoglobinaemia, the presence of methaemalbumin (formed as a result of haemolysis of red cells containing methaemoglobin) imparts a brown colour to the plasma, while the presence of free methaemoglobin may give the urine a similar colour.

The major clinical manifestation of congenital methaemoglobinaemia is cyanosis. Acute toxic methaemoglobinaemia causes symptoms of anaemia and may lead to vascular collapse and death. Methaemoglobinaemia, except when due to a haemoglobinopathy, can be treated with methylene blue or ascorbic acid, agents which reduce the abnormal derivative back to haemoglobin.

### *Sulphaemoglobin*

Sulphaemoglobin, a group of poorly characterized derivatives of haemoglobin, is often formed together with methaemoglobin. It is also incapable of carrying oxygen but cannot be converted back to haemoglobin.

### *Carboxyhaemoglobin*

Carboxyhaemoglobin (COHb) is formed from haemoglobin in the presence of carbon monoxide, the affinity of the pigment for this gas being some 200 times greater than for oxygen. Because of this, only small quantities of carbon monoxide in the inspired air can result in the formation of large amounts of COHb and hence greatly reduce the oxygen-carrying capacity of the blood. Small amounts of COHb (less than 2%) are commonly present in the blood of urban dwellers and greater amounts (up to 10%) may be found in the blood of tobacco smokers.

### *Haematin*

Haematin is oxidized ($Fe^{3+}$) haem. It is released from methaemoglobin when red cells containing this pigment are haemolyzed but can be formed from free haem in severe intravascular haemolysis. Haematin combines with albumin in the blood stream to form methaemalbumin.

Methaemalbuminaemia is sometimes a feature of acute haemorrhagic pancreatitis.

These various derivatives of haemoglobin can be detected by their spectral characteristics, and quantified when necessary.

# PORPHYRINS

Protoporphyrin IXα, which combines with iron to form haem, is the end-product of a series of complex reactions. The first step that is unique to this pathway is the combination of glycine and succinyl-CoA to form δ-aminolaevulinic acid (ALA), a reaction catalyzed by the enzyme ALA synthase (*Fig. 17.2*). Two molecules of ALA then condense to form porphobilinogen (PBG), in a reaction catalyzed by PBG synthase (also known as ALA dehydratase).

The first porphyrins (strictly, porphyrinogens, *see below*) are formed when four molecules of PBG condense together. The initial product of this reaction, catalyzed by hydroxymethylbilane synthase (PBG deaminase) is hydroxymethylbilane. In the presence of uroporphyrinogen III cosynthase, this is converted to uroporphyrinogen III. In the absence of this enzyme, hydroxymethylbilane is converted non-enzymatically to uroporphyrinogen I. A series of enzyme-catalyzed reactions through isomers of the III series leads to the formation of protoporphyrin IXα. Haem is formed when iron is incorporated into the molecule in a reaction catalyzed by ferrochelatase.

The porphyrinogens are themselves unstable and become oxidized to their corresponding porphyrins when they are excreted in faeces or urine. Porphyrinogens and porphyrin precursors are colourless. Porphyrins are dark red in colour and intensely fluorescent. The major sites of porphyrin synthesis are the liver and the erythroid bone marrow.

The rate-limiting step in this sequence of reactions is the first, catalyzed by ALA synthase, which is susceptible to inhibition by the end-product, haem.

## The porphyrias

These are a group of inherited diseases in which a partial deficiency of one of the enzymes of porphyrin synthesis leads to decreased formation of haem and thus, by releasing ALA synthase from inhibition, results in the formation of excessive quantities of porphyrin precursors (ALA and PBG) or porphyrins. When precursors are produced in excess, the clinical manifestations are primarily neurological (the precursors are neurotoxins). When porphyrins themselves are the major product, the predominant feature is photosensitivity; the porphyrins absorb light and become excited, inducing the formation of toxic free radicals. The porphyrias are diagnosed on the basis of their clinical features and the pattern of porphyrins and precursors present in blood and excreted in faeces and urine.

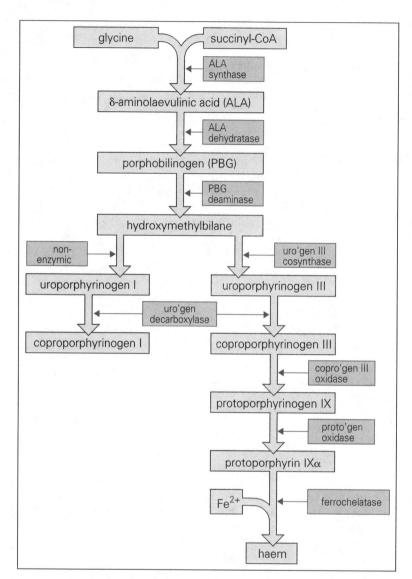

**Fig. 17.2** The biosynthesis of porphyrins. PBG deaminase is also known as hydroxy-methylbilane synthase and ALA dehydratase as PBG synthase.

The porphyrias are classified as acute or non-acute, according to their clinical presentation, and hepatic or erythropoietic, depending on the major site of abnormal metabolism (*Fig. 17.3*). All the porphyrias are rare. Cutaneous hepatic porphyria is the most common but many cases are probably not inherited. Of the purely genetic types, acute intermittent porphyria is the most common, with a prevalence in the United Kingdom, where it occurs more frequently than in many countries, of only 1–2 cases per 100,000 of the population. Unusually for inherited metabolic diseases, their mode of inheritance is autosomal dominant, with the exception of congenital erythropoietic porphyria and ALA dehydratase deficiency porphyria (autosomal recessive). The features of the porphyrias are summarized in *Fig. 17.4*. The genes for the enzymes involved in porphyrin synthesis have been identified and cloned but the porphyrias are genetically heterogenous; this hinders the application of molecular biological techniques to the identification of carriers and to screening for porphyrias.

## Acute porphyrias

Acute intermittent porphyria (AIP) is the commonest of these. Photosensitivity is never a feature of AIP although it may occur in patients with hereditary coproporphyria and variegate porphyria.

| Classification of the porphyrias | | |
|---|---|---|
| **acute** | acute intermittent porphyria | **hepatic** |
| | hereditary coproporphyria | |
| | variegate porphyria | |
| **chronic** | cutaneous hepatic porphyria | |
| | congenital erythropoietic porphyria | **erythropoietic** |
| | erythropoietic protoporphyria | |

**Fig. 17.3** Classification of the porphyrias. In addition to these conditions, an acute porphyria known as aminolaevulinic dehydratase deficiency porphyria has been described, but is exceedingly rare.

| Classification and characteristics of the porphyrias | | | | | | | | |
|---|---|---|---|---|---|---|---|---|
| condition | deficient enzyme | inheritance | course | erythroid/ hepatic | sympto-matology | abnormal porphyrin concentrations | | |
| | | | | | | red cells | urine | stools |
| **ALA dehydratase deficiency porphyria** | ALA dehydratase | AR | acute | E | N | proto | **ALA** | |
| **acute intermittent porphyria** | PBG deaminase | AD | acute | H | N | | ALA, **PBG** | |
| **hereditary coproporphyria** | copro'gen oxidase | AD | acute | H | N, P | | ALA, PBG **copro-** | copro- |
| **variegate porphyria** | proto'gen oxidase | AD | acute | H | N, P | | ALA, PBG **copro-** | copro- **proto-** |
| **cutaneous hepatic porphyria** | uro'gen decarboxylase | variable† | chronic | H | P | | **uro-** | isocopro- |
| **congenital erythropoietic porphyria** | uro'gen III cosynthase | AR | chronic | E | P | uro-* copro-* | **uro-*** copro-* | copro-* |
| **erythropoietic protoporphyria** | ferrochelatase | AD | chronic | E | P | **proto** | | proto |

\* type I isomers    †AD in some families    N = neurological    P = photosensitizing

**Fig. 17.4** Features of the porphyrias. The most important abnormalities are in bold; the changes shown for the acute porphyrias may only be present during an attack.

## Clinical features

These conditions share the characteristics of acute attacks separated by long periods of complete remission. The clinical features of acute attacks are summarized in *Fig. 17.5*. Abdominal pain and psychiatric disturbances are nearly always present; peripheral neuropathy occurs in some 60% of patients. They can be precipitated by various factors, including many drugs (*Fig. 17.5*); most frequently implicated are barbiturates, oral contraceptives and alcohol. These probably act by increasing the activity of ALA synthase, in many cases by increasing the synthesis of hepatic cytochrome P450 and hence the demand for haem, thereby decreasing intrahepatic haem concentrations and releasing the enzyme from inhibition. Some drugs, notably the sulphonamides, inhibit PBG deaminase directly. Whatever the cause, the resulting increased activity of the metabolic pathway increases the formation of metabolites before the enzyme block.

Hormonal factors are also extremely important; symptoms rarely occur before puberty and may fluctuate in relation to menstruation or pregnancy. Women are affected more commonly than men. In some 90% of individuals who inherit the defective gene for AIP, the disease remains clinically latent throughout adult life. In those in whom attacks do occur there is an additional (acquired) enzyme deficiency, of steroid 5α-reductase, which may alter the metabolism of endogenous steroids in favour of the formation of epimers that induce ALA synthase.

## Diagnosis

In all acute porphyrias, excessive ALA and PBG are excreted in the urine during an acute attack. In suspicious circumstances, such as unexplained acute abdominal pain, peripheral neuropathy or psychosis, the urine can be tested for PBG by a simple screening test, which if positive will indicate the need to carry out further investigations (*see Fig. 17.4*) to establish the precise diagnosis. When an acute porphyria has been diagnosed, blood relatives should be screened for latent disease, and if necessary advised concerning the avoidance of precipitating factors. It is important to appreciate that the concentrations of porphyrins and their precursors in the blood, urine and faeces may be normal except during an attack, with the result that it may be necessary to measure the defective enzyme itself to establish who is at risk.

## Management

Once the diagnosis of acute porphyria has been made, every effort must be made to prevent attacks by the avoidance of precipitating factors. During an attack, any such features must be identified and treated appropriately. General supportive measures include maintenance of fluid and electrolyte balance, adequate carbohydrate intake (intravenous glucose is often beneficial) and physiotherapy. Pain can be safely relieved with narcotic analgesics. Intravenous infusion of haematin, which decreases the activity of ALA synthase, has been used with success.

| Acute attacks of porphyrias | | |
|---|---|---|
| **Clinical features** | | **Factors involved** |
| **Gastrointestinal**<br>abdominal pain<br>vomiting<br>constipation<br><br>**Peripheral neuropathy**<br>pain, stiffness and muscle weakness<br>  (limb and girdle muscles > trunk;<br>  upper limbs > lower;<br>  proximal > distal)<br>paraesthesiae, numbness | **Central nervous system**<br>seizures<br>depression<br>hysteria<br>psychosis<br><br>**Cardiovascular**<br>sinus tachycardia<br>systemic hypertension | anaesthesia<br>drugs<br>pregnancy<br>premenstrual<br>infection<br>stress<br>starvation<br>alcohol |

**Fig. 17.5** Clinical features and factors involved in acute attacks of porphyria; gastrointestinal, neuropsychiatric and cardiovascular derangements are all common.

## CASE HISTORY 17.1

A 19-year-old woman was admitted to hospital with colicky abdominal pain, which had started suddenly 12 h before. She had vomited several times but had not opened her bowels since the pain started. Her abdomen was tender on examination but was otherwise normal. Her pulse was 140/min and her blood pressure was 160/100 mmHg. After she had been taken to the ward for observation, a nurse in the emergency room noticed that a specimen of the patient's urine, which had been collected for routine testing, had become a deep red colour although it had been normal when first passed. On being informed of this, the admitting doctor questioned the patient further and examined her more carefully. She said that she had also noticed cramping pains in her arms and was found to have bilateral wrist drop.

### Investigations

screening test for urinary
   porphobilinogen:              strongly positive

quantitative analysis of urine:
| | |
|---|---|
| porphobilinogen | very high |
| δ-aminolaevulinic acid | very high |
| uroporphyrin | slightly raised |
| coproporphyrin | slightly raised |

### Comment

Acute porphyrias may present as an acute abdomen; systemic hypertension and sinus tachycardia are often present. They are of course a very uncommon cause of abdominal pain and the diagnosis may be missed, at least initially. In this case the nurse's observation of the changed colour of the urine was crucial and led to the presumptive diagnosis of an acute porphyria being made, supported clinically by the evidence of neuropathy and also by the positive screening test for PBG. There was no evidence of photosensitivity and the very high urinary excretion of porphyrin precursors, with only slightly increased excretion of intact porphyrins, favours a diagnosis of acute intermittent porphyria rather than variegate or hereditary coproporphyria, both of which are anyway much less common.

The patient's symptoms and signs resolved rapidly with appropriate treatment. It transpired that she had started taking an oral contraceptive pill a few days before. The diagnosis was later confirmed by the demonstration of a reduced red cell hydroxymethylbilane synthase activity; she was advised to use an alternative method of contraception and told which drugs she should avoid. She remained well thereafter and no problems arose when she underwent elective surgery (cholecystectomy) three years later, nor during a subsequent pregnancy.

## Non-acute porphyrias

Erythropoietic protoporphyria and congenital erythropoietic porphyria are both very rare. Photosensitivity occurs with both but is much more severe with the latter, causing extensive blistering and leading to tissue destruction and scarring.

Cutaneous hepatic porphyria (known as porphyria cutanea tarda and symptomatic porphyria) also presents with photosensitivity. The initial lesion is just erythema but this progresses to the formation of vesicles and bullae, and eventually to scarring and pigmentation. This porphyria can be inherited (familial, type II) (15–20% of cases) or acquired (sporadic, type I). In both types there is an approximately 50% reduction in hepatic uroporphyrinogen decarboxylase activity in the liver; in type II, this deficiency occurs in all tissues. Although the acquired type can develop spontaneously, it is more frequently seen in association with excessive alcohol ingestion (often with liver disease) (90% of cases) or as a consequence of exposure to hepatotoxins or drugs.

### Management

Management involves the identification and removal of precipitating factors; venesection to remove excess iron from the liver (iron inhibits uroporphyrinogen III cosynthase and uroporphyrinogen decarboxylase); avoidance of direct sunlight, and the use of barrier creams to protect the skin.

## Other causes of porphyrinuria

Increased urinary porphyrin excretion can occur in conditions other than the porphyrias. In patients with liver disease, particularly with cholestasis, the normal biliary excretion of porphyrins is impaired and there is increased urinary excretion – just as occurs with bilirubin. Porphyrinuria can also result from acquired defects in haem synthesis, as for example in lead poisoning. Lead inhibits ALA dehydratase (*see Fig. 17.2*) and, to a lesser extent, coproporphyrinogen oxidase and ferrochelatase. As a result, the urinary excretion of ALA and coproporphyrin, and red cell protoporphyrin content may all be increased in lead poisoning. However, the measurement of blood lead concentration is to be preferred for the diagnosis of both lead poisoning and occupational overexposure to lead (see *Chapter 20*).

# IRON

The total iron content of the adult body is approximately 4 g (70 mmol), of which some two-thirds is in haemoglobin. Iron stores (mainly spleen, liver and bone marrow) contain about one-quarter of the body's iron. Most of the remainder is in myoglobin and other haemoproteins; only 0.1% of the total body iron is in the plasma where it is almost all bound to a transport protein, transferrin.

## Iron absorption and transport

The mean daily intake of iron is about 20 mg (0.36 mmol), but less than 10% of this is absorbed. The regulation of iron absorption is not fully understood. It is determined by the state of the body's iron stores, being increased when they are depleted and decreased when they are adequate. It is also increased when erythropoiesis is increased (irrespective of the state of the iron stores).

The main site of iron absorption is the proximal small bowel. Iron is more readily absorbed in the $Fe^{2+}$ form but dietary iron is mainly in the $Fe^{3+}$ form. Gastric secretions are important in iron absorption in that they liberate iron from food (although haem can be absorbed intact) and promote the conversion of $Fe^{3+}$ ions to $Fe^{2+}$. Ascorbic acid and other reducing substances facilitate iron absorption while phytic acid (in cereals), phosphates and oxalates form insoluble complexes with iron and decrease its absorption.

Once absorbed into the intestinal mucosal cells, iron is either transported directly into the blood stream, or else combines with apoferritin, a complex iron-binding protein, to form ferritin. This iron is lost into the lumen of the gut when mucosal cells are shed. In iron deficiency, the apoferritin content of mucosal cells decreases and a greater proportion of absorbed iron reaches the blood stream.

In the blood, iron is transported bound mainly to transferrin, each molecule of which binds two $Fe^{2+}$ ions. Transferrin is normally about one-third saturated with iron. In tissues, iron is bound in ferritin and haemosiderin. Free iron is very toxic and protein binding allows iron to be transported and stored in a non-toxic form.

Iron is lost from the body in faeces (non-absorbed and shed mucosal iron), by desquamation of skin and, in

women, by menstrual blood loss. Endogenous iron loss in males is about 1 mg (18 μmol)/24 h. Very little iron is excreted in the urine.

## Diagnostic tests for iron status

Iron status may require assessment when iron deficiency or overload is suspected or when the distribution or metabolism of iron is thought to be abnormal. Haematological tests used in this context include measurement of haemoglobin and red cell indices. Iron stores can be assessed directly by examination of the bone marrow, but measurement of plasma ferritin concentration is the best non-invasive test for iron deficiency. It is rarely necessary to use biochemical tests merely to substantiate a diagnosis of iron deficiency, since this is by far the commonest cause of microcytic, hypochromic anaemia and the diagnosis is confirmed by a response to iron therapy.

### Plasma iron

The plasma iron concentration is of little value in the investigation of iron metabolism, except in relation to haemochromatosis and in the diagnosis and management of iron poisoning. A fall in plasma iron concentration is a late feature of iron deficiency, although a raised plasma iron is usually present in iron overload. However, the concentration of iron in the plasma of normal individuals fluctuates considerably; differences of more than 20% can occur within a few minutes, and of 100% from one day to the next. Considerable catamenial variation occurs in women. Many conditions, including infection, trauma, chronic inflammatory disorders (especially rheumatoid arthritis) and neoplasia, are associated with low plasma iron concentration (but normal iron stores), while others, for example hepatitis, cause an increase in concentration.

### Plasma total iron-binding capacity

Measurement of iron-binding capacity is effectively a functional measurement of transferrin concentration. Knowing the plasma iron, the transferrin saturation can then be calculated; it is normally about 33%. Although plasma total iron-binding capacity is increased in iron deficiency, many other factors can affect it while the saturation, dependent as it is upon the (highly variable) plasma iron concentration, is itself highly variable. While it is true that low saturation is characteristic of iron deficiency, it also occurs in other conditions, such as pregnancy and chronic disease, in the absence of iron deficiency. The transferrin saturation is, however, a valuable screening test for idiopathic haemochromatosis (it is usually increased to 100% in this condition) but is not useful otherwise.

## Plasma ferritin

Although plasma ferritin concentration is more difficult to measure than iron or iron-binding capacity, it is by far superior to them for the assessment of body iron stores. The only known cause of a low plasma ferritin concentration is a decrease in body iron stores; concentrations below 20 µg/L indicate depletion, and below 12 µg/L suggest a complete absence of stored iron. However, ferritin is an acute phase protein and patients with iron deficiency may have plasma ferritin concentrations within the reference range when they are acutely ill. In patients with anaemia and chronic disease, the plasma ferritin concentration will indicate whether there is also iron deficiency and whether iron stores are adequate to meet the increased demand for incorporation into haemoglobin if the underlying condition can be treated successfully. Plasma ferritin concentration is increased in iron overload, for example, in haemochromatosis, but may also be increased in some patients with liver disease and certain types of cancer, due to release of the protein from tissues. Raised concentrations should therefore be interpreted with caution, but a normal concentration militates against iron overload.

## Iron deficiency

This may be due to inadequate intake, impaired absorption, excessive loss or a combination of these. The anaemia that develops is hypochromic and microcytic and if there is an obvious cause of iron deficiency, further investigation of the anaemia is not required. If the cause of an anaemia is in doubt, the finding of a low plasma ferritin concentration will indicate iron deficiency.

## Iron overload

This can occur with increased intestinal absorption of iron: either acutely, as in iron poisoning, or chronically, as is seen in peoples who traditionally cook their food in iron pots (Bantu siderosis). Increased parenteral iron administration occurs unavoidably in patients given repeated blood transfusions for the treatment of refractory anaemias and can also lead to overloading of the body's iron stores (haemosiderosis or acquired haemochromatosis). The excess iron is deposited mainly as haemosiderin in reticuloendothelial cells in the liver and spleen where it is relatively innocuous, but with time parenchymal deposition may lead to hepatic fibrosis and myocardial damage.

### Hereditary (primary) haemochromatosis

The most severe iron overload is seen in patients with hereditary or primary haemochromatosis. This condition is characterized by excessive intestinal iron absorption. Its molecular basis is not known. The mode of inheritance is autosomal recessive, and there is a strong link with the histocompatibility antigen HLA-A3 (present in approximately 70% of patients but only 28% of the normal population) and to a lesser extent with HLA-B14. It is thought that about 0.5% of caucasoids are homozygous for haemochromatosis, making it a common inherited disease. It is probably underdiagnosed; all patients with chronic liver disease should be investigated for haemochromatosis unless some other cause is readily apparent. It could also be argued that males developing diabetes in middle life should be screened for haemochromatosis.

The phenotypic expression in homozygotes depends upon the availability of dietary iron and overall iron turnover. Thus the condition is commoner in men than in women (because of menstrual iron loss), and when it does occur in women, does so on average at a later age. Even in men it is uncommon before the age of 40; although the defect is present from birth, it is only when the body becomes massively overloaded with iron that clinical features develop. Furthermore, the prevalence in homozygotes in countries with a high dietary content of available iron is greater than where the dietary content is low.

---

### CASE HISTORY 17.2

A 45-year-old man presented with weight loss, lassitude and weakness. His skin was noticeably bronzed, although it was winter and he had not been out of the country. On examination, he was found to have hepatosplenomegaly, rather sparse body hair and small testes. On further questioning, he admitted that he had lost his libido and become impotent.

### Investigations

| | |
|---|---|
| urine | positive for glucose |
| blood glucose (fasting) | 10 mmol/L |
| | |
| serum: iron | 70 µmol/L |
| iron-binding capacity | 67 µmol/L |
| ferritin | 5000 µg/L |
| testosterone | 9 nmol/L |
| luteinizing hormone | 2 U/L |

### Comment

Skin pigmentation is virtually always present in idiopathic haemochromatosis, though it develops insidiously and may go unnoticed by the patient. It is a result of increased melanin deposition (and iron in advanced cases). Deposition of iron in the pancreas causes islet cell destruction and diabetes. Parenchymal iron deposition in the liver leads to cirrhosis which may be complicated by hepatoma formation; the liver disease is often exacerbated by excessive alcohol ingestion. Both primary and secondary hypogonadism can occur; in this case, the low luteinizing hormone level suggests that the hypogonadism is secondary to pituitary damage. The joints are often involved and deposition of iron in the myocardium can cause arrhythmias and cardiac failure.

The total iron-binding capacity is normal in this case but may be decreased as a result of the impaired ability of the liver to synthesize transferrin. It is, however, fully saturated with iron with the result that the plasma iron concentration is always elevated. Plasma ferritin concentration is massively elevated; values of several thousand micrograms per litre are typical of idiopathic haemochromatosis (mean normal 100 μg/L in males). The diagnosis of haemochromatosis can be confirmed by demonstration of the massive excess of parenchymal iron in a sample of liver obtained by percutaneous biopsy.

The families of patients with haemochromatosis should be screened to detect homozygotes for the defective gene, who are at risk of developing the condition and can be given prophylactic treatment. Treatment of homozygotes before the onset of overt disease has been shown to prevent the development of cirrhosis and reduce the (otherwise considerable) risk of hepatocellular carcinoma. HLA typing and iron studies can be used for screening. Heterozygotes are not at risk; the results of iron studies in them may be normal but some can be detected by HLA typing.

MANAGEMENT AND PROGNOSIS

The mainstay of treatment of idiopathic haemochromatosis is repeated venesection; with each unit of blood, 200–250 mg of iron are removed from the body. It is often possible to do this as often as once a week without rendering the patient anaemic. Plasma iron and ferritin concentrations are used to monitor treatment and once the excess iron has been removed, further accumulation can be prevented by less frequent (two- to three-monthly) venesection. Diabetes and heart failure are treated by conventional means, and hormonal deficiencies by appropriate replacement. Untreated, the prognosis is poor, but it is considerably improved by removal of the excess iron. There is often an improvement in cardiac and hepatic functions, but the diabetes, hypogonadism and joint disease are not affected.

Desferrioxamine, an iron-chelating agent, is valuable in patients receiving multiple blood transfusions for refractory anaemia and who are at risk of developing iron overload. Desferrioxamine has to be infused intravenously; unless this is performed daily, the rate of removal of iron is much slower than with venesection.

## SUMMARY

Haemoproteins consist of a haem molecule (a tetrapyrrole ring linked to an $Fe^{2+}$ ion) bound to a protein. In haemoglobin, the protein consists of two pairs of identical polypeptide chains and four haem molecules; it is the latter which are responsible for binding oxygen. Haemoglobin contains two-thirds of the body's iron. Iron is essential for normal haemopoiesis and iron deficiency is an important cause of anaemia. Many genetically determined variants of haemoglobin are known including haemoglobin S, responsible for sickle cell anaemia; some of these variants are of no clinical consequence but others, like HbS, can cause severe disease. Haemoglobin can undergo chemical changes in the blood, for example, binding carbon monoxide and forming carboxyhaemoglobin which is incapable of transporting oxygen.

The synthesis of the tetrapyrrole ring of haem involves a complex metabolic pathway from glycine and succinyl-CoA through intermediates known as porphyrinogens. Inherited metabolic disorders are known affecting each of the enzymes of the haem synthetic pathway and are collectively called porphyrias. These conditions are classified into the acute porphyrias (whose effects are primarily neurological), for example, acute intermittent porphyria, and the chronic (with primarily cutaneous manifestations) such as cutaneous hepatic porphyria. The neurological features are due to the accumulation of porphyrin precursors, whereas the accumulation of porphyrins themselves causes photosensitivity and hence leads to skin damage.

The porphyrias are also classified into hepatic and erythropoietic porphyrias, according to the major site of the enzyme abnormality. With the exceptions of congenital erythropoietic porphyria and ALA dehydratase deficiency porphyria, which are autosomal recessive, the porphyrias are unusual among inherited metabolic disorders in having an autosomal dominant mode of inheritance. Although cutaneous hepatic porphyria may be inherited, it is often acquired, such as when it occurs with excessive alcohol intake. Each porphyria gives rise to a characteristic pattern of porphyrins and metabolites in blood, urine and faeces which can be used to make the diagnosis.

Dietary iron is absorbed in the proximal small intestine, more readily in the $Fe^{2+}$ form. Almost all the iron in the plasma is protein-bound to transferrin. Iron deficiency can be due to inadequate intake or malabsorption, or excessive loss of iron, and gives rise to a microcytic, hypochromic anaemia. The plasma iron concentration is an unreliable guide to the body's iron status; measurement of plasma ferritin concentration (ferritin is a primarily intracellular iron-binding protein) is the best biochemical test of iron status.

Free iron is highly toxic and iron poisoning, particularly in children, can be fatal. Chronic iron overload occurs in haemochromatosis, a genetically determined disorder characterized by excessive absorption of dietary iron which becomes deposited in many tissues of the body, including cardiac muscle, endocrine organs and parenchymal cells of the liver. Clinical features of haemochromatosis include skin pigmentation, cirrhosis, cardiomyopathy and impaired endocrine function. The condition is best treated by repeat-ed venesection to remove iron from the body. In haemosiderosis, in which iron accumulates, for example as a result of repeated blood transfusion for refractory anaemia, the excess iron is deposited in reticuloendothelial cells and there is much less tissue damage.

## FURTHER READING

Cavill J, Jacobs A & Wormwood M (1986) Diagnostic methods for iron status. *Annals of Clinical Biochemistry*, **23**, 168–171.

Elder G H, Smith S G & Smyth S J (1990) Laboratory investigation of the porphyrias. *Annals of Clinical Biochemistry*, **27**, 395–412.

Finlayson N D C (1990) Hereditary (primary) haemochromatosis. *British Medical Journal*, **301**, 351–352.

Scriver C R, Beaudet A L, Sly W S & Valle D (1994) *The Metabolic Basis of Inherited Disease*. 7th edn. New York: McGraw-Hill Book Company.

# 18. Hyperuricaemia and Gout

## INTRODUCTION

Uric acid is the end-product of purine nucleotide metabolism in humans. At physiological pH, uric acid is 98% ionized and is therefore present mainly as the urate ion. In the extracellular fluid (ECF), where sodium is the predominant cation, uric acid effectively exists as a solution of its sodium salt, monosodium urate. This salt has a low solubility, the ECF becoming saturated at urate concentrations little above the upper limit of the reference range. In consequence, there is a tendency for crystalline monosodium urate to form in subjects with hyperuricaemia.

The most obvious clinical manifestation of this process is gout, in which crystals form in the cartilage, synovium and synovial fluid of joints. Other manifestations include renal calculi and tophi (accretions of sodium urate in soft tissues). A sudden increase in urate production, typically seen as a complication of the treatment of haematological malignancy, can lead to widespread crystallization in the urinary collecting system, causing acute obstruction and the syndrome of acute urate nephropathy (*see Chapter 19*).

## URIC ACID METABOLISM

Purine nucleotides are essential components of nucleic acids; they are intimately involved in energy transformation and phosphorylation reactions and act as intracellular messengers. There are three sources of purines in man: the diet, degradation of endogenous nucleotides and *de novo* synthesis (*Fig. 18.1*). Since purines are metabolized to uric acid, the body urate pool (and hence plasma concentration) depends on the relative rates of both urate formation from these sources and urate excretion. Urate is excreted by both the kidneys and the gut, renal excretion accounting for approximately two-thirds of the total. Urate secreted into the gut is metabolized to carbon dioxide and ammonia by bacterial action (uricolysis).

Urate handling by the kidney is complex (*Fig. 18.2*). It is filtered at the glomeruli and is almost totally absorbed in the proximal convoluted tubules; distally, both secretion and reabsorption occur. Normal urate clearance is about 10% of the filtered load. In normal subjects, urate excretion increases if the filtered load is increased. In chronic renal failure, the plasma concentration rises only when the glomerular filtration rate falls below about 20 mL/min.

Dietary purines account for about 30% of excreted urate.

The introduction of a purine-free diet reduces plasma urate levels by only 10–20%.

The metabolic pathways leading to uric acid synthesis are shown in outline in *Fig. 18.3*. *De novo* synthesis leads to the formation of inosine monophosphate (IMP), which can be converted to the nucleotides adenosine monophosphate (AMP) and guanosine monophosphate (GMP). Nucleotide degradation involves the formation of the respective nucleosides (inosine, adenosine and guanosine); these are then metabolized to purines. The purine derived from IMP is hypoxanthine, which is converted by the enzyme xanthine oxidase first to xanthine and then to uric acid. Guanine can be metabolized to xanthine (and so to uric acid) directly, but adenine cannot. However, AMP can be converted to IMP by the enzyme AMP deaminase and, at the nucleoside level, adenosine can be converted to inosine. Thus, surplus GMP and AMP can be converted to uric acid and excreted.

However, the excretion of uric acid represents the waste of a metabolic investment since purine synthesis requires considerable energy expenditure. Pathways exist whereby purines can be salvaged and converted back to their parent nucleotides. For guanine and hypoxanthine, this is accompanied by the enzyme, hypoxanthine–guanine phosphoribosyl transferase (HGPRT), and for adenine by adenine phosphoribosyl transferase (APRT).

## URIC ACID IN PLASMA

Plasma urate concentrations are, in general, higher in men than in women, tend to rise with age (Fig. 18.4), and are usually elevated in people in the higher socioeconomic groups and in the obese. There is considerable variation in plasma urate concentrations between different ethnic groups.

In adult males in the United Kingdom, the upper limit of the reference range is usually taken as 0.42 mmol/L. In an aqueous solution of pH 7.4, at 37°C, and with an ionic strength similar to that of plasma, the solubility of monosodium urate is 0.57 mmol/L; in plasma, the presence of protein appears to reduce this somewhat. The risk of gout increases with increasing plasma urate concentrations (*Fig. 18.5*). Undoubtedly, many factors are involved in the precipitation of monosodium urate crystals in connective tissue; gout may not necessarily occur with hyperuricaemia (indeed, 85% of patients with hyperuricaemia remain asymptomatic throughout life) but hyperuricaemia is a prerequisite for the development of gout. Gout can be precipitated by a sudden change (either increase or decrease) in urate concentration. When urate concentration has fallen rapidly in a hyperuricaemic individual (for example, as a result of a change in diet, decrease in alcohol consumption or treatment with a hypouricaemic drug), the plasma urate concentration may not be elevated when the patient presents with gout. The solubility of monosodium urate declines rapidly with decreasing temperature and this may, to some extent, explain the tendency for the more peripheral joints, which have lower intra-articular temperatures, to be more frequently affected.

## HYPERURICAEMIA

Hyperuricaemia may occur due to increased formation of uric acid, decreased excretion, or a combination of both. Some causes of increased formation are given in *Fig. 18.6*.

When hyperuricaemia is due to decreased excretion, it is renal excretion that is usually affected. Indeed, in hyperuricaemia the total amount of urate removed by uricolysis in the gut is increased. Reference to Fig. 18.2 will show that decreased renal urate excretion could result from decreased filtration or tubular secretion. Plasma urate only rises late in chronic renal failure, but many factors can affect tubular function and thereby cause hyperuricaemia; the more important of these are given in Fig. 18.6. Excessive alcohol ingestion probably increases *de novo* purine synthesis (and some alcoholic beverages contain high concentrations of purines), but any increase in lactate production due to alcohol may also impair urate excretion.

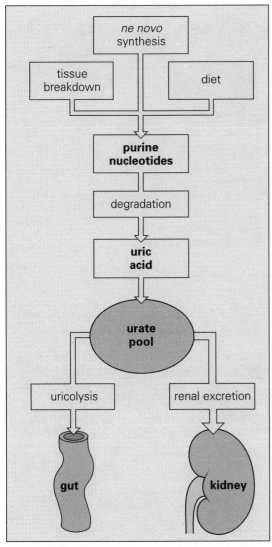

**Fig. 18.1** Sources and excretion of urate.

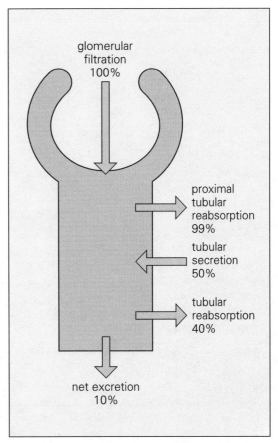

**Fig. 18.2** Urate excretion in the kidney.

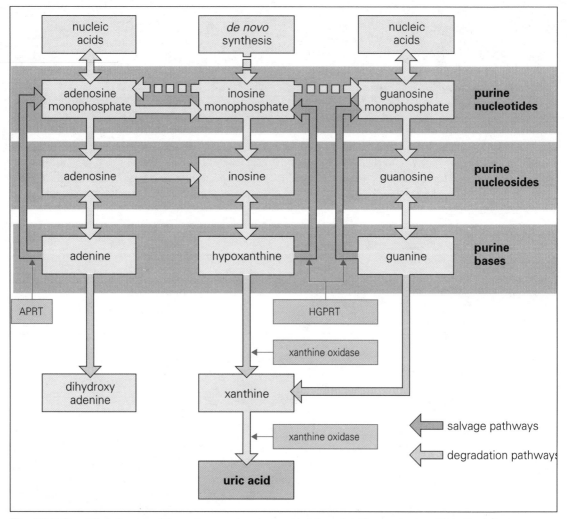

**Fig. 18.3** Simplified diagram of the pathways of purine nucleotide metabolism and uric acid synthesis in man. APRT = adenine phosphoribosyl transferase; HGPRT = hypoxanthine–guanine phosphoribosyl transferase.

**Fig. 18.4** Mean plasma urate concentrations in men and women.

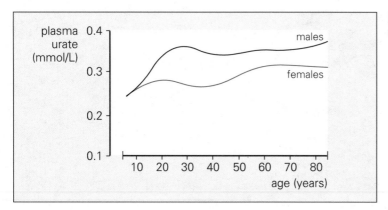

| Plasma urate (mmol/L) | Risk of developing gout (%) | |
|---|---|---|
| | males | females |
| < 0.41 | 2 | 3 |
| 0.42–0.47 | 17 | 17 |
| 0.48–0.53 | 25 | * |
| > 0.54 | 90 | * |
| *insufficient data; such levels are exceptional in females | | |

Fig. 18.5 Risk of developing gout in relation to plasma urate concentration.

| Causes of hyperuricaemia | |
|---|---|
| Increased urate formation | Decreased renal urate excretion |
| **Primary**<br>increased purine synthesis:<br>  idiopathic<br>  inherited metabolic disease<br><br>**Secondary**<br>excessive dietary purine intake<br>disordered ATP metabolism:<br>  alcohol<br>  tissue hypoxia<br>increased nucleic acid turnover:<br>  malignant disease<br>  psoriasis<br>  cytotoxic drugs | **Primary**<br>idiopathic<br><br>**Secondary**<br>chronic renal disease<br>increased renal reabsorption/<br>decreased secretion:<br>  thiazide diuretics<br>  salicylates (low doses)<br>  lead<br>  organic acids (e.g., lactic<br>  acid, hence alcohol) |

Fig. 18.6 Causes of increased formation of uric acid and reduced uric acid excretion by the kidneys. Note that salicylates reduce uric acid excretion at low doses only; at high doses (>4 g/day) aspirin is uricosuric as it blocks the tubular reabsorption of uric acid.

## Gout

Gout is customarily defined as primary (idiopathic) or secondary (when a condition known to cause hyperuricaemia is present). However, gout is uncommon when hyperuricaemia develops secondarily to other conditions. The tendency for hyperuricaemia and gout to be familial has led to investigation for a causal inherited metabolic defect. Although there are a few rare conditions in which such a defect does lead to hyperuricaemia, none has been found in the great majority of cases of primary gout. Some 90% of patients appear to excrete urate at a rate inappropriately low for the plasma concentration, while about 10% have excessive urate production. Dietary factors and alcohol ingestion exacerbate hyperuricaemia in about half the cases, but while their amelioration may reduce the plasma urate levels somewhat, these usually remain elevated. Gout is rare in premenstrual women, in whom mean plasma levels of urate are much lower than in men of corresponding age (see Fig. 18.4), but the incidence increases markedly after the menopause.

### CASE HISTORY 18.1

An obese 55-year-old male was awoken from sleep, after spending the evening at a business dinner, by excruciating pain in his left first metatarsophalangeal joint. He was unable to put his foot to the floor. The affected joint was hot, swollen, red and extremely tender. He was treated with indomethacin and the symptoms resolved rapidly. One year previously he had had an episode of renal colic but had declared himself to be busy to be too investigated in connection with this.

**Investigations**

serum urate             0.78 mmol/L

**Comment**

This is the classic presentation of gout. The onset is often sudden, nocturnal and monoarticular. In 70% of cases the metatarsophalangeal joint of the great toe is the first to be affected. The classical signs of inflammation were present and hyperuricaemia was confirmed. In this case, the previous episode of renal colic may well have been due to a renal urate stone. Gout is more common in men than women and is associated with higher social class, driving (type A) personality, obesity, hypertriglyceridaemia, hypertension and excessive food and alcohol intake.

## Diagnosis

The diagnosis of gout is primarily clinical but is supported by the demonstration of hyperuricaemia. The diagnosis is confirmed by the presence of tophi or of monosodium urate crystals in the synovial fluid. These crystals are typically needle-shaped, 2–10 μm long and are seen within neutrophils. They show strong negative birefringence when viewed with polarized light.

The differential diagnosis includes other crystalline arthropathies and septic arthritis.

## Pathogenesis

Monosodium urate crystals forming in joints are engulfed by neutrophil leucocytes but damage the lysosomal membranes of these cells, so causing cellular disruption. The generation of superoxide free radicals and release of lysosomal enzymes into the joint precipitates an acute inflammatory reaction. The release of interleukin-1 from monocytes and tissue macrophages also provides an inflammatory stimulus.

## Management

Anti-inflammatory drugs (of which indomethacin is the most efficacious) are used to treat acute gout, but have no effect on the hyperuricaemia. This can be treated by dietary measures, avoidance of alcohol and, if possible, of relevant drugs (especially diuretics). Urate-lowering drugs, of which the most widely used is allopurinol, are used for long-term treatment when there have been recurrent acute attacks of gout; when there is renal damage or renal calculi with hyperuricaemia; in tophaceous gout, or if plasma urate concentrations persistently exceed 0.6 mmol/L. Allopurinol is an inhibitor of xanthine oxidase and thus inhibits the synthesis of urate from xanthine. It decreases plasma urate concentration and urinary urate excretion; urinary xanthine excretion is increased, but xanthine is more water-soluble than urate.

Starting treatment with hyperuricaemic drugs may precipitate an acute attack of gout and they should not be taken during or for several weeks after an acute episode.

## Stages of gout

Four stages in the natural history of gout have been described (*Fig. 18.7*). Asymptomatic hyperuricaemia (i) can be present for years before an acute attack (ii) is precipitated, for example, by trauma or dietary indiscretion. Symptom-free periods of months or years follow ('intercritical gout', iii) punctuated by acute attacks leading, if untreated, to chronic tophaceous gout. Since the introduction of allopurinol, tophaceous gout, once common, is now rarely seen. It tends to occur mainly in elderly women treated with diuretics for many years (in particular thiazides, which inhibit renal tubular secretion of urate) rather than as a sequel to recurrent attacks of acute gout.

## Rare causes of hyperuricaemia

There are a number of rare, inherited metabolic diseases associated with hyperuricaemia and gout (*Fig. 18.8*). In all of them, hyperuricaemia results from increased uric acid synthesis.

# HYPOURICAEMIA

This is uncommon and clinically inconsequential. It may be due to either decreased urate synthesis or increased excretion and so is seen in congenital xanthine oxidase deficiency (xanthinuria), severe liver disease and renal tubular disorders such as the Fanconi syndrome. It can also result from excessive medication with allopurinol and the use of uricosuric drugs such as probenecid.

# OTHER CRYSTALLINE ARTHROPATHIES

Gout is not the only crystalline arthropathy. The deposition of calcium pyrophosphate in joints may mimic gout clinically (pseudogout) and chondrocalcinosis (calcium deposition in

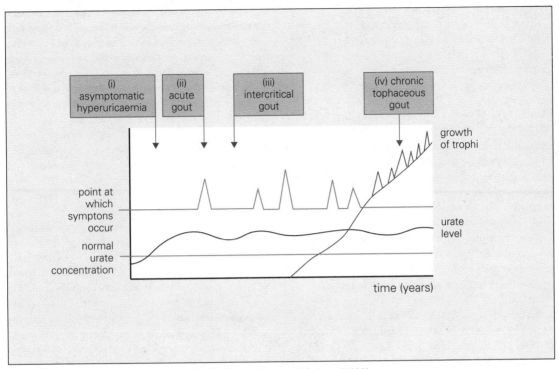

**Fig. 18.7** The natural history of gout. Modified from Dieppe & Calvert (1983).

| Major inherited metabolic diseases associated with hyperuricaemia | |
| --- | --- |
| **Enzyme abnormality** | **Consequence** |
| hypoxanthine–guanine phospho-ribosyl transferase deficiency (Lesch–Nyhan syndrome and less severe variants) | decreased activity of salvage pathway decreases purine reutilization and thus increases uric acid synthesis |
| glucose 6-phosphatase deficiency (glycogen storage disease type I) | (i) increased metabolism of glucose 6-phosphate through pentose phosphate pathway increases formation of ribose 5-phosphate, a substrate for purine nucleotide synthesis<br><br>(ii) hyperlactataemia decreases uric acid secretion in renal tubules |
| phosphoribosyl pyrophosphate synthetase (PRPP synthetase) variant (with increased activity) | PRPP is a substrate for purine nucleotide synthesis and also activates the rate limiting enzyme |

**Fig. 18.8** Inherited metabolic diseases associated with hyperuricaemia.

joint cartilage) may be present. The condition may be familial but most cases occur in association with hyperparathyroidism, haemochromatosis or other metabolic disorders. The rhomboid-shaped crystals formed show weak positive birefringence when viewed with polarized light. The deposition of hydroxyapatite in joints has also been described.

## SUMMARY

Uric acid is the end-product of the metabolism of purines. These substances are components of nucleotides which in turn are components of nucleic acids. They also have an essential role in energy transformations, act as intracellular messengers, and are involved in neurotransmission.

The pathological significance of uric acid is related primarily to its low solubility. At concentrations little above those in which it is normally present in body fluids, uric acid can be precipitated in the form of monosodium urate crystals. In joints this causes gout, an acute inflammatory arthritis, and can lead to chronic, destructive joint disease; in the kidneys, renal damage can occur and uric acid can be precipitated from the urine to form calculi; with long-standing hyperuricaemia, accretions of urate known as tophi can form in soft tissues.

The concentration of uric acid in the plasma depends upon the relative rates of its formation and excretion. Formation in turn depends upon the rate of purine turnover which is dependent upon the balance between dietary purine intake, *de novo* synthesis and degradation. Excretion takes place through the kidneys (about two-thirds) and gut (where uric acid is broken down by bacterial action).

Hyperuricaemia can occur secondarily to many conditions, in some of which there is increased urate formation (e.g., malignant disease, especially haematological malignancies) and in others, decreased excretion (e.g., renal failure). Gout, however, is more frequently seen in patients who do not suffer from such conditions and in these cases is known as primary or idiopathic gout. There is frequently a family history of the condition but although a small number of rare inherited metabolic disorders are known in which an enzyme defect leads to excessive urate synthesis, in the majority of patients no such defect is demonstrable. About 10% of patients with idiopathic gout appear to have excessive urate production; in the remainder, the rate of urate excretion appears to be inappropriately low for the rate of production. Dietary factors and alcohol often exacerbate hyperuricaemia.

Patients with acute episodes of gout require treatment with analgesics and anti-inflammatory drugs; in the long term, plasma urate levels can be reduced by dietary modification and the use of allopurinol, an inhibitor of xanthine oxidase, the enzyme responsible for the synthesis of uric acid. This drug thus reduces the formation of uric acid and instead xanthine, which is far more soluble, becomes the principal end-product of purine metabolism.

Pseudogout can resemble gout clinically. This condition is due to the deposition of crystals of calcium pyrophosphate in joints. These can be distinguished from monosodium urate crystals by using polarizing microscopy.

## FURTHER READING

Dieppe P & Calvert P (1983) *Crystals and Joint Disease.* London: Chapman & Hall.

Scriver C R, Beaudet A L, Sly W S & Vallee D (1994) *The Metabolic Basis of Inherited Disease.* 7th edition. New York: McGraw-Hill Book Company.

# 19. Metabolic Aspects of Malignant Disease

## INTRODUCTION

The clinical signs and symptoms in patients suffering from cancer are often directly related to the physical presence of the tumour. For example, the tumour may destroy essential normal tissue, cause obstruction of ducts, or exert pressure on nerves. Systemic manifestations, including cachexia and pyrexia, are also frequently present and indeed may be the only evidence of the presence of a tumour. In some patients, the clinical features may be those of an endocrine syndrome. This would be expected with a tumour of endocrine tissue such as a malignant insulinoma (producing hypoglycaemia) or an adrenal carcinoma (producing Cushing's syndrome), but often occurs with tumours not obviously of endocrine origin.

In many cases, there is good evidence that such syndromes are due to the secretion of a hormone by the tumour. This has been termed *ectopic* hormone secretion since the hormone is not secreted from its normal site, while *eutopic* hormone secretion describes secretion from the endocrine gland. However, it seems likely that in many cases these tumours arise from cells normally capable of hormone secretion, but which are present in only very small numbers in the non-neoplastic tissue. 'Aberrant' rather than 'ectopic' hormone secretion may be a more accurate description of this phenomenon. Tumours can be associated with other systemic manifestations, for example, a cerebellar syndrome, arthropathy, etc.; the term 'paraneoplastic syndromes' encompasses all the systemic manifestations of cancer not directly related to the physical presence of the primary tumour, whether or not they are due to a hormone.

This chapter discusses paraneoplastic syndromes, certain familial endocrine syndromes and also tumour markers, substances whose presence is a reflection of the presence of tumours, and whose concentrations can be measured as an aid to the diagnosis or monitoring of malignant disease.

## PARANEOPLASTIC ENDOCRINE SYNDROMES

### Origins and classification

These syndromes are due to the secretion of peptide hormones or other humoral factors, which are coded for by genes and translated from m-RNA. All somatic cells contain a full complement of genes, and aberrant hormone secretion could be explained either by novel expression of a gene that is not normally expressed in the cells from which the tumour arises, or by re-expression of a gene that is expressed during development in a stem cell from which the tumour cells are derived. The fact that these syndromes tend to be associated with certain tumours, notably small cell carcinoma of bronchus, and that some tumours give rise to predominantly only one syndrome, favours the second explanation.

Small cell carcinoma of bronchus is an example of an APUD tumour. This term, derived from 'amine precursor uptake and decarboxylation', was originally used to describe tumours of neuroectodermal origin sharing similar amine-handling characteristics. In fact, the major products of most of these tumours are low molecular weight peptides (many of them hormones). Some of the cells of the APUD series are shown in *Fig. 19.1*. However, paraneoplastic syndromes also occur in association with tumours that do not arise from APUD cells and, apart from their ability to secrete hormones, no single distinctive property has been shown to be common to all non-endocrine tumours associated with these syndromes.

Hormone secretion by tumours does not always cause an endocrine syndrome. This may be because insufficient is secreted to cause a persistently raised plasma concentration (particularly since normal secretion of the hormone may be suppressed), or because the principal secretory product is an inactive precursor of the hormone.

Some tumours associated with aberrant hormone secretion are shown in *Fig. 19.2*. The most frequently encountered paraneoplastic endocrine syndromes are dilutional hyponatraemia, hypercalcaemia and Cushing's syndrome. Calcitonin secretion is though to be common, but is clinically silent.

### Cushing's syndrome

Cushing's syndrome is the condition which results when tissues are exposed to supraphysiological concentrations of glucocorticoids. It is discussed in detail in *Chapter 8*.

---

**CASE HISTORY 19.1**

A retired warehouseman presented with muscle weakness and back pain. He had also lost 5 kg in

---

weight in the previous two months and had recently been passing more urine than usual. He had smoked 25–30 cigarettes a day for many years but had generally enjoyed good health. On examination, in addition to the weakness and signs of weight loss, he was found to have glycosuria and was hypertensive, but his appearance was otherwise normal and no abnormal physical signs were elicited.

### Investigations

serum: sodium 144 mmol/L
       potassium 2.2 mmol/L
       bicarbonate 39 mmol/L
blood: glucose 10.2 mmol/L

*High-dose dexamethasone suppression test:*
plasma cortisol:
  (0900 h) 1520 nmol/L
  (0900 h) after dexamethasone
  2 mg, 4 times daily for 2 days 1500 nmol/L
plasma ACTH 460 ng/L
  (normal <80 ng/L)

A discrete mass was present in the left lower zone on chest radiography.

### Comment

The greatly elevated plasma cortisol and ACTH concentrations are typical of ectopic ACTH secretion. Plasma ACTH concentration changes are generally much higher than those seen in Cushing's disease, except when a carcinoid or thymic tumour is responsible. Since ACTH secretion is not under normal feedback control, the hypercortisolaemia is not suppressed by dexamethasone.

With ectopic ACTH secretion, the clinical presentation is typically dominated by the metabolic sequelae of excessive cortisol secretion, as in this case. These include hypokalaemia with alkalosis, which exacerbates the physical weakness due to steroid-induced myopathy; glucose intolerance, sometimes sufficient to cause frank diabetes, and hypertension. Osteoporosis predisposes to crush fractures of the vertebrae and the presence of secondary tumour deposits may also give rise to back pain. The classic somatic manifestations of Cushing's syndrome are often absent, a reflection of the very rapid progression of the condition in most cases. ACTH-secreting carcinoid and thymic tumours are an exception; the clinical syndrome in these cases may closely resemble Cushing's disease even to the extent that ACTH secretion, and hence that of cortisol, is suppressible by dexamethasone.

| Endocrine cells of the APUD series | |
|---|---|
| **Cell/tissue** | **Hormone** |
| hypothalamus | oxytocin, vasopressin; releasing/inhibitory hormones |
| anterior pituitary | TSH, ACTH, FSH, LH, prolactin, growth hormone |
| pancreatic islets | insulin, glucagon |
| pancreatic islet and non-islet | somatostatin, VIP, pancreatic polypeptide |
| gastric endocrine | gastrin, glucagon |
| intestinal endocrine | e.g., secretin, cholecystokinin, enteroglucagon |
| thyroid C cells | calcitonin |
| parathyroid | parathyroid hormone |

**Fig. 19.1** Endocrine cells of the APUD series and the hormones they produce.

| Some non-endocrine tumours associated with hormone secretion | | |
| --- | --- | --- |
| **Tumour** | **Hormone** | **Syndrome** |
| small cell carcinoma of bronchus* | ACTH (and precursors) vasopressin hCG | Cushing's syndrome dilutional hyponatraemia gynaecomastia |
| squamous cell carcinoma of bronchus | PTHrP | hypercalcaemia |
| breast carcinoma | calcitonin | none |
| carcinoid tumours* | ACTH vasopressin | Cushing's syndrome dilutional hyponatraemia |
| renal adenocarcinoma | PTHrP | hypercalcaemia |
| mesenchymal tumours | insulin-like growth factors | hypoglycaemia |
| *known or possible APUD tumours | | |

**Fig. 19.2** Non-endocrine tumours frequently associated with aberrant hormone secretion. Renal adenocarcinomas may secrete erythropoietin, causing polycythaemia, but this is not ectopic secretion since this hormone is a normal product of the kidney. PTHrP = PTH-related peptide.

Ectopic secretion of ACTH by non-endocrine tumours is common. Evidence of it has been found in up to 50% of patients with small cell bronchial carcinomas, though massive secretion, giving rise to the typical features as shown by this case, is uncommon. ACTH is produced by post-translational modification of the precursor, pro-opiomelanocortin (POMC), and both this precursor, and other products of the POMC gene (see p. 106), may be secreted in some cases.

With bronchial carcinomas, the prognosis is usually very poor unless the tumour is suitable for surgical excision. As discussed on p. 131, drug treatment may provide symptomatic relief.

### Ectopic antidiuretic hormone (ADH) secretion

A case of this syndrome is described in Case History 2.3. The secretion of ADH (vasopressin) by the tumour is uncontrolled and thus likely to be greater than the body's normal requirements, resulting in water retention with dilutional hyponatraemia. When this is mild and develops slowly, it is often asymptomatic; however, severe hyponatraemia is associated with water intoxication, which can be fatal. The symptoms (drowsiness, confusion, fits and coma) may mimic those of cerebral metastases. Ectopic ADH secretion is most commonly seen with small cell carcinomas of the bronchus but other tumours may be responsible, e.g., carcinoid tumours and pancreatic adenocarcinomas. A similar syndrome results from the inappropriate secretion of ADH that can occur in a variety of non-malignant diseases (see p. 23).

### Tumour-associated hypercalcaemia

Hypercalcaemia is common in malignant disease. When bony metastases are present, dissolution of calcium from bone by the secondary tumour may be a contributory factor. However, hypercalcaemia often occurs in the absence of metastases, suggesting that a humoral factor is responsible.

**CASE HISTORY 19.2**

An elderly man presented with loin pain and increasing thirst. Examination of the urine showed haematuria but no glycosuria.

Secretion of PTHrP may contribute to hypercalcaemia even when bony metastases are present. In general, there is a poor correlation between the extent of metastatic bone involvement and the severity of hypercalcaemia. Also, although hypercalcaemia can affect renal function adversely and decrease calcium excretion, it would be expected that if renal function were normal, the suppression of PTH secretion from the parathyroids would result in decreased renal tubular calcium reabsorption. This would allow the excretion of the calcium mobilized from bone. PTHrP, like PTH, stimulates tubular calcium reabsorption, and decreases calcium excretion.

Hypercalcaemia is common in haematological malignancies, particularly myeloma, and is due to the release of osteoclast-activating cytokines (e.g., interleukin-1, tumour necrosis factor (TNFβ)) by the tumours. Osteoclasts may also be activated by prostglandins produced by tumour metastases in bone, for example, metastases from breast carcinoma.

## Tumour-associated hypoglycaemia

This condition is discussed in detail in *Chapter 11*. It is only rarely due to ectopic insulin secretion by non-β cell tumours. Tumour-associated hypoglycaemia, which is usually associated with large mesenchymal tumours, is probably due to the secretion of insulin-like growth factors (somatomedins) by the tumours.

## Other paraneoplastic endocrine syndromes

Gynaecomastia may occur in patients with bronchial carcinomas, due to secretion of human chorionic gonadotrophin (hCG). Precocious puberty may develop in male children with hepatic tumours secreting hCG, but this is very rare. Secretion of erythroprotein is responsible for the polycythaemia which can occur in association with uterine fibromyomata and the rare tumour, cerebellar haemangioblastoma. Secretion of erythropoietin by adenocarcinomas of the kidney can cause polycythaemia but this is not ectopic secretion, since the kidney is the normal source of this hormone.

Paraneoplastic syndromes are common, but it must be remembered that an endocrine syndrome in a patient with a tumour may be due to coexistent endocrine disease and not necessarily to the secretion of a hormone or other factor by the tumour.

## OTHER METABOLIC COMPLICATIONS OF MALIGNANT DISEASE

Metabolic complications in patients with malignant disease are not always due to aberrant hormone secretion. They may be due to some other effect of the tumour, or develop as a consequence of treatment.

Renal failure can occur for many possible reasons. Causes include obstruction of the urinary tract, hypercalcaemia, direct infiltration of the kidneys (e.g., by lymphoma), Bence Jones proteinuria (in myeloma), antibiotics, cytotoxic drugs and the tumour lysis syndrome. This latter is the result of massive necrosis of tumour cells during the treatment of tumours with cytotoxic drugs. Features include hyperkalaemia, hyperuricaemia, hyperphosphataemia and hypocalcaemia. It is particularly likely to occur with large, chemosensitive tumours such as some lymphomas and leukaemias, and can cause acute renal failure. Preventative measures include the maintenance of adequate hydration, giving allopurinol to inhibit uric acid synthesis and careful monitoring of fluid and electrolyte status.

Hypomagnesaemia (often accompanied by hypokalaemia) is a particular complication of treatment with cisplatin, a cytotoxic drug. Massive wasting of potassium can occur in patients requiring treatment with amphotericin for fungal infections which can develop as a result of the immunosuppressive effect of some tumours and cytotoxic drugs.

## CANCER CACHEXIA

Cachexia, a syndrome of weakness and generalized wasting, is a common feature of malignant disease. Its characteristics are summarized in *Fig. 19.3*. Its causes are imperfectly understood. Deficient food intake, due either to mechanical obstruction of the alimentary tract or to the anorexia that is often present in malignant disease, may be partly responsible, and there may also be loss of protein from ulcerated mucosa or due to blood loss.

The tumour itself requires nitrogen and energy for growth which will be met from body stores if intake is inadequate. Associated infection may cause pyrexia, and increase energy requirements.

The metabolism of many tumours is primarily anaerobic; lactate is produced which is converted back to glucose in the liver and kidney. This represents a waste of energy, since glycolysis results in the net formation of only two molecules of ATP per molecule of glucose, while gluconeogenesis, the reverse process, consumes six.

Cachexia can be seen in patients both with large or widespread tumours and with small tumours. Indeed, it may be the presenting feature of malignancy. In many cases, there is evidence that the production of a humoral factor, cachectin (now identified as the cytokine, tumour necrosis factor-$\alpha$), is in part responsible. This is a normal product of macrophages and may be produced by activated macrophages within tumour tissue or possibly by tumour cells themselves. Among many other effects, this increases the body's energy expenditure.

In the majority of cases, the pathogenesis of cancer cachexia is probably multifactorial; contributory factors are indicated in *Fig. 19.3*. Management is difficult. Nutritional support may be beneficial, but the condition is rarely completely reversible unless the underlying tumour can be treated successfully.

| Cancer cachexia | |
|---|---|
| **Characteristics** | **Pathogenic factors** |
| anorexia and early satiety | anorexia, obstruction causing decreased food intake |
| weight loss | loss of protein (e.g., from ulcerated mucosa) |
| muscle weakness | malabsorption |
| non-specific anaemia | infection |
| pyrexia | consumption of nutrients by tumour |
| | abnormal metabolism by tumour |
| | secretion of cachectin, causing increase in metabolic rate |
| | treatment with cytotoxic drugs |

**Fig. 19.3** Characteristics and pathogenesis of cancer cachexia.

## CARCINOID TUMOURS

Carcinoid tumours arise from the enterochromaffin cells of the gut, cells of the APUD series; 90% of these tumours are found in the appendix and ileocaecal region but they also occur elsewhere in the gut, gallbladder, biliary and pancreatic ducts, and in the bronchi. They are of low-grade malignancy; while they frequently invade local tissue, distant metastases are rare.

The carcinoid syndrome is a result of the liberation of vasoactive amines, such as serotonin, and peptides from the tumour into the circulation. It is usually only seen with bronchial tumours, which liberate their products directly into the systemic circulation, or when tumours in the gut have metastasized to the liver. Since the greater part of the gut is drained by the portal circulation, the secreted products of tumours in the gut pass to the liver where they are inactivated. However, the secreted products of hepatic metastases reach the systemic circulation via the hepatic veins.

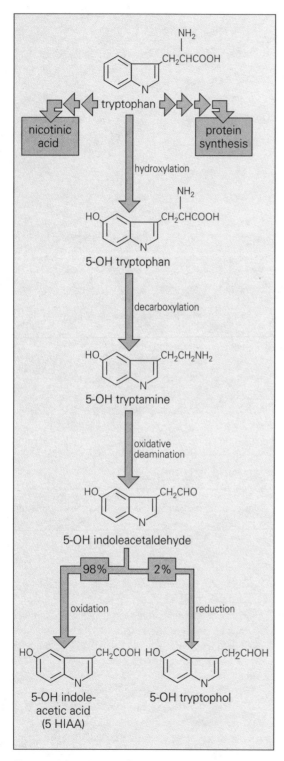

**Fig. 19.4** Metabolism of 5-hydroxindoles.

Serotonin (5-hydroxytryptamine, 5-HT) is synthesized from tryptophan (*Fig. 19.4*). In patients with carcinoid syndrome, 50% of dietary tryptophan (rather than the usual 1%) may be metabolized by this pathway, diverting tryptophan away from protein and nicotinic acid synthesis. (Pellagra-like skin lesions due to nicotinic acid deficiency are an occasional feature of the carcinoid syndrome.) The major amine secreted by intestinal carcinoid tumours (derived from embryonic midgut) is 5-hydroxytryptamine. Bronchial carcinoids (derived from foregut) tend to produce 5-hydroxytryptophan since they often lack the decarboxylase enzyme. All carcinoid tumours may also produce histamine and kinins which are important in the symptomatology of the carcinoid syndrome. Further, the secretion of peptide hormones, e.g., ACTH and calcitonin, is often demonstrable and may contribute to the clinical presentation.

---

### CASE HISTORY 19.3

A 50-year-old woman presented with a history of episodic facial flushing and dizziness, sometimes accompanied by wheezing respiration. These attacks could occur at any time but she was frequently embarrassed by them at meal times.

#### Investigations
urinary 5-hydroxyindoleacetic acid excretion
  270 μmol/24 h (normal 10–50 μmol/24 h)

An isotopic scan of the liver revealed multiple filling defects suggestive of tumour deposits.
  A distorted hepatic vasculature with evidence of tumour circulation was demonstrated on arteriography, but the primary tumour could not be located.

#### Comment
Facial flushing is the commonest clinical feature of carcinoid syndrome and may be provoked by the ingestion of food or alcohol, or by emotional stimuli. It may become continuous and spread to other parts of the body. The vasodilatation causes transient hypotension and patients may complain of dizziness. Other clinical features are listed in *Fig. 19.5* and include intermittent abdominal discomfort, diarrhoea and bronchospasm with wheezing. Right-sided valvular lesions of the heart, particularly pulmonary stenosis, may lead to cardiac failure.

The diagnosis is confirmed by demonstrating an increase in the urinary excretion of 5-hydroxyindoleacetic acid. This is usually more than twice the upper limit of normal and may be much greater. Foodstuffs containing serotonin (bananas, tomatoes) or drugs such as reserpine which stimulate endogenous serotonin release, must be avoided during collection.

## Management

Carcinoid tumours are difficult to manage. Once metastases have developed, surgical removal is usually not possible though partial resection may be palliative since the tumours are usually slow-growing. The best available medical treatment is with somatostatin analogues; these cause symptomatic relief and may cause some tumour regression. Interferon has also been used with some success. Hepatic metastases may be destroyed by hepatic arterial embolization. Partial symptomatic relief may be provided by serotonin antagonists, e.g., methysergide, or *p*-chlorophenylalanine, an inhibitor of tryptophan 5-hydroxylase.

## PLURIGLANDULAR SYNDROMES

The pluriglandular syndromes, also known as syndromes of multiple endocrine neoplasia (MEN), are familial disorders with an autosomal dominant inheritance, in which tumours (benign or malignant) or hyperplasia develop in two or more endocrine glands. These syndromes are uncommon, but it is important to recognize that a patient presenting with certain endocrinopathies could have one of these syndromes. The glands affected in the pluriglandular syndromes are shown in *Fig. 19.6*. Although the syndromes are inherited, the predominant features vary in different members of the same family; thus one person may present with recurrent peptic ulceration due to a gastrinoma (Zollinger–Ellison syndrome), while a sibling may have urinary calculi as a result of hyperparathyroidism.

## TUMOUR MARKERS

Tumour markers are substances which can be related to the presence or progress of a tumour. They include substances, including enzymes, other proteins and smaller peptides, which are secreted into body fluids by tumours, and antigens expressed on cell surfaces. Clinical chemistry laboratories are usually only involved in the measurement of tumour markers falling into the first category.

---

**Clinical features of the carcinoid syndrome**

**Gastrointestinal**
discomfort, hyperperistalsis
    and borborygmi
diarrhoea
nausea and vomiting
colicky pain

**Cardiovascular**
flushing
pulmonary stenosis (may lead to
    right heart failure and occasionally
    mitral stenosis)

**Respiratory**
bronchospasm
variable rate and depth of breathing

**Other**
pellagra
manifestations of secretion of other
    hormones

**Fig. 19.5** Clinical features of the carcinoid syndrome.

---

**Glands affected in multiple endocrine neoplasia**

MEN type I
parathyroids
pancreatic islets
anterior pituitary
adrenal cortex
thyroid (follicular cells)

MEN type IIa
thyroid (medullary cell carcinoma)
adrenal medulla (phaeochromocytoma)
parathyroids

MEN type IIb
thyroid (medullary cell carcinoma)
adrenal medulla (phaeochromocytoma)
parathyroids (rarely)
various somatic abnormalities:
    Marfanoid habitus
    mucosal neuromata
    pigmentation

**Fig.19.6** Glands affected in multiple endocrine neoplasia (MEN).

The ideal secreted tumour marker could be used for:
- Screening
- Diagnosis
- Prognosis
- Monitoring treatment
- Follow-up to detect recurrence.

Although some markers are reliable for some of these purposes, probably only one (chorionic gonadotrophin, a marker for choriocarcinoma) is widely used for all. The development of monoclonal antibody techniques has led to the discovery and subsequent investigation of many new tumour markers in recent years, but overall the number of markers which are of proven clinical value remains small.

## α-Fetoprotein

α-Fetoprotein is a glycoprotein of molecular weight 67,000 Da. It is synthesized by the yolk sac and the fetal liver and gut. In the fetus, it is a major plasma protein; in adults, the normal concentration is less than 15 μg/L. Increased plasma concentrations of α-fetoprotein are seen in normal pregnancy. Its use in the diagnosis of neural tube defects is discussed in *Chapter 16* .

α-Fetoprotein is a valuable marker for hepatocellular carcinomas and testicular teratomas. Overall, primary liver cancer is uncommon in the United Kingdom, and therefore population screening for the condition cannot be justified. However, some groups of patients – notably those with cirrhosis, persistence of hepatitis B virus and haemochromatosis – are at particularly high risk and selective screening using α-fetoprotein measurement may be of value. It is insufficiently sensitive for diagnostic purposes, and also lacks specificity, in that its plasma concentration can be modestly elevated in cirrhosis, and in other abdominal malignancies. It is not helpful in assessing prognosis. However, in histologically confirmed liver cancer, serial measurements of α-fetoprotein are of considerable value in monitoring the response of the patient to treatment. The normal hepatic regeneration that occurs following partial hepatic resection often engenders an increase in α-fetoprotein concentration, but this is only transient.

---

### CASE HISTORY 19.4

A two-year-old boy presented with progressive abdominal swelling. On examination, the liver was found to be massively enlarged. Ultrasound and radiological examinations suggested the presence of a tumour, and histological examination of tissue obtained by percutaneous needle biopsy showed this to be a hepatoblastoma.

### Investigations

serum α-fetoprotein      33,000 kU/L

A partial hepatectomy was performed but complete removal of the tumour was not possible because of its extent. The child was therefore started on a course of cytotoxic therapy.

### Comment

Such a massively elevated concentration of α-fetoprotein in a child is effectively diagnostic of hepatoblastoma. The change in serum α-fetoprotein is shown in *Fig. 19.7*. Partial hepatectomy produced a temporary fall in α-fetoprotein but continued growth of the tumour resulted in a further increase. Cytotoxic treatment produced a sustained decline in α-fetoprotein levels, and this corresponded to clinical remission.

---

In patients with testicular teratomas, α-fetoprotein measurements are valuable in assessing prognosis, in staging and in monitoring therapy. A very high concentration indicates a massive tumour load and a poor prognosis (a mortality rate greater than 40% if α-fetoprotein concentration is greater than 1000 kU/L). A rapid fall to normal after orchidectomy implies that the disease was limited to the testis. Remission is achieved in 80% of patients with metastatic teratoma of the testis, using a combination of surgery and chemotherapy.

The efficacy of treatment can be assessed from the decline in plasma α-fetoprotein which reflects the decrease in tumour mass. Once a patient is in remission, repeated measurements are essential; a rise in concentration will be due to recurrence of the tumour and indicates the need for further treatment or a change in the chemotherapeutic regimen. It should be appreciated that plasma concentrations of α-fetoprotein within the 'normal' range are compatible with the presence of tumour; a rise in concentration, even if within this range, should raise the suspicion of tumour recurrence. On the other hand, tumours may lose the ability to secrete α-fetoprotein and so vigorous clinical assessment remains an important part of the follow-up of these patients.

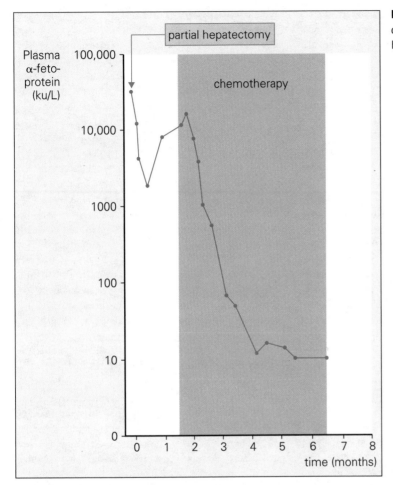

**Fig. 19.7** α-Fetoprotein concentration in a patient with hepatoblastoma.

## Carcinoembryonic antigen (CEA)

This tumour marker is present in elevated concentrations in the plasma of 60% of patients with colorectal cancer, more commonly so with advanced disease (80–100% if hepatic metastases are present) than with tumours confined to the colon. However, elevated concentrations are also found in a variety of non-malignant conditions, including liver disease of various types, pancreatitis and inflammatory bowel disease, and in some people who smoke heavily.

CEA is neither sufficiently specific nor sensitive to be used in screening for colorectal carcinoma. CEA concentrations in plasma correlate poorly with tumour bulk, which limits the usefulness of measurements in monitoring treatment. Following surgical resection of a tumour plasma CEA concentration can be expected to fall. However, while a subsequent rise suggests a recurrence, recurrence is not always heralded by such a rise and even when it is, it may

not affect the clinical outcome since further treatment is rarely of benefit.

## Paraproteins

Paraproteins (*see pp 208–209*) are detectable in either serum or urine in 98–99% of patients with myeloma. Not only is their detection valuable in the diagnosis of this condition, but paraprotein levels correlate well with tumour bulk with the result that the reduction in the amount of paraprotein is a good indicator of the efficacy of treatment.

## Human chorionic gonadotrophin (hCG)

hCG is a hormone produced by the normal placenta, reaching a maximum concentration in plasma by the eighth week of pregnancy. hCG is composed of an α- and β-subunit: the α-subunit is identical to that of luteinizing hormone (LH), follicle stimulating hormone (FSH) and thyroid stimulating hormone (TSH); the β-subunit, however, is specific to hCG and is therefore measured in assays for the hormone. The presence of hCG in the plasma at other times indicates the presence of abnormal trophoblastic tissue or a tumour secreting the hormone ectopically.

β-hCG is an almost ideal tumour marker for choriocarcinoma, a malignant proliferation of chorionic villi which may develop from hydatidiform mole, itself a potentially malignant proliferation of this tissue which occurs in approximately 1 in 2000 pregnancies in the United Kingdom. Hydatidiform mole is treated by uterine curettage, but the patient is at risk of developing choriocarcinoma if removal is incomplete. β-hCG is an extremely sensitive tumour marker; tumours weighing only 1 mg (corresponding to $10^5$ cells) may be detectable. All patients who have had hydatidiform moles must be followed up with regular checks of plasma β-hCG concentration. Should a tumour develop, the marker can be used as an indicator of the response to treatment and, if this is successful, in long-term follow-up thereafter.

hCG is also secreted by approximately 50% of testicular teratomas and should be measured together with α-fetoprotein in the follow-up of patients after treatment of the tumour. Since LH concentrations rise after orchidectomy, it is important that an assay specific to the β-chain of hCG is employed to avoid cross reaction causing an apparent increase in hCG.

## Other hormones as tumour markers

Hormones secreted both eutopically and ectopically can provide useful tumour markers. The measurement, for example, of metabolites of serotonin in the diagnosis of carcinoid syndrome and of catecholamines in phaeochromocytomas, has been discussed elsewhere (*pp. 134, 273*). Calcitonin is a valuable marker, not only for medullary cell carcinoma of the thyroid (eutopic secretion) but in some cases of carcinoma of the breast (ectopic secretion). Medullary cell carcinoma of thyroid is commonly familial and can be part of a pluriglandular syndrome. Calcitonin measurements can be used to screen for this tumour in the families of affected patients. Although basal plasma concentrations of calcitonin may be normal, an excessive rise following provocation, for example, with alcohol, pentagastrin or calcium infusion, is seen in patients with medullary carcinoma.

Ectopic hormonal markers of other tumours, for example, bronchial carcinomas, are of little practical use in the management of patients. They are not present sufficiently frequently to be of use in screening and the response to treatment is, in general, so poor that their measurement provides no practical support to the clinician.

## Markers of prostatic cancer

Prostatic acid phosphatase (PAP) was formerly widely used as a marker to monitor patients with disseminated prostatic carcinoma being treated with oestrogens. Although elevated levels of the enzyme are seen in more than 90% of patients with disseminated disease, they are seen in only about one-third of patients with a tumour confined to the prostate, rendering it unsuitable as a screening test. Most laboratories now prefer the measurement of prostate specific antigen (PSA), a glycoprotein unrelated to PAP, as a marker for prostatic cancer. PSA is detectable in all men, and its plasma concentration increases with age and in benign prostatic hypertrophy, so that it is unsuitable for population screening for prostatic cancer. However, it is a more sensitive marker than acid phosphatase, particularly in early disease, and is also superior for monitoring treatment. Using a cut off of 4 mg/L, specificity is 97% in men over the age of 40, and sensitivity for stage I disease, 67%. The finding of an elevated level of PSA in a patient with prostatism is thus not diagnostic of prostatic cancer but should prompt the patient's admission for biopsy and histological diagnosis.

## Other enzymes as tumour markers

Plasma enzyme activities are often increased in patients with cancer, but this is usually tumour-related rather than tumour-derived – that is, it is a secondary effect of the tumour rather than a result of secretion of an enzyme by the tumour. Examples include the increases in alkaline phosphatase activity seen in patients with biliary obstruction or bony metastases.

Alkaline phosphatase has several isoenzymes, and an increase in the plasma activity of the placental type in plasma occurs in many patients with testicular seminomas and is tumour-derived. Measurement of placental alkaline phosphatase is of value in monitoring the response of such patients to treatment.

Neuron-specific enolase is an isoenzyme of enolase present in nerve and neuroendocrine cells. Small cell carcinomas of bronchus, which are neuroendocrine in origin, frequently secrete this enzyme and when this occurs, patients' response to treatment can be monitored by serial measurements.

## Carbohydrate antigen (CA) markers

These are tumour markers which have been identified as a result of attempts to develop monoclonal antibodies against tumour extracts or tumour-derived cell lines. They are high molecular weight glycoproteins. Many CA markers have been identified and investigated; none has yet been identified

| Some clinically useful tumour markers | | |
|---|---|---|
| **Marker** | **Tumour** | **Uses** |
| α-fetoprotein | hepatoma germ cell | SDMF DPMF |
| β-human chorionic gonadotrophin | germ cell choriocarcinoma | DPMF SDPMF |
| carcinoembryonic antigen | colorectal carcinoma | MF |
| paraproteins | myeloma | DMF |
| calcitonin | medullary thyroid carcinoma | SDMF |
| prostatic specific antigen | prostatic carcinoma | MF |
| CA 125 | ovarian carcinoma | SPM |

S = screening (only in individuals at high risk)
D = diagnosis
P = prognosis
M = monitoring treatment
F = follow-up

**Fig. 19.8** Some clinically useful tumour markers.

which is specific for a particular tumour, or even tissue, and in general, those that are in use clinically are used for monitoring rather than for screening or diagnosis. An exception is CA 125, a marker for ovarian cancer. Ovarian cancer shows a strong familial incidence, and CA 125 measurements can be used in combination with other techniques (e.g., vaginal examination, ultrasonography) to screen for the tumour in relatives of patients, although it should be appreciated that CA 125 can be elevated in patients with other cancers, or with benign conditions, e.g., endometriosis. The CA 125 concentration at the time of diagnosis is of little prognostic significance but serial measurements are valuable in monitoring patients following surgical resection of a tumour. An inadequate fall in concentration during chemotherapy suggests that treatment is being unsuccessful and may prompt a change in treatment to palliative treatment only.

Other tumour markers of this category which are of potential value in monitoring the response of patients to treatment include CA 19-9 for adenocarcinoma of pancreas and possibly colorectal and gastric carcinomas, CA 50 for colorectal carcinoma and CA 15-3 for carcinoma of breast. Plasma CA 19-9 concentrations are elevated in more than 80% of patients with carcinoma of the exocrine pancreas, but only occasionally in benign disease. However, its potential value as a marker is diminished by the fact that pancreatic cancer tends to present late, when no effective treatment is available.

In carcinoma of the breast, both CA 15-3 and mucin-like carcinoma associated antigen (MCA) may help to identify patients who have metastases at the time of diagnosis.

## CONCLUSION

The clinical usefulness of secreted tumour markers for screening and diagnosis is limited to a small number of markers (*Fig. 19.8*) and relatively uncommon tumours. Other markers are of use in monitoring the response of patients to treatment and there is considerable research in progress in this field. Antibodies developed against tumour cell-surface antigens are of considerable value in the differential diagnosis of lymphomas and leukaemias, although their measurement is not usually the responsibility of the clinical biochemist.

## SUMMARY

Patients with malignant disease frequently suffer from disorders not directly attributable to the physical presence of the tumour. These 'paraneoplastic' syndromes include metabolic disorders, notably those in which ectopic hormone secretion occurs. This term refers to the secretion of a known hormone (or a substance with hormone-like activity) by a non-endocrine tumour.

The clinical features produced can closely resemble those seen when a hormone is secreted in excess by its normal tissue of origin (eutopic secretion). Examples include Cushing's syndrome and the syndrome of inappropriate antidiuretic hormone secretion caused by the production of adrenocorticotrophin and antidiuretic hormone (vasopressin), respectively, by small cell carcinomas of bronchus and various other tumours; a syndrome resembling hyperparathyroidism (but in fact rarely due to parathyroid hormone itself) occurring in some patients with squamous cell carcinomas of bronchus and renal adenocarcinomas; and hypoglycaemia which may occur in patients with large mesenchymal tumours, though not due to insulin. Other hormones that have been shown to be secreted by non-endocrine tumours include chorionic gonadotrophin, growth hormone releasing hormone, calcitonin and erythropoietin. The mechanism of ectopic hormone secretion is unclear but it is presumed that selective derepression of the appropriate genes occurs in the tumour cells.

Cancer cachexia, a non-specific syndrome of weight loss, anorexia and weakness, is common in patients with cancer. It is probably multifactorial in origin but the secretion of a humoral substance by the tumour may be partly responsible.

Many tumours capable of secreting hormones are derived from cells of the APUD system (cells of neuroectodermal origin characterized by their ability to take up and decarboxylate amines). Carcinoid tumours are derived from argentaffin cells, themselves members of the APUD family. These tumours are mainly found in the gut; they are of low grade malignancy and may go unnoticed unless metastasis occurs. They tend to secrete 5-hydroxytryptamine (5-HT); this is released into the portal circulation and usually metabolized by the liver but when hepatic metastases are present, 5-HT reaches the systemic circulation and may produce the carcinoid syndrome. The diagnosis is made by demonstrating an increased urinary excretion of the 5-HT metabolite, 5-hydroxyindoleacetic acid.

Some tumours occur in association and this tendency is often inherited. There are several syndromes of multiple endocrine neoplasia. Tumours that may be present in these syndromes include parathyroid adenomas, medullary cell carcinomas, phaeochromocytomas and pancreatic endocrine tumours.

Hormones secreted by tumours are occasionally useful as markers for the presence of the tumour but in general the fact that any particular hormone is also being produced by its normal source and is usually not consistently secreted by a particular tumour vitiates their measurement for this purpose. Some tumours, however, regularly secrete substances which are not usually detectable in the plasma and these may be useful markers both for diagnosis and for following the progress of a malignancy. The best established examples of such tumour markers are α-fetoprotein (for testicular teratoma and hepatocellular carcinoma), β-human chorionic gonadotrophin (choriocarcinoma), prostate-specific antigen (carcinoma of prostate), carcinoembryonic antigen (colorectal carcinoma) and paraproteins (myeloma). Of the many newer tumour markers, CA 125 is of value in patients with ovarian carcinoma, CA 19-9 in exocrine pancreatic cancer and CA 15-3 in carcinoma of breast.

# FURTHER READING

Abe K (ed.) (1980) Endocrinology and cancer. *Clinics in Endocrinology and Metabolism,* **9**, 209–433.

Beastall G H, Cook B, Rustin G J S & Jennings J (1991) A review of the role of established tumour markers. *Annals of Clinical Biochemistry,* **28**, 5–18.

Calman K C (1982) Cancer cachexia. *British Journal of Hospital Medicine,* **27**, 28–34.

Duffy M J (1989) New cancer markers. *Annals of Clinical Biochemistry,* **25**, 379–387.

Gagel R F (ed.) (1994) Multiple endocrine neoplasia. *Endocrinology and Metabolism Clinics of North America,* **23**, 1–233.

Insogna, K L (1989) Humoral hypercalcaemia of malignancy. *Endocrinology and Metabolism Clinics of North America,* **18**, 779–794.

Wilson J D & Foster D W (eds) (1992) *Williams – Textbook of Endocrinology.* 8th edition. Philadelphia: W B Saunders Company.

# 20. Therapeutic Drug Monitoring and Chemical Aspects of Toxicology

## INTRODUCTION

Clinical chemistry laboratories are called upon to measure drugs in body fluids for three main purposes: (i) to provide information relevant to the diagnosis and management of patients suspected to have taken drug overdoses; (ii) to provide such information in patients taking drugs therapeutically; (iii) to screen for the presence of drugs of abuse. This chapter covers these topics and discusses the metabolic sequelae of some common poisonings.

## THERAPEUTIC DRUG MONITORING

The questions that should be addressed when prescribing a drug are summarised in *Fig. 20.1*. All patients treated with drugs should be monitored clinically to assess the efficacy of treatment and to detect any adverse effects; laboratory assessment may also be helpful for these purposes. Thus, it may be possible to measure a particular index of therapeutic

| Prescribing a drug |
|---|
| What effect is it hoped to achieve? |
| Is the drug chosen capable of producing the desired effect? |
| What are the side-effects of the drug and, if they are predictable, do the likely benefits of using the drug outweigh the disadvantages? |
| Are there any special factors in the patient which increase the likelihood of an abnormal response to the drug? |
| How should the effect of the drug be monitored? |
| If the drug is not effective, or produces undesirable effects, why does this happen? |

**Fig. 20.1** Questions that must be addressed when prescribing a drug.

response, for example, the blood glucose concentration in a patient with diabetes treated with insulin, or thyroid function tests in a patient with thyrotoxicosis treated with carbimazole. Additionally, the laboratory may also be asked to monitor for possible toxic effects: for example, proteinuria in patients treated with penicillamine, or abnormalities of thyroid function in patients treated with the iodine-containing antiarrhythmic drug, amiodarone.

An individual's response to a particular drug is dependent upon many factors, for example, age, sex, renal function and the concurrent administration of other drugs. These factors must be borne in mind when deciding what dose of drug to prescribe, but in many cases the optimum dosage can be arrived at by commencing treatment with a standard dose and modifying this as necessary in the light of the observed response.

This approach is suitable for the many drugs whose effects can be assessed reliably, such as hypotensive agents, anticoagulants, insulin and oral hypoglycaemics, but it is not universally applicable. Obviously, optimization of drug dosage in this way is impossible when the effect of treatment is not easily ascertainable. An example is the use of anticonvulsants as prophylaxis in epilepsy. The incidence of seizures prior to treatment is unpredictable in many patients, making it difficult to assess the effect of the drug in preventing them. It is also difficult to adjust dosage on the basis of the therapeutic effect when a drug has a low therapeutic ratio (that is, the dose required to produce a therapeutic effect is close to that at which features of toxicity are seen) especially if the adverse effects are hard to recognize. In such cases, measurement of the concentration of the drug in the plasma may provide valuable objective information.

It is outside the scope of this chapter to discuss in detail the many factors that can influence the relationship between the dose of a drug and the intensity of its effects. Some of these are listed in *Fig. 20.2*. It is reasonable to assume that there will be a greater correlation between the intensity of a drug's effect and its plasma concentration than with the dose of the drug that the patient takes. Despite this, plasma concentrations and tissue effects may correlate poorly since the drug must first travel from the plasma to its site of action, and once there the responsiveness of the tissues may

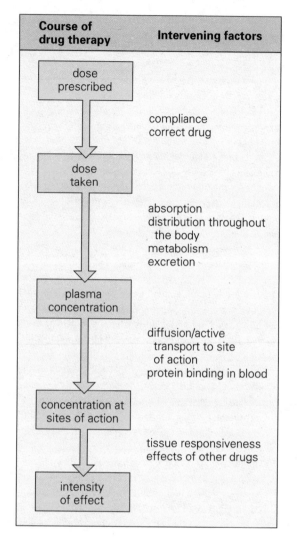

| Course of drug therapy | Intervening factors |
|---|---|
| dose prescribed | |
| | compliance<br>correct drug |
| dose taken | |
| | absorption<br>distribution throughout<br>  the body<br>metabolism<br>excretion |
| plasma concentration | |
| | diffusion/active<br>  transport to site<br>  of action<br>protein binding in blood |
| concentration at sites of action | |
| | tissue responsiveness<br>effects of other drugs |
| intensity of effect | |

not be constant or predictable. Additionally, there may be no correlation at all when a drug is itself inactive (but is metabolized to an active substance in the body) or when it acts irreversibly.

Nevertheless, the correlation between the plasma concentration and pharmacological effect is surprisingly strong for many drugs and provides the rationale for the use of concentration measurement in therapeutic drug monitoring (TDM). It is important that any experimentally determined relationship between plasma drug concentration and the effect of a drug is confirmed in a clinical setting, and that plasma drug concentrations are interpreted in the particular clinical context. The time of sampling in relation to the time of dosage may be critical and the sensitivity of the target organ may vary, being influenced, for example, by genetic factors, nutritional status, the presence of other drugs and the health of the patient.

Even if there is good evidence that measuring the plasma concentration of a particular drug can provide useful information, in individual cases there should always be a rational reason for the request (i.e., a specific question should be asked, the answer to which will influence management); the right specimen (particularly with regard to timing) must be provided; and the analysis must be accurate and its result interpreted correctly. Finally, appropriate action should ensue.

**Fig. 20.2** Factors influencing the relationship between drug usage and the intensity of its effect; the latter is not necessarily directly related to the plasma concentration but may be more closely related to it than the dose prescribed

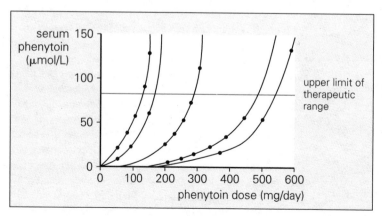

**Fig. 20.3** Relationship between the steady state serum concentration of phenytoin and dose; 80 μmol/L is the upper limit of the therapeutic range. Data for five patients are shown. Redrawn from Richens and Dunlop (1975).

In addition to individualizing the drug therapy, measurements of plasma concentrations of drugs can be useful in the diagnosis of suspected toxicity and in the assessment of compliance.

## Measuring plasma concentration

The most frequently used assays measure total plasma concentration of a drug. With drugs that are protein bound, changes in plasma protein concentration may have a disproportionate effect on the total drug concentration relative to the amount free in the plasma and thus available to tissues. The assay chosen must be specific for the drug itself (or its active metabolite where appropriate) and should not measure inactive metabolites or be affected by other drugs that the patient may be taking.

As with other biochemical measurements, plasma concentrations of drugs are compared with standard data. The term 'reference range' is inappropriate in this context, since healthy people will not be taking the drug. The term 'therapeutic' or 'target' range is used instead. This is the range between the minimum effective concentration of the drug and the maximum safe concentration. Often, only the upper limit is stated, since a drug may be efficacious in some individuals at concentrations below the generally accepted minimum effective concentration. On the other hand, optimum management may sometimes require that a drug's concentration is maintained above the upper limit of the therapeutic/target range. Such ranges are not absolute; for example, hypokalaemia increases sensitivity to digoxin and effectively lowers the upper limit.

In the following section the use of plasma measurements of a few representative and commonly used drugs is discussed to illustrate the general principles of therapeutic drug monitoring.

## MONITORING OF SPECIFIC DRUGS

### Phenytoin

The therapeutic effectiveness of this popular anticonvulsant drug is difficult to assess without monitoring. It has a low therapeutic ratio and the signs of toxicity may mimic the neurological diseases associated with epilepsy. Further, phenytoin has unusual pharmacokinetic properties; the enzyme responsible for the elimination of the drug becomes saturated within the therapeutic range of plasma concentrations. This phenomenon has several important implications. In particular, the relationship between plasma concentration and dose is non-linear (*Fig. 20.3*); thus small increments in dose may lead to disproportionate increases in steady state plasma concentrations. On the other hand,

even if the dose is unchanged, a small decrease in drug-metabolizing enzyme activity, or the presence of other drugs that inhibit phenytoin metabolism, could transform a therapeutic plasma concentration to a toxic concentration. *Fig. 20.3* also indicates the wide variation of doses required to achieve therapeutic plasma levels in different individuals.

---

**CASE HISTORY 20.1**

A young woman developed idiopathic epilepsy at the age of 19 and had three generalized convulsions in 10 days before being started on phenytoin, 150 mg/day. She had a further fit two days after the first dose but thereafter remained fit-free.

**Investigations**

plasma phenytoin (four weeks after
starting treatment)                30 µmol/L

**Comment**

Steady state plasma concentrations of phenytoin may not be reached for three to four weeks. The upper limit of the therapeutic range is 80 µmol/L. The usual procedure when commencing treatment is to give a standard dose of 150–200 mg/day (in adults) and to measure the plasma concentration after three to four weeks. If the patient is well controlled and there are no features of toxicity the same dose may be continued even if, as in this case, the plasma concentration is low in the therapeutic range. A dose increment is not indicated if the patient is fit-free just on the basis of the plasma concentration of the drug. In the well-controlled patient, this initial plasma concentration may be useful later to help ascertain the cause (for example, poor compliance, drug interaction) should seizures recur.

If the patient is not well controlled, increments in dose can be made, guided by measurement of plasma concentrations, to produce a steady state concentration in the therapeutic range. Phenytoin has a long half-life when used chronically and plasma concentrations remain relatively constant throughout the day. For this reason (unusually in therapeutic drug monitoring) the time of sampling in relation to the time the drug was taken is not critical. However, it is essential to leave sufficient time after changing the dose to allow a new steady state to develop. This takes approximately four times the plasma half-life of the drug.

---

The measurement of plasma phenytoin concentration is also useful if adverse effects occur, if there is an unexplained deterioration in the patient's control, and if a drug known to interact with phenytoin has to be prescribed. It is of particular value in children and during pregnancy, when dramatic fluctuations in plasma levels and in epileptic control may occur.

## Other anticonvulsants

The value of measuring the plasma concentrations of some other anticonvulsant drugs is shown in *Fig. 20.4*. The case is proven for carbamazepine but not for any others. The dosage of ethosuximide can often be adjusted on clinical grounds. With sodium valproate, there is no clear safe maximum concentration, there is a poor correlation between plasma concentration and efficacy, and hepatotoxicity, which is anyway rare, cannot be predicted from plasma concentration. Vigabatrin and lamotrigine are new anticonvulsant drugs. TDM of vigabatrin is unlikely to be of value. Plasma concentrations show little relationship to clinical effect, probably because the drug binds irreversibly to its target enzyme ($\gamma$-aminobutyric acid transferase) in the brain. The possible value of TDM for lamotrigine is still being examined.

## Digoxin

Digoxin is frequently used in the management of cardiac failure with atrial fibrillation, a common problem in the elderly. Plasma digoxin measurements are valuable not only in the assessment of the appropriate dose to prescribe, but also in the diagnosis of digoxin toxicity and in assessing patient compliance. Failure to take a prescribed medication (non-compliance) is a common cause of failure to achieve a therapeutic response.

The therapeutic range for plasma digoxin concentration is generally taken as 1.0–2.6 nmol/L. There is a significant increase in plasma concentration following a dose of the drug and a minimum period of six hours should elapse before blood is drawn for assessment of the mean steady state concentration. In practice it is often simplest, and satisfactory for diagnostic purposes, if a blood sample is taken shortly before a dose is due.

While the therapeutic effect is minimal when plasma concentration is below 1 nmol/L and toxicity becomes more common at concentrations above 2.6 nmol/L and is almost invariable if they exceed 3.8 nmol/L, there is in general a rather poor correlation between plasma concentration and therapeutic effect. Furthermore, evidence of toxicity may sometimes be seen in patients whose plasma concentration is below 2.6 nmol/L while others may tolerate levels 50% higher than this without ill effect.

| Therapeutic monitoring for anticonvulsant drugs | | |
|---|---|---|
| **Drug** | **Therapeutic range** | **Monitoring** |
| phenytoin | <80 µmol/L | essential |
| carbamazepine | <42 µmol/L | useful but not essential |
| ethosuximide | <700 µmol/L | useful but not essential |
| phenobarbitone | <170 µmol/L | tolerance makes upper limit imprecise |
| primidone | | metabolized to phenobarbitone (which should be monitored) primidone levels not useful |
| sodium valproate | >700 µmol/L ? | not proven to be useful |
| clonazepam | <285 µmol/L | not proven to be useful |

**Fig.20.4** Therapeutic monitoring of anticonvulsant drugs.

This phenomenon is partly a result of the existence of various factors which alter either the therapeutic response to a given plasma concentration of digoxin or the plasma concentration achieved on a particular dose (*Fig. 20.5*). Hypokalaemia is a particular problem since many patients treated with digoxin are also receiving diuretics, which may cause this (see *Case History 22.2*); also, renal impairment may be a consequence of congestive cardiac failure. It is thus very important to consider the clinical setting when assessing the significance of plasma digoxin concentrations.

Digoxin concentrations are also useful in the diagnosis of digoxin toxicity. This is important because some of the features of toxicity are relatively non-specific (for example, nausea and vomiting), while others include dysrhythmias which could possibly be a complication of the underlying heart disease. It is important that the possible influence of pathological and physiological factors is considered (*see Fig. 20.5*).

If a patient taking digoxin is symptom-free yet has a plasma concentration less than 1 nmol/L, it is likely that the drug is not required, and it may be withdrawn, though under supervision.

## Antidysrhythmics

Methods are available for the measurement of many other drugs used in patients with heart disease, in particular, anti-

| Sensitivity to digoxin |
|---|
| **Stimulatory factors** |
| hypokalaemia<br>hypercalcaemia<br>hypomagnesaemia<br>hypoxia<br>hypothyroidism |
| **Inhibitory factors** |
| hypocalcaemia<br>hyperthyroidism |

**Fig. 20.5** Factors affecting sensitivity to digoxin. In addition, renal impairment and hypothyroidism may increase the plasma concentration of digoxin in relation to the dose taken; hyperthyroidism may decrease the concentration.

dysrhythmics. The arguments relating to the value of plasma concentrations in monitoring treatment are complex and the place of therapeutic drug monitoring is debatable. It is probably useful for procainamide, lignocaine and quinidine, but its role with antidysrhythmics such as amiodarone and verapamil has yet to be established.

## Lithium

Lithium is widely used in the management of acute mania and for prophylaxis in manic-depressive psychosis. The optimum therapeutic plasma concentration varies from patient to patient with an overall range of 0.3–1.3 mmol/L, 12 h after the last dose. Higher concentrations are required to produce a satisfactory effect in acute illness than when the drug is used for prophylaxis. Lithium has a low therapeutic ratio and there are wide interindividual differences in dose requirements, with the result that the monitoring of plasma concentration has become vital to the management of patients on lithium therapy.

Lithium is nephrotoxic and is excreted by the kidneys, and consequently toxicity may be self-perpetuating. Renal handling of lithium is also related to sodium balance and diuretics may cause lithium retention.

Plasma concentrations >1.5 mmol/L should be avoided. In lithium toxicity, dialysis may be required to remove the drug if the concentration exceeds 3.5 mmol/L. Its efficacy can be monitored by plasma lithium measurements.

Blood samples for monitoring lithium treatment should be taken 12 h after the previous dose; up to a week may be needed after dosage is changed before a new steady state is attained.

## Theophylline

This is a bronchodilator, used in the treatment of asthma and neonatal apnoea. Response to theophylline in different patients varies considerably in relation to dosage but correlates well with plasma concentration. The therapeutic range is 55–100 µmol/L (25–80 µmol/L in infants, *see below*); toxicity (principally cardiac dysryhthmias) may occur at higher concentrations. Because patients requiring intravenous theophylline for severe asthma may already be being treated with an oral preparation and thus have the drug in their blood stream, there may be a requirement to measure concentrations rapidly. In infants, in whom the drug is used as a respiratory stimulant, significant metabolism to caffeine occurs; this metabolite is also pharmacologically active and ideally its concentration should be measured as well as that of theophylline.

## Cyclosporin

This is an immunosuppressive drug, widely used following transplant surgery to prevent graft rejection. It is nephrotoxic but toxicity should be avoidable if plasma concentrations are monitored. Measurements may also help to distinguish between drug toxicity and incipient rejection of a grafted kidney, both of which can cause an increase in plasma creatinine concentration.

## Aminoglycoside antibiotics

These agents (for example, gentamicin) are nephro- and ototoxic, but relatively high concentrations are needed for bactericidal effects. They have a short plasma half-life. Toxicity appears to relate to the trough concentration (i.e., that found immediately before a dose); bactericidal action requires a sufficient peak concentration (achieved shortly after a dose has been given) although too high a peak concentration should be avoided. The peak and trough concentrations can be manipulated independently to some extent by altering the dose and the frequency of dosage. Thus, increasing the dose will increase both concentrations but if the peak concentration is satisfactory and the trough too low, the same dose may be given, but at more frequent intervals.

## Other drugs

The use of high doses of methotrexate (a cytotoxic drug) is made safer by the use of TDM. Methotrexate inhibits dihydrofolate reductase and depletes intracellular stores of reduced folate. At high concentrations, this depletion may become potentially harmful to the host as well as the tumour, by causing bone marrow suppression. Marrow damage becomes maximal later than the effect on tumour cells, and can be prevented by the use of leucovorin (folinic acid) 'rescue' treatment if a high plasma concentration of methotrexate suggests that there is a significant risk of its occurring.

In some centres, TDM is practised for erythropoietin. Although successful use of this agent produces an easily measurable response (an increase in haemoglobin), there is a delay before this occurs and TDM can prevent wasteful over-treatment with this expensive drug.

A case can also be made for the measurement of plasma concentrations of antidepressant drugs.

While at present most therapeutic drug monitoring is based on serum or plasma measurements, there is increasing interest in salivary assays. These tend to reflect the plasma concentration of the non-protein bound, that is, free, drug which is directly available to the tissues; the advantage of this technique is that venepuncture is not required.

## CHEMICAL TOXICOLOGY

Poisoning is a common reason for hospital admission. In most cases, the patient has taken an overdose of a prescribed or over-the-counter drug, but poisoning may also be the result of accident (common in children), suicide or homicide and the range of toxic substances is vast, including industrial and domestic chemicals, plants and fungi as well as drugs.

## Management

There are no specific antidotes for most poisons. Management is therefore primarily directed towards the support of vital functions. This may be supplemented by measures to prevent further absorption (e.g., gastric lavage, oral activated charcoal) or to remove the drug from the body. In severe cases the laboratory has an important role in monitoring vital functions, for example, measuring arterial blood gases. Measurement of the plasma concentration of the poison may indicate the need to take steps to increase its elimination and is valuable in monitoring such treatment. For some poisons, specific treatments are available but these may themselves not be without risk to the patient. Plasma concentrations can then be used to indicate whether such treatment is likely to be of value.

Few poisons produce specific physical signs: patients' histories, if available, may not be reliable and mixed drug overdoses are common. There is therefore a need for an analytical service to identify what poisons may have been ingested, particularly if a patient does not respond to conventional management. This presents an entirely different problem for the laboratory since what is required is a screening service capable of identifying any of a large number of toxins, rather than providing quantitative data on a small number (see p 292).

## POISONING WITH SPECIFIC AGENTS

### Paracetamol

A specific antidote is available for paracetamol, the metabolism of which is summarized in *Fig. 20.6*. The major products of its metabolism are harmless glucuronide and sulphate conjugates, which are excreted in the urine together with a small amount of the unchanged drug. Small quantities of a highly hepatotoxic metabolite (*N*-acetyl *p*-benzoquinonimine) are also formed through the action of the mixed function oxidase (cytochrome P450) enzyme system; this is normally detoxified by conjugation with glutathione. However, the glucuronidation and sulphation pathways are saturable and so when an overdose of the drug is taken, a greater proportion is converted to the toxic

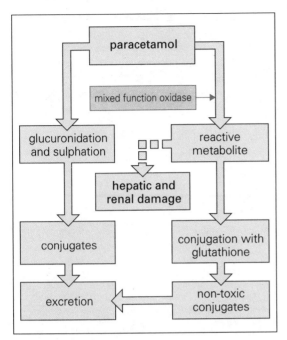

**Fig. 20.6** The metabolism of paracetamol. When the drug is taken in therapeutic doses, all the reactive metabolite formed is detoxified by conjugation with glutathione; when taken in overdose, glutathione supplies are rapidly exhausted and the metabolite accumulates causing cell damage.

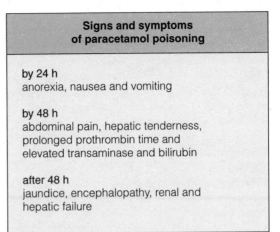

**Signs and symptoms of paracetamol poisoning**

by 24 h
anorexia, nausea and vomiting

by 48 h
abdominal pain, hepatic tenderness, prolonged prothrombin time and elevated transaminase and bilirubin

after 48 h
jaundice, encephalopathy, renal and hepatic failure

**Fig. 20.7** Signs and symptoms of paracetamol poisoning.

metabolite. Glutathione supplies are limited, and if they are insufficient to detoxify this metabolite, liver damage will result. The metabolite is also nephrotoxic, with the possible consequence that renal failure develops as well.

### Clinical features

Paracetamol is an insidious poison since there may be no clinical disturbance during the first 24 h after taking an overdose, except anorexia, nausea and vomiting (*Fig. 20.7*). The conscious state is normal unless a sedative drug has been taken concurrently (compound preparations containing paracetamol and a sedative, such as dextropropoxyphene, are common). If liver damage occurs, abdominal pain with hepatic tenderness will develop and liver function tests become abnormal (prolonged prothrombin time, elevated plasma transaminase activity and bilirubin concentration). The prothrombin time is the best marker of severity. If renal failure occurs, plasma creatinine concentration is a better indicator of renal function than that of urea, since hepatic

urea synthesis may be decreased. With massive overdoses, patients may develop fulminant hepatic failure (*see p. 84*).

It is possible to predict the likelihood of liver damage from the plasma concentration of paracetamol. The blood sample must be taken at least 4 h after ingestion of the drug. The plasma concentration can be used as a guide to patient management, that is, whether to treat the patient with an antidote (*Fig. 20.8*). Unfortunately, the time at which the drug was taken may not be known and it is then wisest to treat the patient actively if the concentration falls within the treatment zone. Patients on treatment with enzyme-inducing drugs, e.g., phenytoin, are at greater risk of developing liver disease. There is no rational basis for the use of an antidote once liver damage has occurred, and it has previously been assumed that measuring plasma paracetamol concentration more than 12–15 h after an overdose is of no value. However, later measurements may be justified to confirm the diagnosis since there is now evidence that treatment with N-acetyl cysteine may be beneficial even 30 h after paracetamol ingestion.

### Management

The most widely used antidotes are N-acetylcysteine (which must be given parenterally) and methionine (given orally). Although it is more expensive, N-acetylcysteine is usually preferred as the absorption of methionine is unpredictable, especially if the patient is vomiting. N-Acetylcysteine is given by intravenous infusion initially at a high dose and then at a lower dose over a period of 20 h. Plasma creatinine

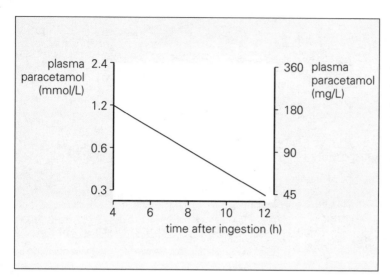

**Fig. 20.8** Plasma paracetamol concentrations and prognosis in paracetamol poisoning. Specific treatment is indicated if the concentration is above the line joining concentrations of 1.2 mmol/L at 4 h and 0.3 mmol/L at 12 h.

concentration and the prothrombin time should be checked before starting and at the end of treatment. Both *N*-acetyl-cysteine and methionine act by promoting hepatic glutathione synthesis, thereby increasing the capacity of the liver to detoxify the active metabolite.

In treating paracetamol poisoning, general emergency measures must not be forgotten. Gastric lavage or administration of an emetic is only of use in the first 4 h after an overdose. The patient must be kept hydrated, preferably using 5% dextrose since there may be a tendency to hypoglycaemia with hepatic damage. Vitamin K should be given prophylactically. Should liver failure develop, close clinical and laboratory monitoring are vital.

## Salicylates

Salicylate poisoning, usually with aspirin (acetylsalicylic acid) is common. It can produce profound metabolic disturbances and though there is no specific antidote, measures can be taken to increase the excretion of the drug which, though effective, are not without hazard in themselves. The upper limit of the therapeutic range of plasma salicylate concentration is approximately 2.5 mmol/L (35 mg/100 mL), but tinnitus, an early symptom of toxicity, may become apparent at lower concentrations.

The effects of salicylates which lead to metabolic disturbances are summarized in *Fig. 20.9*, and include stimulation of the respiratory centre, a non-respiratory acidosis, uncoupling of oxidative phosphorylation and a central emetic effect.

**CASE HISTORY 20.2**

A 20-year-old male student was brought into hospital in a confused state, having been found at home by his flatmate with an empty bottle of aspirin tablets on his desk.

On admission, he was hyperventilating and sweating profusely. He was pale but not anaemic. He was not grossly dehydrated but the inside of his mouth was dry and there was a smell of ketones on his breath. His pulse was 112/min, blood 110/60 mmHg and temperature 39.5°C.

**INVESTIGATIONS**

| serum: | | |
|---|---|---|
| | sodium | 131 mmol/L |
| | potassium | 3.2 mmol/L |
| | bicarbonate | 10 mmol/L |
| | urea | 10 mmol/L |
| | glucose | 3.2 mmol/l |
| | salicylate | 3.9 mmol/L |

| arterial blood: | |
|---|---|
| hydrogen ion | 62 nmol/L (pH 7.20) |
| $P_{CO_2}$ | 3.5 kPa (26 mmHg) |
| prothrombin time | 18 s (control 14 s) |

**Comment**
The results are consistent with the metabolic effects of salicylates described above. There is an acidosis,

compensated to some extent by hyperventilation (see Chapter 3). The initial acid–base disturbance (in adults, but usually not in children) is a respiratory alkalosis due to direct stimulation of the respiratory centre. This is usually overwhelmed by the developing acidosis, but during the alkalotic phase any compensatory renal excretion of bicarbonate will deplete the capacity of the body to buffer excess hydrogen ions, thus making the acidosis more dangerous.

Patients who have taken overdoses of salicylates are rarely comatose; irritability is an early feature and later hallucination and delirium may occur. Tinnitus may be a prominent feature. The prothrombin time may be prolonged, as in this case, due to decreased hepatic synthesis of clotting factors. Salicylates also inhibit platelet aggregation. However, although gastric erosions may occur, due directly to the action of salicylate on the gastric mucosa, severe bleeding is uncommon in aspirin overdosage. Nevertheless, prophylactic vitamin K is often administered.

### Management

There is no specific antidote to aspirin. It is metabolized by hydrolysis to salicylic acid, the active form of the drug, which is excreted unchanged in the urine; other metabolites include various inactive conjugates. The conjugation pathways are saturable, and once they are saturated, urinary excretion becomes the major route for elimination of the drug. If the urine is acidic, salicylic acid is not ionized and, though filtered by the glomeruli, is reabsorbed by the tubules. If the urine is alkaline, salicylic acid ionizes; its tubular reabsorption is decreased and urinary excretion is enhanced. This is the rationale for alkalinization using sodium bicarbonate infusions in the treatment of salicylate poisoning. However, this process is in itself potentially dangerous and requires careful monitoring. It should not be attempted if the patient already has a systemic alkalosis or if the urine pH exceeds 8, the aim being to maintain a urine pH greater than 7.5 during treatment. Potassium supplements are required (hypokalaemia may hinder effective alkalinization of the urine); dehydration and hypoglycaemia must be corrected, and fluid balance, blood glucose, arterial hydrogen ion concentration and urine pH must be monitored. It is often advocated that a high intravenous fluid input is maintained to promote a diuresis, but fluid overload must be avoided. It is far more important to ensure adequate alkalinization of the urine.

Aspirin is absorbed only slowly from the gut so gastric lavage is always worth attempting in overdose unless specifically contraindicated. The decision whether to embark on active treatment should be based on clinical grounds but guided by laboratory data. Maintenance of adequate hydration and general supportive measures are important for all patients. Alkalinization should be undertaken if plasma salicylate concentration exceeds 3.6 mmol/L (50 mg/100 mL) in adults and 2.2 mmol/L (30 mg/100 mL) in children more than 6 h after the overdose. If the initial concentration exceeds 6.5 mmol/L (90 mg/100 mL) and if there is renal impairment or if other therapeutic measures fail, haemoperfusion or haemodialysis will usually be necessary. Plasma salicylate levels should be measured during treatment as an indication of its efficacy.

## Iron

Iron poisoning, although much less common now than in the past, still occurs and can cause severe illness especially in young children. Iron causes necrosis of the gastrointestinal mucosa with resultant haemorrhage and fluid and electrolyte loss. Patients may develop encephalopathy and renal failure with circulatory collapse, and acute liver necrosis may develop in those who survive these complications.

Severe poisoning is indicated by plasma iron levels in excess of 90 µmol/L in a child, or 145 µmol/L in adults. Management involves the use of desferrioxamine, an iron-chelating agent, to promote iron excretion, together with appropriate supportive measures.

## Lead

Acute lead poisoning is very uncommon but chronic poisoning occurs more frequently. In children the source may be old paint or toys, and cosmetics and patent medicines imported from the Indian subcontinent. In adults most cases are associated with occupational exposure (e.g., battery manufacture, smelting, ship-breaking), and lead poisoning is a notifiable industrial disease. Lead is concentrated in erythrocytes and in persons who are not occupationally exposed to the metal, a blood concentration of greater than 1.5 µmol/L should be followed up. In lead workers, the presently accepted upper limit for blood lead is 3.4 µmol/L. Symptomatic lead poisoning is usually associated with concentrations in excess of 5 µmol/L, but in children symptoms may be present at lower concentrations.

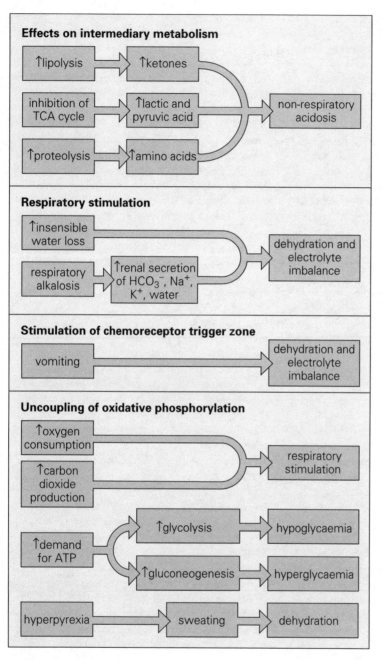

**Fig. 20.9** Pathophysiology of salicylate poisoning.

### Tests

Although blood lead measurement is the screening method of choice for excessive exposure, other tests may sometimes be useful. Lead interferes with several steps in porphyrin synthesis (*see p. 257*) and porphyrinuria (due mainly to coproporphyrin III) may be present in lead poisoning although this is not a very sensitive test. An excess of δ-aminolaevulinic acid in the urine is also characteristic but not specific. An excess of protoporphyrin in erythrocytes is a more sensitive indicator of excessive exposure to lead but again is not specific, also occurring in iron deficiency. However, the results of these tests may indicate a need to measure blood lead concentration itself, which may involve sending the blood sample to a specialized laboratory if the assay is not available locally.

Chemical pathology laboratories are becoming increasingly involved in screening for other industrial toxins, especially heavy metals. Specialized laboratories should be able to provide an analytical service for cadmium and mercury as well as lead.

### Clinical features and management

Lead poisoning causes nausea, vomiting and severe abdominal colic. In the nervous system, encephalopathy with convulsions and impairment of consciousness may lead to coma and death. In severe cases, usually due to acute lead poisoning, active treatment with a chelating agent, e.g., calcium versenate or dimercaprol, given parenterally, is required. In milder cases, oral penicillamine is useful, while for asymptomatic persons whose blood concentration indicates excessive exposure to lead, the source of lead should be identified and removed or the exposed person removed from the source.

## Alcohol

Although there is no specific antidote to ethanol, drug overdose is often complicated by the simultaneous ingestion of alcohol. It potentiates the action of many drugs and measurement of blood alcohol concentration may provide the explanation for an unexpected delay in a patient's recovery from drug overdose.

Blood alcohol measurements may also be of value in the management of patients with head injuries, when the effects of alcohol may make it difficult to assess the severity of any brain damage due to the injury itself.

### Clinical features and effects

Chronic alcoholism is now a major health problem in many areas of the world. In addition to its well-known harmful effects on the liver, chronic alcohol ingestion can damage many organs and tissues in the body. Metabolic sequelae include hypertriglyceridaemia, hypoglycaemia, hypogonadism, hyperuricaemia, a form of Cushing's syndrome, thiamin deficiency and cutaneous hepatic porphyria. Measurement of blood alcohol concentration may be of value in establishing a diagnosis of alcoholism.

It has been suggested that the finding of an ethanol concentration of greater than 65 mmol/L (300 mg/100 mL) at any time is diagnostic; in a patient who is asymptomatic, the concentration suggested is 33 mmol/L (150 mg/100 mL). The combination of a raised plasma $\gamma$-glutamyl transferase and increased mean red cell volume is a characteristic and sensitive index of excessive alcohol intake, although not an entirely specific one. Better laboratory tests are urgently required;

measurement of desialotransferrin is promising but not ideal and has not yet been introduced in many laboratories.

---

### CASE HISTORY 20.3

A garage mechanic was admitted to the emergency room unconscious, having been found in this state at home by his flatmate. He had been acutely depressed since the death of his girlfriend in a road traffic accident two weeks before. On examination, he was unrousable. Temperature, blood pressure and pulse were normal but he was hyperventilating.

#### Investigations

serum: (multi-channel autoanalyzer 'profile')

| | |
|---|---|
| sodium | 138 mmol/L |
| potassium | 5.2 mmol/L |
| bicarbonate | 4 mmol/L |
| urea | 7.0 mmol/L |
| creatinine | 110 µmol/L |
| glucose | 4.5 mmol/L |
| calcium | 1.5 mmol/L |
| osmolality | 326 mmol/kg |

(phosphate, protein, 'liver function' tests were within reference limits)

paracetamol, salicylate: not detected

blood: hydrogen ion     104 nmol/L

       $P\text{co}_2$           2.0 kPa

urine: negative for glucose and ketones

#### Comment

There is a severe non-respiratory acidosis; diabetic ketoacidosis is excluded by the normal glucose and lack of ketonuria. The calculated osmolarity is approximately 288 mmol/L, giving an 'osmotic gap' of 38 mmol/L, suggesting the presence of some other osmotically active substance(s) in the blood. A lactate concentration this high in lactic acidosis would be exceptional. The substance could be ethanol (although the acidosis of ethanol poisoning is usually a ketoacidosis) or some other alcohol. The clue to the diagnosis is provided by the low calcium concentration. The combination of severe acidosis and hypocalcaemia is characteristic of ethylene glycol poisoning. This substance is metabolized to various organic acids, including oxalic acid, which combines with calcium to form insoluble calcium oxalate.

---

## Other poisons

The possibility of poisoning should always be investigated in a comatose patient when no cause is obvious. Measurement of plasma osmolality, and comparison with the calculated value, may sometimes reveal the presence of a foreign substance in the blood, as this case history demonstrates.

## SCREENING FOR DRUGS

It has been pointed out that when a toxin does not have a specific antidote, precise knowledge of its plasma concentration does not contribute to patient management. Nevertheless, qualitative rather than quantitative measurement of a toxic agent may be desirable. If a patient is admitted to hospital unconscious for no readily discernible reason, identification of a drug may help to eliminate other possible causes. It may also draw attention to possible specific complications or suggest treatment, e.g., haemofiltration or dialysis, to remove the drug from the body.

Screening for drugs is also necessary in cases of suspected brain death. Symptoms of apparent brain death may be due to the presence of CNS-depressant drugs and it is vital that this possibility is eliminated before true brain death is diagnosed.

In cases of suspected homicide, the identification of any poisons present is vital and must be carried out by suitably qualified personnel whose testimony would be accepted in court if they were to be called upon as witnesses.

It is not practical for all laboratories to provide facilities for screening for all possible toxins. In the United Kingdom, there is a network of poisons reference laboratories providing advice and an analytical service for such purposes. Also, it is often more efficient to concentrate screening for drugs of abuse in specialized laboratories. Samples for drug screening should be collected after consultation with the nearest laboratory.

Urine is in general more useful for screening than blood, as many drugs and their metabolites are cleared rapidly from the blood but will be present in high concentration in the urine. Urine and blood samples, stomach contents and any tablets or material that may have been ingested should be collected, carefully labelled and, if analysis is not going to be performed immediately, stored in a refrigerator or deep-frozen.

Patterns of usage both of therapeutic drugs, 'recreational' drugs and drugs of abuse are always changing. As a result, laboratories must keep their repertoire of drug tests under constant review, so that they are able to offer an appropriate analytical service.

## SUMMARY

A knowledge of the concentration of a drug in the plasma can be of considerable assistance when deciding the appropriate drug dose to prescribe. This is particularly likely when the drug has a low therapeutic ratio (i.e., when the range of plasma concentrations over which the maximum beneficial effect is seen is only a little less than that at which it becomes toxic) and when it is difficult to assess the effect clinically. For drug concentrations to be used rationally for this purpose, it is essential that there is a predictable and defined relationship between concentration and effect. For many drugs, however, such therapeutic monitoring is unnecessary, as for example when the effect can readily be assessed clinically or by clinical or laboratory measurements, or when a drug of low toxicity has a virtually guaranteed effect when given in a standard dose. It is of no value when the effect of a drug is due to a metabolite, unless the concentration of the metabolite can be measured.

Therapeutic drug monitoring is an established technique in relation to the use of phenytoin, lithium, digoxin, aminoglycoside antibiotics, aminophylline and cyclosporin A. It is also used for certain antidysrhythmic drugs and for anticonvulsants other than phenytoin, but the rationale for therapeutic drug monitoring in some of these cases is open to argument and results should be interpreted and used with caution.

Measurement of drug concentrations in body fluids are also valuable in the investigation and management of patients who have taken overdoses of drugs or have been poisoned. Whilst the management of many forms of drug overdosage and poisoning is essentially conservative with the result that identification of the substance is of little direct use in management, for those drugs for which specific antidotes exist, or for which it is possible to take measures to promote their excretion, measurement of plasma concentrations can be very helpful. Thus the decision to treat paracetamol overdosage with N-acetylcysteine is based on whether the untreated patient would develop hepatic failure; this can be predicted from the plasma paracetamol concentration provided that the time of the drug overdose is known. With regard to salicylate overdosage, although there is no specific antidote, the excretion of the drug can be accelerated by alkaline diuresis and the plasma concentration provides a guide to whether this is necessary.

Specific measures are also available to increase the rate of elimination of iron and lead from the body, and the concentrations of these substances in plasma (iron) or blood (lead) can help decide whether or not to use such measures. Exposure to lead is an occupational hazard in certain industries and measurement of either blood lead concentration or erythrocyte protoporphyrin concentration can be used to detect individuals who have had excessive exposure.

Patients who have taken drug overdoses or been poisoned, frequently develop metabolic problems, the management of which requires the close cooperation of the clinical chemistry laboratory. Salicylate overdosage, for example, can result in profound disturbances of acid–base, glucose and electrolyte metabolism. Serial measurements of the plasma concentration of a drug will indicate the efficacy of any treatment designed to increase its excretion.

## FURTHER READING

Aronson S K, Hardman M & Reynolds D J M (1993) *ABC of Monitoring Drug Therapy.* London: BMJ Publishing Group.

Hallworth M C & Capps N (1994) *Therapeutic Drug Monitoring and Clinical Biochemistry.* London: ACB Ventura Publications.

Paton A P (ed.) (1993) *ABC of Alcohol.* London: BMJ Publishing Group.

Proudfoot A T (1993) *Acute Poisoning.* 2nd edition. Oxford: Butterworth–Heinemann.

# 21. Clinical Nutrition

## INTRODUCTION

An adequate intake of nutrients is essential for normal growth and development and for the maintenance of health. These nutrients include proteins, to supply amino acids, energy substrates (carbohydrates and fat), inorganic salts, vitamins, and other essential nutrients such as essential fatty acids. The daily requirements for these nutrients are determined by many factors, including age, sex, physical activity and the presence of disease; if an individual's requirements are not met, he is at risk of developing a clinical deficiency syndrome.

Excessive intake of nutrients can also be harmful. Obesity is a common condition in the developed world and is related to an intake of energy substrates in excess of the body's requirements. There is much evidence linking several common diseases, including coronary heart disease, hypertension and some cancers, with a relative excess or insufficiency of one or more components of the diet.

This chapter discusses the pathology of some specific deficiency syndromes, with particular reference to the role of the laboratory in their diagnosis and management. This role is also discussed in relation to patients suffering from, or at the risk of, generalized malnutrition. Nutritional support for these patients may be provided enterally (that is, into the alimentary tract, either by mouth or through a feeding tube) or parenterally (intravenously, bypassing the gut). Such treatment requires close cooperation between the clinician and the laboratory.

## VITAMIN DEFICIENCIES

Vitamin deficiency states can arise as a result of:
- Inadequate intake (with normal requirements).
- Impaired absorption.
- Impaired metabolism (if metabolism is necessary for function).
- Increased requirements.
- Increased losses.

The biochemical functions of most vitamins are well understood, but while the deficiency syndrome may obviously relate to the known function (e.g., osteomalacia in vitamin D deficiency) this is not always the case (e.g., beriberi and Wernicke's encephalopathy in thiamin deficiency). And although the clinical presentation of individual vitamin deficiency states is usually characteristic, in generalized malnutrition, multiple deficiencies can occur and cause a complex clinical presentation.

The classical deficiency syndromes are the end result of a process in which deficiency of a vitamin leads first to mobilization of body stores, then to tissue depletion, biochemical impairment (subclinical deficiency) and eventually to frank deficiency. The functions of vitamins are almost entirely intracellular, and their plasma concentrations do not necessarily reflect intracellular concentrations and thus functional availability.

It follows that plasma concentrations of vitamins may be unreliable as indicators of the body's vitamin status. In deficiency states, plasma levels tend to fall before tissue levels. On the other hand, if a vitamin is administered to a deficient patient, a rise in plasma concentration to normal is not necessarily indicative of adequate replacement.

In practice, the best means of assessing a patient's vitamin status depends upon the vitamin in question. The range of techniques that can be used is illustrated by the following examples.

## WATER-SOLUBLE VITAMINS

### Vitamin $B_1$ (thiamin)

Thiamin pyrophosphate is a cofactor in the metabolism of pyruvate and 2-oxoglutarate to acetyl-CoA and succinyl-CoA respectively, and in a reaction of the pentose shunt pathway catalyzed by the enzyme transketolase. The body contains only about 30 times the daily requirement of this vitamin. Subclinical thiamin deficiency may be unmasked in malnourished patients given glucose intravenously, which increases the metabolic requirement for the vitamin.

Deficiency of vitamin $B_1$ causes beriberi; one of the manifestations of this is Wernicke's encephalopathy, characterized by memory loss and nystagmus, and seen in the United Kingdom chiefly in chronic alcoholics whose diet is poor.

Other features of thiamin deficiency include peripheral neuropathy, muscle weakness, dementia and cardiac failure. Wernicke's encephalopathy responds rapidly to thiamin and since the vitamin is cheap and non-toxic this therapeutic response can be used to make the diagnosis. Laboratory tests for deficiency are seldom necessary.

It may, however, be necessary formally to document deficiency in nutritional research. One method involves administration of a glucose load and measurement of the plasma pyruvate concentration. An excessive rise is seen in thiamin deficiency because the vitamin is a cofactor for the conversion of pyruvate to acetyl-CoA. However, the most sensitive method, which will detect subclinical deficiency, is measurement of transketolase in a red cell haemolysate, the enzyme activity being measured both with and without the addition of thiamin pyrophosphate to the reaction mixture. Enzyme activity may be normal in subclinical deficiency but is increased by the addition of the coenzyme. If the deficiency is clinically obvious, the basal enzyme activity will be low.

---

### CASE HISTORY 21.1

An elderly lady, resident in a private nursing home, complained of difficulty in walking, with paraesthesiae and numbness in her legs. The physical signs were consistent with a peripheral neuropathy.

There had been suggestions that residents were not fed adequately and the doctor took a blood sample for measurement of transketolase before giving his patient vitamin supplements.

#### Investigations
red cell transketolase activity:
  without added thiamin pyrophosphate
                2.0 mmol/h/$10^9$ red cells
  with added thiamin pyrophosphate
                2.4 mmol/h/$10^9$ red cells

#### Comment
The patient's symptoms showed some improvement with the vitamin supplements. Red cell transketolase activity (measured by the decrease in substrate concentration as it is metabolized) was at the lower limit of normal and increased by 20% in the presence of thiamin pyrophosphate. This is consistent with mild thiamin deficiency; an increase of up to 14% is considered normal, while an increase of greater than 25% is clear evidence of deficiency. Peripheral neuropathy is a common clinical problem; thiamin deficiency is but one of many causes.

---

An analogous technique can be used for assessing riboflavin status (by measurement of the red cell enzyme glutathione reductase with and without the vitamin) and pyridoxine (using red cell alanine or aspartate transami-

nases). Deficiency of each of these vitamins (manifest in both cases principally by angular stomatitis, cheilosis and dermatitis) is uncommon in developed countries but may sometimes be seen in alcoholics and grossly malnourished individuals.

## Nicotinic acid

Nicotinic acid is the precursor of nicotinamide. This is a constituent of the coenzymes nicotinamide adenine dinucleotide (NAD) and its phosphate (NADP) which are essential to glycolysis and oxidative phosphorylation.

Part of the body's nicotinic acid requirement is met by endogenous synthesis from tryptophan. The deficiency syndrome, pellagra, can result from either an inadequate dietary intake of nicotinic acid or decreased synthesis. The latter may be a feature of the carcinoid syndrome, in which there is increased metabolism of tryptophan to hydroxyindoles with consequently less available for nicotinic acid synthesis, and of Hartnup disease, a rare inherited disorder of the epithelial transport of neutral amino acids, due to decreased intestinal absorption of tryptophan from the gut.

Nicotinic acid status can be assessed either by a microbiological assay of the vitamin in plasma or by measurement of its urinary metabolites.

## Folic acid

A derivative of folic acid is vital to purine and pyrimidine (and hence nucleic acid) synthesis. Folic acid deficiency is relatively common; its most usual manifestation is as a macrocytic anaemia. This vitamin is now usually measured in haematology departments by immunoassay, although microbiological assays were widely used in the past. The concentration in red cells reflects the body's folate status more accurately than that in plasma.

Tests involving the chemical measurement of formiminoglutamate, an intermediate in the degradation of histidine which requires tetrahydrofolate for its further metabolism, are now obsolete.

## Vitamin B$_{12}$

Vitamin B$_{12}$ comprises a number of closely related substances called cobalamins which are essential to nucleic acid synthesis. Deficiency of the vitamin causes a megaloblastic anaemia and, in severe cases, subacute combined degeneration of the spinal cord.

Dietary deficiency of this vitamin is rare except in strict vegetarians (vegans) and considerable amounts are stored in the liver, with the result that deficiency is not common even with severe malabsorption (unless very long-standing). Vitamin B$_{12}$ deficiency is most commonly seen in pernicious anaemia. This is an autoimmune disease, in most cases of which there is a lack of intrinsic factor essential for the absorption of the vitamin from the gut.

Vitamin $B_{12}$ is measured in plasma by immunoassay, usually in departments of haematology. Tests of vitamin $B_{12}$ absorption are discussed in *Chapter 6*.

## Vitamin C (ascorbic acid)

Ascorbic acid is essential for the hydroxylation of proline residues in collagen and thus for the normal structure and function of this protein. It acts by maintaining the iron in the hydroxylating enzyme in the reduced ($Fe^{2+}$) state, i.e., acting as an antioxidant. It also facilitates the intestinal absorption of dietary non-haem iron by keeping it in the $Fe^{2+}$ state. Subclinical deficiency of ascorbic acid is quite often present in elderly housebound people. The concentration of ascorbate in plasma reflects recent dietary intake and is a poor index of tissue stores of the vitamin. These are better assessed by determination of ascorbate concentration in leucocytes. In practice, this is seldom necessary, since ascorbic acid is cheap and non-toxic, so a therapeutic trial of vitamin supplementation is the simplest procedure to confirm suspected vitamin C deficiency.

---

**CASE HISTORY 21.2**

An 80-year-old widow was admitted to hospital with bronchopneumonia and obvious self-neglect. She lived alone but had several cats, and a neighbour who had called the doctor said that most of the woman's pension was spent on her pets. On examination, she was seen to have widespread perifollicular haemorrhages and a clinical diagnosis of scurvy was made. She was given ascorbic acid (11 mg/kg body weight/day) and her urinary ascorbate excretion was measured. Only after eight days of treatment was there any increase from the initial very low level.

**Comment**

In a person with normal tissue ascorbate stores, ascorbate ingested in excess of requirements is rapidly excreted in the urine. In a patient with ascorbate deficiency, the vitamin is retained until tissue stores are replenished; in severe deficiency this can take more than a week but it should be noted that this test provides only retrospective confirmation of the diagnosis.

---

## FAT-SOLUBLE VITAMINS

### Vitamin A

This vitamin is a constituent of the retinal pigment rhodopsin. It is also essential for the normal synthesis of mucopolysaccharides and growth of epithelial tissue. Mild deficiency causes night blindness while in more severe cases degenerative changes in the eye may lead to complete loss of vision. The normal liver contains considerable stores of the vitamin and deficiency is rarely seen in affluent societies. It is, however, an important cause of blindness in many areas of the world.

Vitamin A is present in the diet and can also be synthesized from dietary carotenes. It can be measured in plasma, in which which it is transported bound to prealbumin and a specific retinol-binding globulin. A low binding protein concentration can cause the plasma concentration of vitamin A to be low and impair its delivery to tissues even when hepatic stores of the vitamin are adequate. Measurements of vitamin A status are rarely required in practice, since deficiency is rare in the Western World. In areas where deficiency is endemic, the diagnosis is usually obvious clinically and the facilities required to provide laboratory confirmation of the diagnosis are often not available.

### Vitamin D

Vitamin D is obtained from endogenous synthesis, by the action of ultraviolet light on 7-dehydrocholesterol in the skin to form cholecalciferol (vitamin $D_3$), and from the diet. Dietary vitamin D is largely vitamin $D_2$ (ergocalciferol); the only important dietary sources are fish and some margarines, which are artificially fortified with vitamin D. Vitamins $D_2$ and $D_3$ undergo the same metabolic changes in the body and have identical physiological actions. For this reason, the terms cholecalciferol and vitamin D are frequently used to refer to both forms of the vitamin.

In most individuals, endogenous synthesis is the major source of vitamin D. Privational (dietary) vitamin D deficiency is seen most commonly in people who also have decreased endogenous synthesis, such as the elderly housebound. It is also seen in immigrants from the Indian subcontinent, particularly women, in whom the effects of poor intake may be exacerbated by decreased exposure to sunlight due to their traditional clothing. Breast milk contains relatively little vitamin D and infants are at risk of vitamin D deficiency particularly if premature (the vitamin is transported across the placenta mainly in the last trimester of pregnancy) or if the mother is vitamin D-deficient.

Cholecalciferol itself has little physiological activity. It is hydroxylated first in the liver to 25-hydroxycholecalciferol

| Trace elements in the human body | |
|---|---|
| **Element** | **Function** |
| chromium | deficiency causes glucose intolerance |
| cobalt | component of vitamin B12 |
| copper | cofactor for cytochrome oxidase |
| fluorine* | present in bone and teeth |
| iodine | component of thyroid hormones |
| iron | component of haem pigments |
| manganese | cofactor for several enzymes |
| molybdenum | cofactor for xanthine oxidase |
| selenium | cofactor for glutathione peroxidase |
| silicon* | present in cartilage |
| tin* | ? |
| zinc | cofactor for many enzymes |

**Fig. 21.1** Trace elements in the human body. * indicates elements which are present, but are not known to be essential.

(25-HCC, calcidiol) and then in the kidney to 1,25-dihydroxycholecalciferol (1,25-DHCC, calcitriol). These metabolites are transported in the circulation by a specific binding protein. Calcitriol is a hormone of vital importance in calcium homoeostasis; its actions and the control of its production are discussed in *Chapter 12*.

Vitamin D status can be assessed in the laboratory by measurement of the plasma concentration of calcidiol, the major circulating metabolite. This undergoes seasonal variation, being higher in the summer than in the winter.

Decreased synthesis or dietary deficiency of vitamin D causes rickets in children and osteomalacia in adults. Other causes include disordered metabolism of cholecalciferol and malabsorption. The clinical biochemistry of rickets and osteomalacia is considered in more detail in *Chapter 12*.

## Vitamin K

Vitamin K is required for the γ-carboxylation of glutamate residues in coagulation factors II (prothrombin), VII, IX and X. This process confers physiological activity by permitting the binding of calcium to the proteins. Vitamin K deficiency results in an increase in the prothrombin time, a functional assay of relevant coagulation factor activity. These factors are synthesized in the liver and the prothrombin time is also used as a test of liver function. Its most frequent use is in the monitoring of patients on anticoagulant treatment with antagonists of vitamin K, e.g., warfarin.

## Vitamin E

Vitamin E (tocopherol) is an important antioxidant, particularly in cell membranes, protecting unsaturated fatty acid residues against free radical attack. Clinical deficiency may occur in severe malabsorption, particularly in infants. Manifestations include haemolytic anaemia and neurological dysfunction.

There is some evidence that a high intake of vitamin E confers some protection against coronary heart disease, possibly by preventing the oxidation of LDL cholesterol.

## TRACE ELEMENTS

The maintenance of normal health requires provision in the diet not only of adequate protein, energy substrates and vitamins, but also of various inorganic salts and trace elements. Trace elements in the body are by definition present in concentrations less than 100 parts per million (ppm); they are shown in *Fig. 21.1*. None is required in more than milligram quantities per day while the daily requirement for some is measurable in micrograms. Consequently the 'essential' status of some of these trace elements is difficult to confirm.

### Trace element deficiency

Deficiencies of trace elements can occur for the same general reasons as vitamin deficiencies.

The commonest trace element deficiency is that of iron; it is common even in affluent societies, particularly in women during the reproductive years. Iodine deficiency causes goitre and, if severe, hypothyroidism; it is now uncommon in the developed world but is still a problem in some areas. Deficiency of other trace elements is uncommon except under special circumstances. These include severe malnutrition, artificial feeding (especially if prolonged), prematurity and the presence of excessive losses (such as with enterocutaneous fistulae or severe diarrhoea). Multiple deficiencies may occur in these conditions, confusing the clinical picture and making diagnosis difficult.

## Laboratory assessment

Unfortunately, the laboratory assessment of the body's trace element status is difficult, as specialized equipment and considerable technical expertise are required. Measurements are often made in plasma, but these may not accurately reflect the concentration of a trace element at its (usually intracellular) site of action. Although a low plasma concentration may not indicate deficiency in the tissues, such deficiency is usually accompanied by a low plasma concentration, with the result that if a low concentration is found, it is reasonable to provide appropriate supplementation. Trace element deficiency should be anticipated in patients at risk and steps taken to prevent the occurrence of a deficiency syndrome.

## Zinc

Zinc is a trace element of particular importance. It is essential for the activity of many enzymes, including several involved in nucleic acid and protein synthesis. The clinical manifestations of zinc deficiency include dermatitis and delayed wound healing; there is, however, no evidence that zinc supplementation accelerates wound healing in patients who are not deficient. Zinc deficiency is a well-recognized potential complication of artificial (particularly parenteral) nutrition if insufficient supplementation is provided. Patients who are catabolic, for example, following trauma or major surgery, lose large amounts of zinc in the urine and are at risk of becoming depleted. Severe deficiency is seen in the condition acrodermatitis enteropathica, in which there is a defect in intestinal zinc absorption.

Plasma zinc concentrations must be interpreted with caution; blood should be collected in the fasting state since zinc concentrations may fall by up to 20% following a meal. Low plasma concentrations are not exclusive to zinc deficiency; they are also seen in conditions such as malignant disease and chronic liver disease without associated clinical evidence of tissue deficiency. Plasma zinc concentrations fall during an acute phase response, as a result of uptake by the liver. Finally, because zinc is extensively bound to albumin, plasma zinc concentration should be considered in relation to that of albumin.

## Copper

Copper is also essential for the activity of certain enzymes, notably cytochrome oxidase and superoxide dismutase. In the blood, 80–90% of copper is present in caeruloplasmin. Copper deficiency is uncommon; manifestations include anaemia and leucopenia. Wilson's disease, a disorder characterized by excessive tissue deposition of copper, is discussed in *Chapter 5*.

## Selenium

Selenium is required as a prosthetic group for the enzyme glutathione peroxidase which, together with the tocopherols (vitamin E) is part of the antioxidant system which protects membranes and other vulnerable structures from oxidative attack by free radicals. These highly reactive species can be generated (for example) as a result of the activation of phagocytic cells or exposure to ionizing radiation. Selenium deficiency is usually only seen as a result of a low intake (it is endemic in some parts of China which have a low soil selenium content) and has been reported in patients on long-term parenteral nutrition. The most obvious clinical feature is myopathy (especially cardiomyopathy). Selenium can be measured in plasma but measurement of red cell glutathione peroxidase activity provides a better measure of tissue selenium status.

# PROVISION OF NUTRITIONAL SUPPORT

Patients requiring nutritional support should be fed enterally whenever possible; this is more natural, cheaper and less hazardous than parenteral feeding. Parenteral nutrition is, however, required in patients with intestinal failure, e.g., due to gut resection or a fistula, and sometimes in those with a very high energy requirement (such as following severe burns) when it may be impossible to provide adequate nutrition by the enteral route alone.

Nutritional support may be required for patients who are already malnourished, as a result of, for example, severe small bowel disease or a stenosing carcinoma of the oesophagus. In such patients it is necessary both to correct existing deficits and to supply continuing needs. It is far better, when possible, to introduce nutritional support before serious deficiencies have developed and the need should be anticipated by identifying patients at risk.

The diagnosis of severe malnutrition does not require the aid of the laboratory since it is clinically obvious. A plasma albumin concentration of below 30 g/L is often held to be an index of malnutrition, but the plasma albumin can be low for many other reasons (*see p. 204*) and may be higher than this in a malnourished patient with dehydration. Other plasma proteins show no advantage over albumin as indices of nutritional status. Even combinations of biochemical and anthropometric (e.g., weight, skinfold thickness) data in 'prognostic nutritional indices' appear not to be superior to skilled clinical assessment in determining which patients are likely to benefit from nutritional support. However, the laboratory will be required to provide data for monitoring malnourished patients and it is important to be aware of both the value and the limitations of such data.

## Laboratory monitoring of parenteral nutrition

Patients fed parenterally are given an intravenous infusion of glucose, a fat emulsion, amino acids, vitamins and inorganic salts. The appropriate quantities of all these constituents are usually compounded together in a single container under sterile conditions, and infused continuously over 24 h, or sometimes overnight.

Patients receiving parenteral nutrition require careful clinical monitoring. Fluid status should be assessed both clinically and by means of fluid balance charts to ensure that the patient is not over-hydrated or under-hydrated, especially if there are abnormal losses. Short-term changes in weight usually reflect changes in fluid status but weighing the patient may be impracticable.

### Plasma potassium and glucose

Plasma potassium and glucose concentrations must be measured daily in patients receiving parenteral nutrition. The urine should be checked for glucose every 6 h when parenteral nutrition is started; glucose intolerance is common and usually causes glycosuria. When glucose intolerance does occur, blood and plasma measurements should be made more frequently to monitor the effect of any changes in glucose or insulin input. Hypoglycaemia is usually only a problem if parenteral feeding is stopped suddenly.

### Sodium

Mild hyponatraemia (sodium concentration 125–135 mmol/L) is common in patients receiving parenteral nutrition. It is often multifactorial in origin and is not on its own an indication for increasing the sodium input. Measurement of urinary sodium excretion is useful if there is hyponatraemia; when it is due to sodium depletion and renal function is normal, the urine will contain little sodium. Spurious hyponatraemia (see p. 20) due to the infusion of lipid emulsions should not be a problem in practice. If, during continuous lipid infusion, the plasma is more than faintly opalescent to the naked eye, the lipid is not being cleared adequately and the rate of administration should be decreased. Significant spurious hyponatraemia only occurs if the plasma is frankly lipaemic. Hypernatraemia is much less common than hyponatraemia and is usually due to lack of water rather than excess of sodium. The cause of hypernatraemia should always be determined and treated appropriately.

### Plasma creatinine and urea

If the patient has a good urinary output it is unnecessary to measure the plasma creatinine concentration more than twice a week. However, urea should be measured more frequently, especially after starting a patient on parenteral nutrition. If the input of amino acids exceeds the body's ability to utilize them for protein synthesis, there will be an increase in urea formation and plasma urea concentration may increase.

### Plasma bicarbonate

Unless required for other purposes, there is rarely any need to measure plasma bicarbonate or assess acid–base status in patients on TPN.

### Plasma proteins

Plasma albumin concentration is frequently decreased in patients requiring nutritional support. Because the plasma half-life of albumin is long, and many factors influence its concentration, it is of little value in monitoring patients except that in the short-term it may indicate a change in fluid balance. Transferrin has a shorter half-life, but its usefulness in this context is limited because its concentration increases in iron deficiency and because it is an acute phase protein. The plasma levels of prealbumin (half-life two days) and retinol-binding protein (half-life 12 h) are reduced in malnutrition and increase rapidly when adequate nutritional support is provided. In practice, however, such measurements add little to what is often obvious clinically.

### Liver function tests (LFT)

Patients on TPN frequently develop abnormalities of LFTs, for example an increase in alkaline phosphatase, in the absence of any other cause. Rarely, a cholestatic jaundice may occur. The pathogenesis is multifactorial: causes include over-provision of energy substrates (fat or carbohydrate), leading to hepatic fat deposition, and biliary sludging due to decreased secretion of bile. The abnormalities are always reversible in adults, but occasionally lead to progressive liver damage in children.

### Other measurements in plasma

The frequency of monitoring of other analytes will be determined by the clinical circumstances. In general, it is advisable to measure plasma calcium and phosphate twice weekly. Hypophosphataemia is a serious potential complication of parenteral nutrition.

In practice, given the availability of multichannel analyzers, the tendency is to measure all these analytes daily, even though this may not be strictly necessary. Many patients receiving nutritional support are seriously ill or have existing deficiencies or increased losses of nutrients, factors that may necessitate more frequent monitoring.

| Metabolic complications of parenteral nutrition |
|---|
| hyperglycaemia |
| hypokalaemia/hyperkalaemia |
| hyponatraemia/hypernatraemia |
| hypophosphataemia |
| abnormal liver function tests |
| acidosis |
| hypoglycaemia (rebound) |
| **long-term parenteral nutrition** |
| metabolic bone disease |
| deficiency states |

**Fig. 21.2** Metabolic complications of parenteral nutrition, listed in approximate order of frequency.

However, in patients on parenteral nutrition who are otherwise well, biochemical measurements can be made less frequently.

Plasma magnesium and zinc need not be measured more often than weekly unless a deficiency is identified which requires correction. Measurements of other trace elements are seldom required in patients on short-term (e.g., perioperative) TPN, but will be required in patients on long-term TPN, e.g., for short gut syndrome. Most such patients live at home. They are usually nutritionally stable and require monitoring only every six weeks to two months.

### Haematological measurements
Regular haematological measurements must be performed and will give an indication of haematinic deficiencies.

### Urine analysis
Nitrogen balance can be assessed from a comparison of known nitrogen input with nitrogen excretion. A crude estimate of nitrogen excretion is provided by urinary urea excretion (this being the major route of nitrogen excretion) provided that the plasma urea is constant and that there are no unusual losses. Measurements of urinary sodium and potassium output may be misleading unless considered together with the plasma concentrations, input and the patient's renal function. A high urinary sodium excretion will usually be due to excessive sodium administration and so is not on its own an indication for increasing sodium input. However, a low urinary sodium excretion is usually indicative of sodium depletion except in patients who are stressed. Urinary potassium excretion must also be interpreted with regard to intake. Potassium balance is negative

in patients who are catabolic, but becomes positive when new tissue is being laid down.

In a patient with stable renal function, 24-hour urinary creatinine excretion, being related to muscle bulk, can provide an index of the body's protein status. As with other such indices, serial, rather than isolated, measurements are more useful.

Some of the commoner metabolic complications of parenteral nutrition are summarized in *Fig. 21.2*.

## SUMMARY

Nutritional disorders can be due to a deficiency or an excess of nutrients. Deficiency syndromes include those due to the lack of a single nutrient and those in which there is generalized deficiency; some essential nutrients can be harmful if taken in excess and, if an individual's total energy intake is greater than his requirements, obesity will develop.

Specific laboratory methods are available for the diagnosis of deficiencies of individual water-soluble vitamins but, with the exception of those for folic acid and vitamin $B_{12}$, they are rarely required in clinical practice. Among the fat-soluble vitamins, vitamin A deficiency is rare in the developed world but vitamin D deficiency, leading to rickets and osteomalacia, occurs relatively frequently, particularly in the elderly, premature infants, patients with malabsorption and in certain racial groups. The diagnosis can be confirmed by demonstrating a low plasma concentration of 25-hydroxycholecalciferol. Vitamin K deficiency leads to impairment of blood clotting with prolongation of the prothrombin time; plasma measurements of the vitamin itself are not required for diagnosis.

Deficiencies of minerals required in large amounts by the body (for example, sodium, potassium, calcium, magnesium) can usually be inferred from clinical observation and measurement of their plasma concentrations. It is more difficult to diagnose deficiencies of trace elements, such as zinc, manganese and copper, since plasma levels may not accurately reflect the body's status with regard to these elements.

Patients with generalized malnutrition show characteristic, though not specific, biochemical abnormalities, for example, low plasma concentrations of albumin, transferrin and certain other proteins and decreased urinary creatinine excretion. There may also be evidence of specific deficiencies of vitamins or minerals. These patients require nutritional support. This should be enteral wherever possible, that is, using the gut either by supplementation of the diet or by tube feeding. In patients with intestinal failure, however, feeding must be parenteral. This entails the infusion of nutrients intravenously and is a potentially hazardous procedure. There is a risk of metabolic complications, for example, hyperglycaemia, hypophosphataemia and hypo- or hyperkalaemia, but these should be preventable by frequent biochemical monitoring. Biochemical and clinical monitoring are also necessary to assess nitrogen balance and to follow the patient's response to treatment.

## FURTHER READING

Labbé R F (1993) Nutrition support. *Clinics in Laboratory Medicine,* **13**, 313–530.

Marshall W J & Mitchell P E G (1987) Total parenteral nutrition and the clinical chemistry laboratory. *Annals of Clinical Biochemistry,* **24**, 327–336.

Neale G (1988) *Clinical Nutrition.* London: Heinemann Medical Books.

Sax H C & Souba W W (1993) Enteral and parenteral feeding: guidelines and recommendations. *The Medical Clinics of North America* **77**, 863–938.

Woolfson A M J (ed.) (1986) *Biochemistry of Hospital Nutrition.* Edinburgh: Churchill Livingstone.

# 22. Clinical Chemistry at the Extremes of Age

## OLD AGE: INTRODUCTION

The investigation and management of illness in the elderly poses a number of special problems, for both the physician and the clinical biochemist. These include:

- Different patterns of disease.
- Different presentation of disease.
- Decline in normal functions with age.
- Different reference ranges.

Many conditions are more common in the elderly than in younger adults; examples of such conditions of particular interest to the clinical biochemist include diabetes mellitus (*see Chapter 11*), Paget's disease of bone (*see p 198*) and thyroid diseases (*see pp 144-149*). Further, the presentation of diseases in the elderly may be different from that normally seen in younger people. Thus myocardial infarction may present with confusion, consequent on a reduction in cerebral blood flow, rather than chest pain; the presenting feature of diabetes mellitus may be one of its complications,

for example ischaemic ulceration, rather than polyuria and thirst. *Case Histories 22.1 to 22.4* provide more detailed examples of these problems.

The functions of some organs decline with age and such decline may be accelerated by even mild disease. The glomerular filtration rate decreases with age and so does the creatinine clearance. However, the plasma creatinine concentration changes little, because creatinine production also falls with age; this reflects a decrease in muscle mass and often also in meat consumption. Despite the fall in the glomerular filtration rate, renal function remains sufficient for normal homoeostasis although it may not be adequate to allow complete excretion of a drug or to sustain any further decrease in glomerular filtration without a failure of homoeostasis.

## REFERENCE RANGES

Such changes in normal function mean that the reference ranges applicable to healthy adults may not be applicable to the elderly, while the increased incidence of many diseases with increasing age makes it difficult to obtain data on normal people. Ideally, laboratories should construct age-related reference ranges for age-dependent analytes (*Fig. 22.1*), but in practice this is not always done.

This problem is exemplified by the enzyme alkaline phosphatase. Common causes of raised activity of this enzyme in the plasma of the elderly include malignant disease with metastasis to bone or liver, osteomalacia and Paget's disease of bone. In the United Kingdom, the incidence of Paget's disease exceeds 5% in people aged over 60. Many cases are mild and clinically silent, being discovered only after a raised plasma alkaline phosphatase has been found, often as part of a biochemical screening test. Asymptomatic patients with Paget's disease do not require treatment, but theoretically screening programmes are only worthwhile if abnormal results are followed up. How extensively this can be done is governed by economic factors. The practice in many laboratories is to assume that, in the absence of any clinical or other laboratory evidence of disease, an alkaline phosphatase of up to one and a half times the upper limit of normal for young adults does not justify further investigation in an elderly subject.

| Plasma constituents showing age-dependent changes in concentration | |
|---|---|
| cholesterol | increases progressively during adult life |
| glucose | increases (glucose tolerance decreases with age) |
| alkaline phosphatase | increases |
| urate | increases |
| total protein | decreases (slight decrease probably related to decreased protein intake) |
| albumin | decreases (as total protein) |

**Fig. 22.1** Plasma constituents showing age-dependent changes in concentration.

## SCREENING

The higher prevalence of many diseases in the elderly provides some of the justification for screening programmes. If a condition has a high prevalence in a population, the predictive value of a positive test is much higher than if it is low (*see Chapter 1*). Such screening may be carried out in general practice, at over-60s clinics, in geriatric assessment centres or on admission to hospital. The biochemical tests which should form part of such a screen (*Fig. 22.2*) reflect the diseases that are of particular concern in this age group, some of which have been mentioned above. Plasma potassium is included since diuretics are commonly prescribed for the elderly and, according to the type used, may cause hypokalaemia or hyperkalaemia. The possible influence of inter-current disease on tests of thyroid status must be borne in mind. The results of such tests may erroneously suggest thyroid disease in a patient who is ill for some other reason (sick euthyroid syndrome) and it is best to avoid doing these tests at such a time.

| Biochemical tests used to screen for disease in the elderly | |
|---|---|
| **Analyte** | **Common abnormalities** |
| plasma potassium | hypokalaemia (diuretic and purgative-induced) hyperkalaemia (potassium-sparing diuretic with poor renal function) |
| plasma creatinine | increased (renal impairment) |
| plasma calcium | hypercalcaemia (hyperparathyroidism) hypocalcaemia (osteomalacia) |
| plasma alkaline phosphatase | increased (osteomalacia, Paget's disease and malignancy) |
| plasma glucose | increased (diabetes mellitus) |
| plasma TSH and fT4 | hypothyroidism and hyperthyroidism |
| faecal occult blood | carcinoma of the large bowel |

**Fig. 22.2** Biochemical tests used to screen for disease in the elderly.

### CASE HISTORY 22.1

A general practitioner was called to see a previously fit man in an old people's home. The patient had become acutely short of breath two hours before, soon after his breakfast, and developed a cough with frothy white sputum. He also complained of dizziness, but denied chest pain.

On examination, he had widespread crepitations throughout his lung fields; his blood pressure was 120/70 mmHg but had been 150/90 mmHg when checked by the doctor two months previously.

He was given a diuretic, with considerable symptomatic relief ensuing. An ECG showed changes consistent with a very recent myocardial infarct. The doctor took a blood sample for measurement of creatine kinase activity and was surprised when the laboratory telephoned him to say that this was normal.

**Comment**

The breathlessness, cough and crepitations are classic features of left ventricular failure. A likely cause of this, and the fall in blood pressure, was myocardial infarction; chest pain does not always occur, particularly in the elderly. The general practitioner should not have been surprised that the creatine kinase was normal – the blood had been taken too soon after the presumed infarction. He was advised by the clinical biochemist to take a further blood sample; this was timed at 26 hours after the onset of symptoms and the creatine kinase was clearly raised at 280 IU/L.

### CASE HISTORY 22.2

An elderly lady presented with an exacerbation of congestive cardiac failure. She was being treated with digoxin and a thiazide diuretic.

### Investigations

serum:  digoxin       3.2 nmol/L
(12 hours after previous dose)
potassium      3.0 mmol/L
urea           11.2 mmol/L
creatinine      160 µmol/L

### Comment

Drug interactions are an important cause of ill-health at all ages, but particularly in the elderly. An exacerbation of cardiac failure in a patient treated with digoxin should raise the suspicion of digoxin toxicity. The serum concentration here is compatible with this and digoxin toxicity is enhanced by hypokalaemia; thiazide diuretics are an important cause of this. The elevated serum creatinine concentration indicates impaired renal function; this can impair the excretion of digoxin and lead to its accumulation in the plasma (*see also Case History 2.7*).

### CASE HISTORY 22.3

A 70-year-old woman presented with a painful ulcer on the sole of her left foot. On examination her foot felt cold and appeared ischaemic; no pulses were palpable below the femorals on either side.

Her urine contained a trace of glucose and a biochemical screen revealed a random plasma glucose concentration of 15 mmol/L although she denied any thirst or polyuria.

### Comment

The patient's random plasma glucose concentration is diagnostic of diabetes mellitus. The classic thirst and polyuria of diabetes may not always be present, particularly in the elderly, in whom the renal threshold for glucose is often elevated as a result of a decreased glomerular filtration rate. This may just be a feature of declining renal function with age, but can be exacerbated by renal disease which can develop as a complication of diabetes.

### CASE HISTORY 22.4

An elderly lady was admitted to hospital after she had fallen at home and fractured her femur. She was a recluse and rarely went out, depending on a home help to do her shopping.

In addition to the fracture a radiograph showed typical features of osteomalacia.

### Investigations

serum:  calcium               1.75 mmol/L
phosphate          0.70 mmol/L
alkaline phosphatase   440 IU/L
albumin                 30 g/L

Her fracture was treated by replacement arthroplasty. After her operation, a medical student took a detailed history from the patient and discovered that she had recently developed constipation and had passed some fresh blood *per rectum*. He found her liver to be enlarged and a barium enema revealed a stenosing carcinoma of the sigmoid colon. A laparotomy was performed and the tumour was resected, but the liver was seen to contain several metastatic tumour deposits. Measurement of alkaline phosphatase isoenzymes showed an increase in both the bone and the liver isoenzyme.

### Comment

The low serum calcium (even when the low albumin is taken into account), slightly reduced phosphate (a reflection of secondary hyperparathyroidism) and raised alkaline phosphatase (reflecting increased osteoblastic activity) are typical of osteomalacia. This is more common in the elderly and both poor nutrition (the low albumin would be consistent with this) and decreased endogenous synthesis of vitamin D (due to lack of exposure to sunlight) may be important in its pathogenesis. The plasma 25-hydroxycholecalciferol concentration is usually low. Typical radiological features are not always present; the definitive technique for making the diagnosis is histological examination of a bone biopsy, but this is a specialized, invasive procedure and in practice the diagnosis is often confirmed by the response to a therapeutic trial of vitamin D. Any patient may be suffering from more than one disease, but such an occurrence is more common in the elderly.

Other case histories of particular relevance may be found *on pp 22, 48 and 143.*

## CHILDHOOD: INTRODUCTION

Just as the elderly present particular problems for the clinical biochemist, so, too, do children. The most obvious of these relates to the size of the blood sample. For the very young it is essential to employ analytical methods that will use the smallest possible amount of plasma and this usually means providing special equipment. Small quantities of capillary blood can be conveniently collected by pricking the heel, but this should be done by experienced personnel and the results obtained may be affected by haemolysis or by contamination with tissue fluid.

Complete, accurately timed collections of urine are very difficult to obtain in children. It is usually more reliable to relate the concentrations of urinary constituents to urine creatinine concentration.

Many conditions present exclusively, or predominantly, in the neonatal period; examples include many congenital diseases and inherited metabolic disorders (see *Chapter 16*). Other disorders may become apparent at any time during childhood, in particular disorders of growth and of sexual differentiation and development.

Paediatric medicine no longer begins with the birth of the child. It is now becoming possible to treat some fetal disorders *in utero*, and the clinical biochemist will be required to provide an appropriate service to support this.

In a book of this size, it is possible only to outline some of the more important areas where paediatric medicine and clinical biochemistry interact. The reader seeking more detailed information is referred to the *Further Reading* section.

## REFERENCE RANGES

The reference ranges for certain analytes are different in the newborn from the adult (*Fig. 22.3*) and may vary through childhood; the concentrations of some analytes, in particular phosphate and calcium, are affected by the diet. A result should always be interpreted in the light of the reference range appropriate to the child's age. The age-related changes in plasma alkaline phosphatase are discussed in *Chapter 15*; and in immunoglobulins in *Chapter 13*. Creatinine clearance must be corrected for surface area in a child, since it increases as the child grows.

## SCREENING

The well-established programmes for neonatal screening for phenylketonuria and congenital hypothyroidism are discussed in *Chapter 16*. Presently, the rapid increase in the

| Common analytes having different reference ranges in children | |
|---|---|
| **Analyte** | **Difference** |
| plasma potassium | mean and upper limit higher in newborn |
| plasma calcium | higher at birth; normal adult levels by 72h |
| plasma phosphate | higher at birth, then falls but remains higher than adult levels throughout childhood; rises at puberty then falls to adult level |
| plasma alkaline phosphatase | as phosphate |

**Fig. 22.3** Common analytes with different reference ranges in children.

identification of mutations responsible for many inherited metabolic diseases, together with development of techniques for obtaining and analyzing fetal DNA, is increasing the availability of reliable antenatal screening, particularly in high-risk pregnancies (i.e., where there is a strong family history of a particular disorder).

## CHILDHOOD DISORDERS

### Neonatal hypoglycaemia

This important condition is discussed in *Chapter 11*. It is particularly likely to occur in low birth weight infants, both premature and 'small-for-dates'; babies born to diabetic mothers; and babies who are ill or who have feeding problems. In such babies, blood glucose measurements should be made every four hours for the first 48 hours and at appropriate intervals thereafter to monitor treatment if hypoglycaemia has occurred. Persistent hypoglycaemia or requirement for glucose infusion at a rate exceeding 10 mg/kg body weight/min to prevent hypoglycaemia should prompt a search for metabolic and endocrine causes (*see Fig. 11.13*).

### Neonatal hypocalcaemia and hypomagnesaemia

The clinical signs of hypoglycaemia include irritability, twitching and convulsions. If the baby's blood glucose concentration is not low, hypocalcaemia, which presents with similar signs, should be suspected.

Plasma calcium, which is higher than normal adult levels at birth (up to 3.00 mmol/L), falls rapidly, then rises to reach adult levels by the third or fourth day of life. The transient, physiological hypocalcaemia is rarely symptomatic but tends to be exaggerated and may be symptomatic in pre-term infants, infants born to diabetic mothers and following birth asphyxia. It can be prevented by giving adequate calcium; if the baby is not feeding normally, intravenous calcium may be required.

Hypocalcaemia occurring after the first 2–3 days of life is uncommon. Causes are shown in *Fig. 22.4*. Most of these conditions are discussed in *Chapter 14*. Hypocalcaemia is a potential complication of exchange blood transfusion (clotting of donor blood is prevented by chelating calcium ions) and can be prevented by giving calcium during a transfusion.

Hypocalcaemia is often accompanied by hypomagnesaemia, and magnesium supplements should be given together with calcium in treating hypocalcaemia. If magnesium is not given, hypocalcaemia is often resistant to treatment. Isolated hypomagnesaemia is rare; it most frequently occurs in the infants of diabetic mothers.

## Jaundice

Most babies become mildly jaundiced shortly after birth. This 'physiological' jaundice is due to immaturity of the hepatic conjugating enzymes, to normal postnatal haemolysis and to enterohepatic circulation of bilirubin (conversion of bilirubin to urobilinogen in the gut cannot occur until the gut becomes colonized with bacteria). In physiological jaundice, the bilirubin is primarily unconjugated and its plasma concentration rarely exceeds 100 µmol/L; the jaundice is never present at birth and does not persist beyond 14 days of life. Physiological jaundice can be exacerbated by various factors, including dehydration, hypoxia, prematurity and birth trauma leading to bruising or a cephalohaematoma.

At high concentrations of unconjugated bilirubin (> 350 µmol/L) there is a risk of kernicterus developing. Since unconjugated bilirubin is bound to albumin the risk is greater if the plasma albumin concentration is decreased or bilirubin is displaced from albumin, for example, by hydrogen ions in acidosis, by certain drugs or by high concentrations of free fatty acids. Unconjugated hyperbilirubinaemia can be treated by increasing water intake, phototherapy or exchange transfusion as appropriate, and of course by treatment of the underlying cause if this can be ascertained and treatment is feasible. Circumstances which should prompt investigation of neonatal jaundice are given in *Fig. 22.5*.

Causes of unconjugated hyperbilirubinaemia in the newborn are given in *Fig. 22.6*.

There are also many causes of conjugated hyperbilirubinaemia in infants; some of these are listed in *Fig. 22.7*.

---

**When to investigate neonatal jaundice**

present at birth or appears during first
    24 h of life
persists beyond 14 days of life
total plasma bilirubin concentration > 250 µmol/L
conjugated hyperbilirubinaemia
jaundice associated with other signs or
    symptoms of disease

**Fig. 22.5** Circumstances in which neonatal jaundice should be investigated.

---

**Causes of unconjugated hyperbilirubinaemia in the newborn**

**Increased haemolysis**
rhesus blood group incompatibility
ABO blood group incompatibility
red cell enzyme defects:
    glucose 6-phosphate dehydrogenase
      deficiency
    pyruvate kinase deficiency

**Decreased conjugation**
Crigler–Najjar syndrome
hypothyroidism
breast milk jaundice (a benign condition seen
    in some breast-fed infants and thought to be
    due to interference with bilirubin
    conjugation by free fatty acids)

**Fig. 22.6** Causes of unconjugated hyperbilirubinaemia in the newborn.

---

**Causes of hypocalcaemia in infancy**

high phosphate intake (unmodified cows' milk)
vitamin D deficiency
hypoparathyroidism
Di George syndrome
pseudohypoparathyroidism
blood transfusion (exchange transfusion)
hypomagnesaemia

**Fig. 22.4** Causes of hypocalcaemia in infancy excluding transient neonatal hypocalcaemia.

## CASE HISTORY 22.5

A female baby was born at 38 weeks' gestation by spontaneous vaginal delivery to a primigravid woman. The baby appeared normal at birth but was slow to feed and frequently vomited after feeds. On the third day after birth, she was noticed to be jaundiced. On examination, she was found to have an enlarged liver and bilateral cataracts.

### Investigations

serum: bilirubin (total)    168 μmol/L
            (direct)     45 μmol/L
       aspartate aminotransferase122 IU/L
       alkaline phosphatase   244 IU/L
urine:   Clinitest            positive

### Comment

Direct-reacting bilirubin is conjugated bilirubin, and its presence in the plasma is pathological. The elevated transaminase activity with normal (for age) alkaline phosphatase is typical of 'neonatal hepatitis' – a term used to denote hepatic inflammation with patent bile ducts – the causes of which include infection (congenital and acquired) and various metabolic disorders. The presence of cataracts and the presence of a reducing substance suggest a diagnosis of galactosaemia (see page 240). The child was started on a galactose-free feed and improved clinically. The diagnosis was confirmed by the finding of a low erythrocyte galactose 1-phosphate uridyl transferase activity.

Biochemical tests do not always reliably distinguish between neonatal hepatitis and extrahepatic biliary atresia. Ultrasonography or an isotopic excretion test may be required.

## Metabolic disorders

Although inherited metabolic diseases are individually rare, they are collectively an important cause of illness in the neonatal period. Conditions which may present at this time include, inter alia, disorders of amino acid, organic acid and carbohydrate metabolism, and urea cycle disorders. If an inherited metabolic disease is suspected, accurate diagnosis is essential. This applies even if there is a fatal outcome as there may be consequences for subsequent pregnancies and parents can be offered genetic counselling or possibly the option of prenatal diagnosis.

### Causes of conjugated hyperbilirubinaemia in the newborn

haemolytic conditions (enterohepatic circulation of bilirubin)
hepatic dysfunction ('neonatal hepatitis') due to:
   infection:
       congenital, e.g., rubella, cytomegalovirus, syphilis
       acquired, e.g., urinary tract infection, septicaemia, hepatitis
   metabolic disorder:
       $\alpha_1$-antitrypsin deficiency
       galactosaemia
       tyrosinaemia
   congenital abnormality:
       biliary atresia

**Fig. 22.7** Causes of conjugated hyperbilirubinaemia in the newborn

The clinical features of metabolic disorders are rarely specific to any one condition; the salt loss and virilization of female infants with steroid 21-hydroxylase deficiency (see p. 134) are exceptional in this respect. Some clinical features, such as severe acidosis and coma, suggest that a metabolic disorder may be present, but in many cases they are non-specific, babies afflicted by such disorders presenting, for example, with vomiting or 'failure to thrive'.

The determination of the precise diagnosis of a metabolic disorder may require complex and lengthy investigation, so it is important to be able to carry out some simple screening tests to indicate whether a metabolic disorder may be the cause of a baby's illness. An appropriate battery of tests is shown in Fig. 22.8. If the results of these are all normal, a metabolic disorder is unlikely; if there are abnormalities, the pattern of these may suggest a possible diagnosis or indicate what further investigations would be appropriate. It is important that the child should, if at all possible, be on a normal diet when these tests are done; potential abnormalities may otherwise be masked. Thus disorders associated with an abnormal pattern of amino acid secretion may be missed if the infant does not have a normal protein intake.

If a baby suspected of having an inherited metabolic disease appears likely to die before a diagnosis has been established, it is essential that samples of blood, urine and skin (for fibroblast culture) are taken during life or immediately post mortem. Making a diagnosis after death will be valuable in counselling and management should another pregnancy be comtemplated. Samples of liver and muscle may also be helpful for this purpose.

| Screening tests for metabolic causes of illness in the newborn | |
| --- | --- |
| **Urine** | |
| reducing substances | bilirubin |
| glucose | sugar and amino acid chromatography |
| ketones | |
| **Blood** | |
| glucose | hydrogen ion |
| **Plasma** | |
| sodium | magnesium |
| potassium | conjugated bilirubin |
| urea | ammonia |
| creatinine | chromatography for amino acids |
| calcium | |
| phosphate | lactate |

**Fig. 22.8** Screening tests for metabolic causes of illness in the newborn

**CASE HISTORY 22.6**

Thirty-six hours after birth, a male infant started vomiting, developed grunting respiration and rapidly became lethargic and unresponsive. He appeared physically normal and was born at term after a normal pregnancy. The parents were first cousins; it was the woman's first pregnancy. A metabolic screen revealed a very high plasma ammonia concentration (> 1000 µmol/L). The plasma urea was at the lower end of the reference range and plasma amino acid chromatography showed an excess of glutamine and alanine. Despite intensive treatment, including peritoneal dialysis, the baby died 72 hours after birth.

**Comment**

Hyperammonaemia is an important cause of both morbidity and mortality in infants. This was a typical presentation of hyperammonaemia; toxic encephalopathy is usually a prominent feature. Although there are many causes of hyperammonaemia (*see Fig. 22.9*), a case as severe as this, without any suggestion of liver disease, and in a child born of a first cousin marriage, should raise the suspicion of an inherited metabolic disorder of the urea cycle. The excess plasma glutamine and alanine with low to

normal urea, are consistent with this. This child's urine was found to contain a high concentration of orotic acid. This pattern of abnormalities suggests deficiency of ornithine carbamoyl transferase and this was confirmed on post-mortem biopsy of the liver.

Consanguineous parents, or a history of a previous neonatal death, should increase one's suspicion that an inherited metabolic disease may be responsible for a child's illness.

| Some causes of hyperammonaemia in infancy |
| --- |
| transient neonatal hyperammonaemia* |
| inherited disorders of the urea cycle* |
| other inherited metabolic disorders* such as organic acidaemias |
| liver disease (including Reye's syndrome) |
| severe systemic illness* (asphyxia, infection, sepsis) |
| parenteral nutrition (excessive amino acid input) |
| sodium valproate therapy |
| *important causes in the newborn |

**Fig. 22.9** Some causes of hyperammonaemia in infancy. Reye's syndrome is a cause of encephalopathy in children, associated with fatty infiltration of the liver and hyperammonaemia; the cause is not known but there is an association with aspirin treatment.

## Failure to thrive

This is a common paediatric problem and some of the causes are shown in *Fig. 22.10*. Where there are no suggestive clinical features, either in the history or on examination, the results of tests listed in *Fig. 22.8*, together with simple haematological tests and a screen for infectious disease, will in many cases provide a starting point for definitive investigation.

## Disorders of sexual differentiation and abnormal puberty

Precocious sexual development, which may become apparent shortly after birth, is rare; some causes are given in *Fig. 22.11*. It is important to distinguish between true precocious puberty, in which the gonads are fully developed and contain gametes, and pseudoprecocious puberty in which they are not. Pseudoprecocious puberty is often amenable to treatment, albeit palliative, whereas true precocity is often not. Delayed puberty is much more common; causes are given in *Fig. 22.12*. Causes of virilization during childhood and adolescence are summarized in *Fig. 22.13*. Many of the conditions listed are rare, but the results of relatively simple tests, for example, the measurement of adrenal and gonadal steroids, and gonadotrophins, are invaluable in formulating a differential diagnosis. The same holds true for disorders of sexual differentiation, examples of which are shown in *Fig. 22.14*. Although also rare, all these conditions are of immense importance to the patients and their parents, and laboratory investigations are vital in their diagnosis and management.

## Disorders of growth

Many disorders can cause retardation of growth including most of the causes of delayed puberty, indicated in Fig. 22.12. Simple laboratory tests can provide important diagnostic information in such cases, but do not obviate the need for accurate clinical and anthropometric assessment. Growth hormone deficiency is rare; its diagnosis is discussed in *Chapter 7*. It can be treated by hormone replacement. The effects and diagnosis of growth hormone excess are also considered in *Chapter 7*.

| Some causes of failure to thrive |
|---|
| malnutrition |
| malabsorption |
| inherited metabolic diseases |
| infection |
| chronic diseases: |
|    renal |
|    hepatic |
|    pulmonary |
|    cardiac |
| psychosocial deprivation |
| hypothyroidism |
| hypopituitarism |

**Fig. 22.10** Some causes of failure to thrive.

| Causes of precocious puberty and pseudoprecocious puberty |
|---|
| **Precocious puberty** |
| idiopathic |
| pineal tumours, hypothalamic hamartomas |
| post meningitis or encephalitis |
| hypothyroidism |
| **Pseudoprecocious puberty** |
| gonadotrophin-secreting tumours |
| congenital adrenal hyperplasia |
| adrenal tumours |
| ovarian and testicular tumours |

**Fig. 22.11** Causes of precocious puberty and pseudoprecocious puberty.

| Causes of delayed puberty |
|---|
| constitutional (idiopathic) |
| chronic systemic illness, |
|    e.g., renal failure, hypothyroidism |
| undernutrition |
| chronic administration of corticosteroids |
| hypothalamic or pituitary insufficiency |
| primary gonadal failure |

**Fig. 22.12** Causes of delayed puberty. Constitutional delayed puberty is by far the commonest cause, reflecting one extreme of the normal range and affecting some 2.5% of all children.

| Causes of virilization in girls |
|---|
| **Adrenal** |
| congenital adrenal hyperplasia |
| Cushing's syndrome |
| adrenal tumours |
| premature adrenarche |
| **Ovarian** |
| ovarian tumours |
| polycystic ovary syndrome |

**Fig. 22.13** Causes of virilization in girls. In boys these adrenal conditions, testicular tumours and ectopic gonadotrophin secretion may cause pseudoprecocious puberty.

## Causes of abnormal sexual differentiation

**Male pseudohermaphroditism**
(genotypic males with incomplete
  masculinization)
decreased testosterone production:
  various inherited enzyme abnormalities
impaired testosterone metabolism:
  5α-reductase deficiency
  androgen insensitivity syndromes
congenital anomalies

**Female pseudohermaphroditism**
(genotypic female with virilization)
*see Fig. 22.13*

**Syndromes of abnormal gonadal differentiation**
Turner's syndrome (45X0 karyotype)
Klinefelter's syndrome (47XXY karyotype)
other chromosomal abnormalities
true hermaphroditism

**Fig. 22.14** Causes of abnormal sexual differentiation.

## SUMMARY

Many biochemical and physiological functions change with age; some of these are related to specific events, in particular puberty and the menopause, but for others the change is more gradual, for example, a decrease in the glomerular filtration rate in the elderly. This must be borne in mind when interpreting the results of biochemical tests in the elderly and ideally such results should be compared with age-related reference ranges. Thus the plasma cholesterol concentration increases throughout adult life as does the plasma urate, and glucose tolerance decreases in the elderly. The presentation of certain diseases may be different in the elderly and the biochemical tests assume a greater importance in diagnosis; furthermore, many diseases occur more frequently in the elderly and it may be justified to screen for thyroid disease, diabetes mellitus and osteomalacia, among others, in elderly people.

In children too, the reference ranges for some biochemical variables are different from those in adults. Examples include plasma phosphate concentration and alkaline phosphatase activity (both higher) and cholesterol and urate (both lower). Many conditions present most frequently, or even exclusively, in childhood; thus many inherited metabolic diseases characteristically present at or soon after birth.

Metabolic problems which occur particularly frequently in the newborn include hypoglycaemia, hypocalcaemia and hypomagnesaemia. Many infants become jaundiced in the first few days of life but in most cases this is benign. This 'physiological' jaundice is due to an increase in unconjugated bilirubin. Conjugated hyperbilirubinaemia is always pathological.

The clinical features of inherited metabolic disorders presenting in infancy and childhood are often non-specific. In children who, for example, fail to thrive or show unusual irritability or lethargy, simple screening tests on urine and plasma should be performed to identify any abnormality which may be due to an inherited metabolic disease.

Disorders of sexual differentiation are uncommon but following clinical assessment, the results of simple laboratory tests (for example, the levels of adrenal and gonadal hormones, gonadotrophins) are often of vital importance in formulating a differential diagnosis, and indicating the course of further investigations. This is also true of delayed puberty, a much more common complaint. There are many causes of growth failure, including systemic disease, social deprivation and malabsorption; relatively few cases are due to growth hormone deficiency. Again, the results of accurate clinical assessment, combined with simple laboratory tests, will often indicate the diagnosis and thus the appropriate mode of treatment.

## FURTHER READING

Clayton B E & Round J M (eds) (1994) *Chemical Pathology and the Sick Child.* 2nd edition Oxford: Blackwell Scientific Publications.

Green A L & Morgan I (1993) *Neonatology and Clinical Biochemistry.* London: ACB Venture Publications.

Hodkinson M (ed) (1984) *Clinical Biochemistry of the Elderly.* Edinburgh: Churchill Livingstone.

# ADULT REFERENCE RANGES

These reference ranges, from the author's laboratory, are provided for the interpretation of data presented in the case histories. Readers should note that reference ranges may differ between different laboratories; this applies particularly to hormones and enzymes. All values are for concentrations (activities in the case of enzymes) in serum or plasma, except where indicated otherwise.

| | | | | |
|---|---|---|---|---|
| acid phosphatase: total | 4–11 IU/L | | follicular phase | 2–8 U/L |
| prostatic | < 4 IU/L· | | post-menopausal | > 15 U/L |
| adrenocorticotrophic hormone (ACTH): at 0900 h | 10–80 ng/L | | glucose:fasting | 2.8–6.0 mmol/L |
| albumin | 35–50 g/L | | γ-glutamyl transferase (γGT) | < 60 IU/L |
| aldosterone: recumbent | 100–500 pmol/L | | growth hormone: | |
| alkaline phosphatase | 30–90 IU/L | | following glucose load | < 2 mU/L |
| | | | following stress | > 20 mU/L |
| alphafetoprotein(AFP) | < 10 kU/L | | haemoglobin: males | 13–18 g/dL |
| ammonia | 10–47 µmol/L | | females | 12–16 g/dL |
| amylase | < 300 IU/L | | hydrogen ion: arterial blood | 35–46 nmol/L (pH 7.36–7.44) |
| aspartate transaminase (AST) | 10–50 IU/L | | hydroxybutyrate dehydrogenase (HBD) | < 250 IU/L |
| bicarbonate total ($CO_2$) | 22–30 mmol/L | | insulin: fasting | 3–15 mU/L |
| bilirubin: total | 3–20 µmol/L | | in hypoglycaemia | < 3 mU/L |
| calcium | 2.2–2.6 mmol/L | | luteinizing hormone (LH): | |
| carbon dioxide ($P_{CO_2}$) (arterial blood) | 4.5–6.0 kPa (35–46 mmHg) | | adult males adult females: follicular phase | 2.0–10 U/L 2.0–10 U/L |
| cholesterol: total | < 5.2 mmol/L* | | post-menopausal | > 20 U/L |
| high density lipoprotein (HDL) | > 1.2 mmol/L* | | magnesium | 0.7–1.0 mmol/L |
| low density protein (LDL) | < 3.5 mmol/L* | | osmolality | 280–295 mmol/L |
| *indicates ideal values *see page 227* | | | oxygen ($P_{O_2}$): (arterial blood) | 11–15 kPa (85–105 mmHg) |
| copper | 12–19 µmol/L | | parathyroid hormone | 10–65 pg/mL |
| cortisol: at 0900 h | 140–690 nmol/L | | phosphate | 0.8–1.4 mmol/L |
| at 2400 h | < 100 nmol/L | | | |
| creatine kinase (total) | <90 IU/L | | potassium | 3.6–5.0 mmol/L |
| creatinine | 60–120 µmol/L | | prolactin | 50–400 mU/L |
| follicle-stimulating hormone (FSH): | | | protein: total | 60–80 g/L |
| adult males females: | 2–10 U/L | | renin (plasma renin activity, PRA): recumbent | 1.2–2.4 pmol/h/mL |

| | | | | |
|---|---|---|---|---|
| sodium | 135–145 mmol/L | triglyceride: fasting | | 0.4–1.8 mmol/L |
| testosterone: adult males<br>adult females | 9–30 nmol/L<br>0.5–2.5 nmol/L | triiodothyronine (T3): total<br>free | | 1.2–2.9 nmol/L<br>3.0–8.8 pmol/L |
| thyroid-stimulating hormone<br>(TSH, thyrotrophin) | 0.3–4.0 mU/L | urea | | 3.3–6.7 mmol/L |
| | | uric acid | | 0.1–0.4 mmol/L |
| thyroxine (T4): total<br>free | 60–150 nmol/L<br>9–26 pmol/L | zinc | | 12–20 µmol/L |

# Index